TRAVELERS'
HEALTH

HOW TO STAY HEALTHY
ALL OVER THE WORLD

TRAVELERS'
HEALTH

HOW TO STAY HEALTHY
ALL OVER THE WORLD

DEVISED AND EDITED BY

Dr. Richard Dawood

RANDOM HOUSE

NEW YORK

Library of Congress Cataloging-in-Publication Data

Travelers' health : how to stay healthy all over the world / devised and edited by Richard Dawood.
      p.   cm.
Rev. ed. of: Travellers' health. Oxford [Oxfordshire] : New York : Oxford University Press, 1992. 3rd ed.
Includes index.
ISBN: 0-679-74608-0
1. Travel—Health aspects.   2. Tropical medicine.   I. Dawood, Richard
M.   II. Travellers' health.   III. Title: How to stay healthy abroad.
RA783.5.T68   1993   92-37815
613.6'8—dc20   CIP

Design by ROBERT BULL DESIGN
Manufactured in the United States of America

98765432

First Random House, Inc., Edition

To the memory of my grandparents,
two proud Americans whose reminiscences
of travel across Continents and Oceans
sowed the seeds of my own wanderlust.

FOREWORD

by Paul Theroux

In many countries you remember your meals, while in other—and I think more interesting—places, you remember your illnesses. For myself, one of the more memorable afflictions detailed in this book is dengue fever, also known as breakbone fever, which is endemic throughout most of the tropical world. I first came across dengue during Peace Corps training in Puerto Rico in 1963; it was common on the island. But I was not bitten. Nor was I bitten in Africa over the next five years. But in 1969, in Singapore, the attractive woman who lived next door came down with a severe case of dengue. One hot night a few days later I fell ill, actually collapsed—my knees buckled, my temperature shot up to 103, my nerves burned in my skin, I felt paralytic. In the following days, I exhibited other symptoms: my hair began falling out, my joints ached, I became depressed and for several days I sobbed uncontrollably. And I hallucinated, fantasizing extravagantly that the mosquito which had bitten the voluptuous woman next door had also bitten me—two feverish people, one mosquito. The expression "virtual sex" was not in my vocabulary then, but my head was full of metaphysical poetry (I was a member of the English Department), and it comes to the same thing—John Donne is the poet of virtual sex, particularly in "The Flea."

> *Mark but this flea, and*
> *mark in this,*
> *How little that which*
> *thou deny'st me is;*
> *Me it sucked first, and*
> *now sucks thee,*
> *And in this flea, our two*
> *bloods mingled be. . . .*

This was precisely my dengue conceit, and it has a scientific basis. An arbovirus infection, dengue involves only humans and mosquitoes. The same mosquito had probably visited the woman and me.

Illness is nearly always dramatic in imaginative literature—look at Tolstoy's "Death of Ivan Ilyich," or Camus's *The Plague,* or Greene's *A Burnt Out Case;* so much of fiction is a fever chart. But illness is very tedious in a travel book. I am proud of the fact that in six lengthy travel books I have never recorded a single instance of my having diarrhea. It is not delicacy on my part, and my stomach is as susceptible as anyone else's—but who wants to read about it? There is a great personal satisfaction in overcoming illness abroad, but no sensible reader of a travel book wants to hear the gory details of your amebic dysentery or bout of malaria or resident jigger.

This reminds me that on leave from Africa in the 1960s I went to a family doctor in South London and told him I suspected I had the larvae of a jigger flea under my toenail. "You Americans," he said. (We are the world over perceived as hypochondriacs and alarmists.) But I swore it was so, and when he dug the horrible squirming maggot out of my toenail he made a face as though he had gouged an extraterrestrial from my body, and had the grace to say, "Blimey."

The principal difference between fleas and flies is wings. Fleas are wingless; they leap from victim to victim on strong hind legs. Flies fly. The tumbu fly referred to in this book I knew in Central Africa as a Putsi fly—*putsi* is "maggot" in the Chichewa language, but "maggot infestation" (*myiasis*) is a painful nuisance by any name. I had succeeded in avoiding this affliction for almost two years when I happened to take a trip up-country in Malawi in 1965. It was October, known in that region, because of its intense heat, as "the suicide month."

All I lacked on this trip was Corporal Jika Chikwawa, lately of the King's African Rifles, who normally did my washing and ironing. One day up-country, I washed a shirt and hung it out to dry. Putsi flies laid eggs on the shirt. I wore the shirt afterward, and the warmth of my body hatched the larvae, which burrowed into my skin, and a day or two later I had boils all over my shoulders and back. At first I had no idea what this hideous outbreak was, and then I popped one of the boils and a maggot wiggled out. My body ached with forty-odd more, nearly all of them out of my reach. I owe it to my friend Bob Maccani, formerly of Likuni (Central Province), now of Los Angeles, for staying up one hot night and holding a match over each boil until the maggot squirmed, and then squeezing the disgusting things out. This book recommends "placing oil over (the maggot's) breathing apparatus." And it adds (and I am sure that Bob Maccani would agree), "This is a rather unpleasant spectacle to witness." I used this putsi-fly episode to good effect in my African short story "White Lies."

In Malawi and Uganda, I had no personal experience of African eye worm, though my students knew it. The strangest aspect of this filarial infection (caused by a fly bite) is that the victim can see the worm "crawling across the surface of the eyes." How to prevent this happening to you? Avoid "the bites of large Chrysops flies, which breed in shaded forest pools and bite in the daytime." Don't swim in Africa is a good general rule. If you do, the chances are excellent that you will emerge from Lake Victoria, Lake Edward, Lake Albert, the Congo river, or your local swimming hole afflicted also with bilharzia (schistosomiasis). And the cure for this parasite—big needles in the butt—is more painful than the illness. Except for splashing in the waves at Mombasa, I never swam in Africa.

Malaria is one of the worst and most persistent problems in the tropics. The prophylactics are not terribly effective, and there are many strains of malaria, which are both cruelly uncomfortable and sometimes fatal. Using a well-made tent with a mosquito net in New Guinea has helped me more than chloroquine. Some countries, this book states, "underreport their cases of many diseases—perhaps so as not to harm their image or their tourist trade." This denial regarding AIDS risk is certainly common throughout East and Central Africa, but no one ought to be fooled by the smiling assurances of African tourist boards. Keep your immune system away from Ugandan or Kenyan prostitutes, an inordinate proportion of whom, according to World Health Organization estimates, carry the AIDS virus. The general population in these and other African countries is also widely infected.

AIDS is avoidable. Malaria can be very hard to avoid. But the trouble with most equatorial fevers is that they are almost impossible to diagnose or name. Many people have malaria and think it's flu—the initial symptoms are often similar. The worst fever I have ever endured was at a leper colony in a hot low-lying place in Malawi called Mua. It was also a mission hospital, run by Dutch White Fathers. I fell ill. One priest told me I might have blackwater fever—which, I was thrilled to learn, is marked by the destruction of blood cells and extensive kidney damage—another said it could be malaria. Yet more priests speculated and prayed for my soul. I assumed it was malaria, and dosed myself with chloroquine. I sweated for three days, hallucinating, my ears ringing. After the fever had broken I could barely walk upright. Diarrhea came next, and I had to negotiate the latrine, a long-drop privy where bats attached themselves to the edge of the toilet seat. When I entered they let go and flapped in loud batty circles in the pit beneath me. The leprosy itself, which was common in Mua—a thousand lepers in this one hospital compound—was not dangerous at all to me, nor to the priests. Leprosy, or Hansen's disease, as it is now called, is "not particularly contagious or infectious" and has a fairly straightforward cure—sulfa drugs. My experience of the leper colony at Mua was a paradox, a sort of golden period of innocence, my Eden almost. It was 1964. I loved this clearing in the jungle: the simplest bush conditions, the lepers from all over the country, many different people brought together by a blight they called *khate*. AIDS was unknown then; we played cards by lamplight and listened to the lepers drumming; the only urgency was the constant bandaging.

Most ailments go with the territory. I remember an American I met in India who boasted of his constipation—he was unique in Delhi, city of squitters and bowel-shattering meals. Cut yourself on coral anywhere in the Pacific and you often end up with a serious infection. One of my most memorable foreign lesions was a septic knee in Hawaii. What we used to call "dhobie itch" or "Rangoon itch" in Singapore (in Rangoon it is probably called Singapore itch), was a fungal infection, and everyone had it, as everyone eventually had sand fly bites or lice of some sort. "Crab lice or bhodhee lice?" an Indian pharmacist asked me much too loudly in the Victoria Chemist Shop on Serangoon Road in Singapore in 1971, and every customer at the shop turned to stare at me.

It is not possible to travel without coming down with something, but no one should stay home for that reason. Apart from terminal boredom, there are plenty of serious ailments available at home. Nits. Lice. Dog bites. Bedbugs. Food poisoning. Botulism. I was made miserable by a paronychia (infection at the base of a fingernail) in South London, and several years later got the same thing in New Guinea. The first I cured with antibiotics; the second, in the Trobriand Islands, I cured by boiling my thumb twice a day for a week, much to the puzzlement of local children. As I write, a funeral is being held for a Seattle youngster who died having eaten nothing more exotic than a hamburger at his local Jack-in-the-Box fast food outlet. Obviously that ought not to deter anyone from traveling to the Pacific Northwest. And simple accidents, the authors note, are much more common than infectious diseases, at home and abroad. Thomas Merton left his Trappist monastery in Kentucky after twenty-seven years of seclusion, only to fall victim to a faulty fan, which electrocuted him in Bangkok. That is a far more common story than, for example, the celebrated cases of Lassa fever—a hideous, often fatal, but rare disease—which tend to mislead potential travelers to West Africa, who are much more at risk from, say, dysentery or injuries sustained from being mugged.

It can be extremely dangerous for a kayaker to perform an Eskimo roll in an English river. In the past decade, many kayakers in England have contracted Weil's disease, also called leptospirosis, from being infected with spirochetal bacteria. It is a fact that these rivers are tainted with large amounts of rat urine. It is not unusual to read of an English kayaker making a so-called wet exit and successfully swimming to shore, only to fall victim to Weil's disease from the short swim. The consequence is often kidney failure, a hookup to a dialysis machine, and a long convalescence—all this from a few minutes splashing in a pretty tributary of the Avon.

It seems to me salutary that the focus of *Travelers' Health* is on prevention, with suggestions for cures. "How to Stay Healthy" is wonderfully emphasized in this book, which is sensible, undramatic, and exhaustive. Every serious traveler ought to own it. I feel confident that the doctors who have contributed to it are not the overweight and chainsmoking golfers who thirty years ago sent me abroad with facetious warnings of potential crocodile bites and beriberi. The enigmatic quack who measured Marlow's head before his Congo journey in *Heart of Darkness* ("I always ask leave, in the interests of science, to measure the crania of those going out there") was until recently a fairly common general practitioner. The literary physicians who make up Dr. Dawood's cohort are a new breed of doctors—not scaremongers and skeptics, but travelers themselves, who know a thing or two about expatriation, rock climbing, and trekking in distant parts of the world.

I can think of only one illness the authors have omitted, and that is kuru, a disease of the nervous system found in eastern New Guinea, principally among the Foré people. The word "kuru" means "trembling"—one of the symptoms. Perhaps it is right to leave it out, since the unique feature of kuru is that it is contracted only by people after they have eaten human brains.

PREFACE

It is perhaps fitting that a book about the health risks of travel should begin with a statistic on the health risks of staying at home. A twenty-year investigation (the Framingham study) has recently concluded that there is a definite link between heart disease and *not* traveling: women who seldom took vacations or never went away at all were twice as likely to suffer a heart attack, or die from heart disease, as women who went on vacation at least twice each year. If you are a careful, responsible traveler, travel *will* be good for your health and well-being, and good for the people and places you visit. This book is written by travelers, for travelers; it contains detailed, practical advice direct from specialists in every branch of travel medicine, and its sole purpose is to help you stay healthy wherever in the world you choose to go.

Travel is now less complicated and more affordable than it used to be. Today's travelers are more adventurous and more sophisticated in their tastes and choice of destination, and more people now travel overseas than ever before. Places that once were remote and difficult to reach have become readily accessible. International health regulations have been relaxed and immunization certificates are seldom necessary: you can travel to some of the world's most dangerous places directly from your nearest airport, without ever having to seek medical advice.

It is tempting to assume that advances in medical technology at home have been matched by progress in combating disease abroad, but that is incorrect. All of the world's major tropical diseases are spreading and are poorly controlled. The cholera epidemic in Latin America has produced 750,000 recorded cases in the past two years, and the speed and extent of its spread reflects the absence of sanitation and safe water supplies in most parts of the developing world. The cholera situation is now deteriorating, with the recent appearance of a new and more dangerous strain. Malaria is on the increase in almost every country where it occurs, and lethal, drug-resistant strains are a serious problem that is also getting worse. Early in 1993 there was an outbreak of yellow fever in East Africa, and as many as 900,000 local people had to be vaccinated before it could be brought back under control. Diphtheria—a disease that western medicine had almost forgotten—has returned with a vengeance in the former Soviet Union. HIV poses public health problems in the developing world that defy description, and is a growing hazard to travelers. Tuberculosis is once more on the increase, and drug resistant strains are widespread. Also on the increase are two diseases that most American travelers have never heard of: dengue fever in South America, and leishmaniasis, which is now killing thousands of people in the Sudan. Although diseases like these do not often affect travelers, they are serious enough to justify careful precautions to prevent them, and their continuing spread is a reflection of the underlying problem, the fact that world poverty is growing, not receding.

The most common travel-related illnesses are more mundane: two-fifths of all Americans who travel abroad suffer from travelers' diarrhea. This is often just a minor inconvenience, suffered in silence, but can easily become a miserable experience that disrupts travel plans, costs money, and results in hospitalization and a prolonged illness. (It typically wastes a tenth of the vacation and can even be responsible for an unwanted pregnancy by reducing absorption of the Pill.) Some travelers have come to regard diarrhea as inevitable or acceptable—the norm; it is none of these. The likelihood of developing travelers' diarrhea has not diminished in 35 years; despite the huge growth in our awareness of health issues that are closer to home, most travelers are still either not getting the information they need to stay healthy or are not putting it into practice. The result is that half of all international travelers experience some kind of adverse effect on their health.

There are many people who could help change this, but who are not doing so. Tour companies and travel agents, for example, are sometimes well aware of the risks at the destinations they serve, but play them down or dismiss them for fear of discouraging business. They argue that they are not physicians and that it is not their responsibility to dispense medical advice. They belittle the problems instead of pointing out the need for skilled advice or directing travelers to suitable sources. A survey of travelers to malarial areas, for example, showed that only 28 percent had received any kind of notification from their travel agent that malaria might be a possible hazard. In Europe, the situation is much the same: a Dutch survey showed that travelers who had used travel agents as their sole source of advice were in fact at greater risk than those who had not troubled to seek advice from any source.

While the industry is lukewarm about including information about health risks and precautions in its brochures, it is rather less casual about including disclaimers of legal liability—they are always there. The larger tour operators also have the power to influence hygiene and safety standards at their resorts and hotels, but do not use it. Organizations such as the International Society of Travel Medicine have tried hard to enlist the support of the industry to improve the quality of health information that travelers receive, but with little success. There are notable exceptions, and there are signs that things may improve in the future; in the meantime, judge your travel agent not just by his or her ability to get you a good deal, but also by the interest that is taken in the health aspects of your trip.

Destination countries are also worried about discouraging tourism or harming their image, and underreport or play down statistics for diseases such as malaria, yellow fever, and HIV infection and reports of violence, making it more difficult for travelers to take steps to protect themselves. Embassies and tourist offices of these nations consistently supply misleading information, either deliberately or through sheer incompetence and lack of care. Surveys repeatedly show that embassies and tourist offices *are not worth consulting* for any kind of health information.

The medical profession does not have an unblemished record either. Doctors in developed countries receive minimal training in hazards outside their own environment and remain largely unfamiliar with them. Many travelers who go to their physicians for advice come away with a prescription for a vaccine or two, and little more, and it is often a matter of luck whether the vaccines are the right ones. Again, there have been signs of improvement. The International Society of Travel Medicine and the American Society of Tropical Medicine and Hygiene are both making strenuous efforts to improve awareness of good medical practice, and to disseminate information about risks and precautions. Increasing numbers of physicians are taking an interest in travel medicine, and more travel clinics have appeared. Some of these clinics provide good service, although others undoubtedly place too much emphasis on the commercial aspects of selling vaccines. A glance through this book will make it clear that vaccines and medication can only protect you

"I cannot for the life of me understand the logic in your telling readers about the pollution problem in Rio de Janeiro. Somehow it seems a very self-destructive task for a publication supposed to encourage, not discourage, world travel. You are doing both your readers and your advertisers a disservice."
—New York advertising agency executive for VARIG, writing to withdraw further advertising from Condé Nast *Traveler* magazine

"We rejoice in the enrichments of travel, but our aim is to give readers the fullest information, frankly and fairly. They know it's a big world, where sometimes it's sunny and sometimes it rains. Isn't travel just as likely to be discouraged when it begins in illusion and ends in frustration and disappointment?"
—Harold Evans, Editorial, Condé Nast *Traveler* magazine

against a small number of diseases, most of which are not common; judge your travel clinic by the attention it devotes to other precautions, which are just as important.

Hazards to travelers' health arise not just from infections and exotic diseases, outbreaks and epidemics; a wide variety of other factors are involved, and this book addresses all of them in detail. The single most frequent cause of death in travelers abroad is accidents, causing 25 times as many deaths as infectious diseases. Some accidents and disasters are indeed indiscriminate, and raise issues of safety and security that concern all of us. Most accidents involving travelers, however, like the majority of travelers' health problems, are preventable or under a considerable degree of individual control. People worry increasingly about the dangers of blood transfusion and other forms of medical treatment abroad; prevention of accidents is the most effective way of reducing these risks as well.

The scope of this book largely reflects the range of problems that I have come across during my own travels—often without having been able to deal with them to my own satisfaction at the time—and many of the subjects considered here have not previously been given detailed attention in books for travelers. A specialist view is presented on each issue, because the range of subjects considered extends beyond the first-hand experience and expertise of any one individual, and because when travelers are most in need of information or advice about health, they need advice that they can trust and depend on, not secondhand myth and theory, or unsubstantiated lists of dos and don'ts.

Throughout the book, we have done our best to avoid the traditional formula of advising readers to "Consult a physician" every time we come across a difficult issue. It is not easy to find a physician in a remote place, or to communicate with one in a foreign country. Merely finding a physician does not guarantee that correct advice or treatment will be given. Some 85 percent of the world's population have never seen a doctor, and never will; medical advice for travel must take account of the fact that travelers to many parts of the world will be in the same position. There are more physicians in the state of California than there are in the whole of Africa.

Like the rest of medicine, travelers' health is not an exact science, and there is no consensus on many crucial issues. A recent survey found visitors from different countries to the same part of East Africa following no fewer than *eighty* different antimalarial regimes (an alarming 30 percent of the visitors were taking no precautions at all). Some of the problems raised in this book have no satisfactory solution, or have solutions that remain a matter of opinion or the subject of debate. The careful reader will therefore detect some differences of opinion between contributors to this book, or may disagree with their conclusions: we hope that this will stimulate and encourage further debate.

What unites all of the experts who have participated in this project, however, is a deeply rooted belief that nowhere on this planet is off limits—on health grounds at least—to travelers who are adequately prepared; that the health problems of travel are preventable, and that understanding the risks is the surest way to avoid them. Not the least reason for doing so is to savor to the fullest the rich experiences that travel has to offer.

—Richard M. Dawood
September 1993

ACKNOWLEDGEMENTS

This project owes much to the assistance and goodwill of many: among them are a large number of colleagues, friends and erstwhile traveling companions who have contributed to my own knowledge of travel medicine; and too many people to name individually who have provided encouragement, advice and practical help with this project since its inception.

I should like to thank again all of the contributors to this book for their wisdom, patience and participation; among them, I would particularly like to mention Dr. D. Peter Drotman, Dr. Hans Lobel, John Becher and Dr. John Naponick, whose advice during the preparation of this edition has been invaluable.

The drawings of insects are by Amanda Callaghan, and the drawings of snakes and other venomous creatures are by Professor David Warrell; I am grateful to Dr. Paul F. Wehrle for advice on diphtheria.

Special thanks also to: Alison Langton and Oxford University Press; my colleagues at Condé Nast *Traveler,* particularly Graham Boynton, Richard Levine, Gary Stoller, Aaron Sugarman, and Thomas J. Wallace; Eve Glasberg; Betsy Wade; Margaret Staats Simmons; Gillian Whitby; Nicole and Joseph Idler; Sophie Hicks; Paul Theroux; and at Random House, Ian Jackman and his colleagues, and above all, Harold Evans.

—Richard M. Dawood

CONTENTS

CONTRIBUTORS

Dr. **James M. Adam,** OBE, OStJ, BSc, MB, ChB, PhD, FRCP
Colonel (Retd) Royal Army Medical Corps
Lately, Consultant Physiologist, National Institute for Medical Research, and Army Medical Services; and Senior Lecturer, Institute of Environmental and Offshore Medicine, Aberdeen University, UK

Andrew N. Agle, MPH
Director of Operations, Global 2000, The Carter Center, Atlanta, Georgia

Dr. **Christopher L. R. Bartlett,** MSc, MB, BS, FRCP, MFPHM
Director, PHLS Communicable Disease Surveillance Center, Colindale, London
Honorary Lecturer, Department of Environmental and Preventive Medicine, The Medical College of St. Bartholomew's Hospital, London

Dr. **Michael R. Barer,** BSc, MB, BS, PhD
Lecturer in Microbiology, University of Newcastle upon Tyne, UK

John A. Becher, RPh
Chief, Drug Service, National Center for Infectious Diseases, Centers for Disease Control and Prevention, Atlanta, Georgia

Dr. **Ronald H. Behrens,** MD, MRCP
Consultant in Tropical and Travel Medicine, Hospital for Tropical Diseases, London
Honorary Senior Lecturer, London School of Hygiene and Tropical Medicine

Dr. **Alan J. Benson,** MSc, MB, ChB, FRAeS
Senior Medical Officer (Research), Royal Air Force Institute of Aviation Medicine, Farnborough, UK

Professor **Herbert A. Brant,** MD, FRCP(Ed), FRCS(Ed), FRCOG
Professor of Clinical Obstetrics and Gynecology, University College Hospital, London

Dr. **Stanley G. Browne,** CMG, OBE, MD, FRCP, FRCS, DTM
Formerly Secretary, International Leprosy Association
Formerly Consultant Adviser in Leprosy to the Department of Health, UK

Dr. **Elphis Christopher,** MB, BS, DObstRCOG, DCH

Senior Medical Officer (Family Planning), Haringey Health Authority, London
Doctor-in-Charge, Psychosexual Problem Clinic, University College Hospital, London

Dr. **Christopher Curtis,** BA, PhD
Medical Research Council, London
London School of Hygiene and Tropical Medicine

Andrew J. S. Dawood, BDS, MSc
Department of Conservative Dentistry, Guy's Hospital, London

Dr. **Richard M. Dawood,** MD(Lond.), FRCR, DTM&H
The Hospital for Sick Children, London

Lt. Col. **John G. Dickinson,** DM(Oxon.), FRCP, DTM&H, RAMC
Formerly Medical Superintendent, Patan Hospital, Kathmandu, Nepal
Professor of Clinical Physiology, Institute of Medicine, Tribhuwan University, Nepal
Consultant Physician, The Duchess of Kent's Military Hospital, Catterick Garrison, North Yorkshire, UK

Dr. **H. Elizabeth Driver,** BSc, MB, BS, DipTox, MRCPath
Consultant, McKenna & Co, London
Honorary Clinical Lecturer, University College and Middlesex School of Medicine
Consultant, Medical Research Council Toxicology Unit, Carshalton

Dr. **D. Peter Drotman,** MD, MPH, FACPM
Assistant Director for Public Health, Division of AIDS/HIV, National Center for Infectious Diseases, Centers for Disease Control and Prevention, Atlanta, Georgia
Clinical Assistant Professor of Community Health, Emory University School of Medicine, Atlanta, Georgia

Dr. **Herbert L. DuPont,** MD
Mary W. Kelsey Professor of Medical Sciences, and Director, Center for Infectious Diseases, University of Texas Medical School and School of Public Health, Houston
Past President, International Society of Travel Medicine

Dr. **Christopher J. Ellis,** FRCP, DTM&H
Consultant Physician, Department of Communicable and Tropical Diseases, East Birmingham Hospital, Birmingham, UK

Dr. **Richard Fairhurst,** MB, BS
Chief Medical Officer, The Travelers Medical Service, London

Chairman, British Association for Immediate Care

Timothy J. ffytche, FRCS
Consultant Ophthalmic Surgeon, Moorfields Eye Hospital, St. Thomas's Hospital and Hospital for Tropical Diseases, London

Dr. Susan Fisher-Hoch, MD
Medical Epidemiologist, National Center for Infectious Diseases, Centers for Disease Control and Prevention, Atlanta, Georgia

Peter Fison, MA, MB, FRCS, FCOphth
Consultant Ophthalmic Surgeon, Sutton Eye Unit, UK
Honorary Senior Lecturer, St. George's Hospital Medical School, London

Dr. William Foege, MD, MPH
Executive Director, Global 2000, The Carter Center, Atlanta, Georgia
Executive Director, Task Force for Child Survival and Development

Dr. Hemda Garelick, PhD
Research Fellow, Department of Medical Microbiology, London School of Hygiene and Tropical Medicine

Dr. David R. W. Haddock, MD, FRCP, DTM&H
Formerly Senior Lecturer in Tropical Medicine, Liverpool School of Tropical Medicine
Formerly Consultant Physician in Tropical Medicine, Liverpool Area Health Authority

Dr. Anthony P. Hall, FACP, FRCP(Ed)
Consultant Physician, Hospital for Tropical Diseases, London
Honorary Senior Lecturer, London School of Hygiene and Tropical Medicine
Member, WHO Expert Advisory Committee on Malaria

Wing Commander **Richard Harding, PhD, BSc, MB, BS, DAvMed, MRAeS, RAF**
Consultant in Aviation Medicine, Royal Air Force Institute of Aviation Medicine, Farnborough, UK

Dr. John Hawk, MD
Head, Photobiology Department, St. John's Institute of Dermatology, London

Basil Helal, MChirOrth, FRCS, FRCSE
Honorary Consultant Orthopedic Surgeon, The London Hospital, the Royal National Orthopedic Hospital, London, and the Enfield Group of Hospitals, UK

Dr. **Donald Hopkins,** MD, MPH
Senior Health Consultant, Guinea Worm Eradication Program
Director, Global 2000, The Carter Center, Atlanta, Georgia
Director, Intermediate Task Force for Disease Eradication

Barbara Hornby
Editor and Writer
Partner, Network Consultants, human resources consultancy and training
organization

Dr. **C. Robert Horsburgh, Jr.,** MD
Medical Epidemiologist, Division of HIV/AIDS, Centers for Disease Control and Prevention, Atlanta, Georgia

Dr. **Arnold F. Kaufmann,** DVM, MS
Chief, Bacterial Zoonoses Activity, Division of Bacterial Diseases, Centers for Disease Control and Prevention, Atlanta, Georgia

Andreas King, BSc
Assistant Editor, *Water & Waste Treatment* Journal, London

Dr. **Gil Lea,** MB, BS
Consultant Medical Advisor, Trailfinders Immunization Centre and Travel Clinic, London
Consultant Epidemiologist, PHLS Communicable Disease Surveillance Center, Colindale, London

Edward L. Lee II, CPP
President, The Lee Group, Inc., Falls Church, Virginia
Editor, *The Latin American Advisor*

Roger Lewis, MA, DipEd
Visiting Professor, National Research Council—IEROSS, Salerno, Italy
Former trustee, "Release," and National Council for the Welfare of Prisoners Abroad, UK

Dr. **Hans O. Lobel,** MD, MPH
Chief, Malaria Surveillance Branch, Centers for Disease Control and Prevention, Atlanta, Georgia

Dr. **P. E. Clinton Manson-Bahr,** MD, FRCP, DTM&H
Lately Senior Lecturer in Clinical Tropical Medicine, London School of Hygiene and Tropical Medicine
Senior Physician Specialist, Colonial Medical Service

Dr. **Martin Mitcheson,** MB, FRCPsych
Clinical Director, Drug Problem Team, Glenside Hospital, Bristol, UK

Dr. **John Naponick,** MD, CM, MPH&TM
Medical Adviser, Association for Voluntary Surgical Contraception, Dhaka, Bangladesh

Air Commodore **Anthony N. Nicholson,** OBE, DSc, FRCP(Edin), FRCPath, RAF
Consultant Adviser in Aviation Medicine
Royal Air Force Institute of Aviation Medicine, Farnborough, UK

Dr. **Peter O. Oliver,** RD, MD, FFOM, DPH
Lately, Group Medical Director, Cunard Steam-Ship Co., Southampton, UK

Peta A. Pascoe, BSc
Principal Scientific Officer, Royal Air Force Institute of Aviation Medicine, Farnborough, UK

Dr. **Robin Philipp,** MB, ChB, FFOM, FFPHM, MCCM(NZ)
Consultant Senior Lecturer in Public Health Medicine
Director, WHO Collaborating Center for Environmental Health Promotion and Ecology, University of Bristol, UK

Nancy J. Piet-Pelon
Cross-cultural Trainer, Population/Family Planning Consultant, AVSC, Dhaka, Bangladesh

Ellen G. Poage, RN, MPH
Case Manager, Shands Home Care, Fort Myers, Florida

Dr. **Thomas J. Quan,** PhD, MPH
Research Microbiologist, Plague Branch, Centers for Disease Control and Prevention, Fort Collins, Colorado

Dr. **Sonia B. Richards,** MD
Epidemic Intelligence Service Officer, Division of HIV/AIDS, Centers for Disease Control and Prevention, Atlanta, Georgia

Surgeon Commander **Simon S. Ridout,** MB, BS, MSc, AFOM, RN
Principal Medical Officer, RNAS Culdrose, Helston, Cornwall, UK

Rod Robinson, BSc, MIBiol, FRES, FRSH
Senior Research Officer, The Medical Entomology Center, University of Cambridge, UK
Publisher, *Media Medica,* Chichester

Dr. **George P. Schmid,** MD
Clinical Research Investigator, Center for Prevention Services, Centers for Disease Control and Prevention, Atlanta, Georgia

Professor **Gordon Seward,** CBE, MDS, FDSRCS, MB, BS, FRCS(Eng), FRCS(Edin), FFARCS
Emeritus Professor of Oral and Maxillo-Facial Surgery in the University of London

Dr. **Stanley Schwartz,** MD
Dermatologist, Fort Myers, Florida

Dr. **Bonita Stanton,** MD
Professor of Pediatrics and Chief, Division of General Pediatrics, University of Maryland at Baltimore

Dr. **Robert Steffen,** MD
Professor, Division of Epidemiology and Prevention of Communicable Diseases, University of Zurich, Switzerland
President, International Society of Travel Medicine

Aaron Sugarman
Senior News Writer, Condé Nast *Traveler* magazine,
New York

Dr. **Theodore Tsai,** MD, MPH
Former chief of Arboviral Disease Branch, Centers for Disease Control and Prevention, Fort Collins, Colorado

Professor **David A. Warrell,** MA, DM, FRCP
Professor of Tropical Medicine and Infectious Diseases, University of Oxford, UK
Honorary Clinical Director, Alistair Reid Venom Research Unit, Liverpool School of Tropical Medicine

Dr. **Tony Waterston,** MD, MRCP, DCH, DRCOG
Consultant Community Pediatrician, Newcastle General Hospital, UK
Formerly Consultant Pediatrician, Godfrey Huggins School of Medicine, Harare, Zimbabwe

Dr. **Peter J. Watkins,** MD, FRCP
Consultant Physician, Diabetic Department, King's College Hospital, London

Louise Weiss
Travel Writer, New York

Dr. **Philip D. Welsby,** FRCP(Ed)
Consultant Physician in Communicable Diseases, The City Hospital, Edinburgh, UK

Dr. **Martin S. Wolfe,** MD
Director, Travelers' Medical Service, Washington, D.C.
Tropical Medicine Specialist, Office of Medical Services, U.S. Department of State and the Foreign Service, Washington, D.C.

Dr. **George B. Wyatt,** MB, FRCP, FFPHM, DCH, DTM&H
Senior Lecturer in Tropical Medicine, Liverpool School of Tropical Medicine
Consultant Physician, Mersey Regional Hospital Board, UK

Professor **Arie J. Zuckerman,** MD, DSc, FRCP, FRCPath
Dean and Director of the WHO Collaborating Center for Reference and Research on Viral Diseases, Royal Free Hospital School of Medicine, London

ABOUT THIS BOOK

- This book contains more information than other books for travelers: is all this information really necessary? For example, all most travelers really *need* to know about rabies is that it is a serious disease, spread by animal bites. If you are so unlucky as to be bitten abroad, however, as I have been, your life may suddenly depend upon detailed information you would probably not want to carry in your head: how to treat the bite, what kind of vaccine to insist on, and what to do. It is not always possible to predict what will happen when you travel, and health information based on a few tips to follow won't always help you. The main objective of this book is to draw together all the health information you might need, direct from the experts who really know. You may not want to read all of it in advance, and you may choose not to follow all of the precautions we suggest, but having the information at least allows *you* to make that choice.

- This book is mainly about prevention, so to get the most from it you should become familiar with it *before* you travel. It will also help you deal with problems that occur while you are traveling, though diagnosis of infectious diseases may be difficult even with skilled medical care and laboratory facilities.

- Don't be put off by the names of strange diseases you have not come across before, or by some of the more technical information we provide; you do not have to know everything, and the important practical points are summarized at the end of each chapter, but I believe it is important for us to try to give you the background information on which our advice is based.

- *If you are traveling only within North America, Northern Europe, and Australasia,* most of the infectious and parasitic diseases referred to in the first half of this book will not be a significant hazard. All travelers should be immunized against tetanus (p. 91), however, and the sections on diarrhea (p. 13), rabies (p. 197), and Chapter 5 on diseases spread by insects (p. 121) may also be relevant to you. There is much more to the subject of health problems in travelers than infectious diseases, as you will see from the second half of this book.

- If you are traveling elsewhere, especially to *Africa, Asia, or Latin America*, the sections on diseases of poor hygiene and diseases spread by insects will be particularly relevant. An indication of the geographical distribution of specific diseases is summarized in Appendix 3.

- Remember that accidents are the commonest cause of death in travelers, and that most accidents are preventable (p. 262); malaria is the most serious infectious hazard that travelers are likely to come across, and full details about prevention appear on pp. 128–130; hepatitis A is common, but is also preventable (pp. 52–53); diarrhea and sunburn are the two problems that most often interfere with travel plans, and they, too, are preventable.

- Depending on the nature of your trip, the risk of other diseases is probably small anyway, but simple precautions can often dramatically reduce or eliminate the risks altogether; this book is for travelers whose health abroad is too important to be left to chance.

WARNING

Every effort has been made to ensure that the information presented in this book is accurate. Advice from a book has its limitations, however, and cannot always take account of the particular circumstances of each individual traveler. Advice offered here is not intended to be a substitute for skilled medical care, when such care is available.

TRAVELERS'
HEALTH

HOW TO STAY HEALTHY
ALL OVER THE WORLD

INTRODUCTION: STAYING HEALTHY ABROAD

INTRODUCTION: STAYING HEALTHY ABROAD

Prevention is the only strategy for staying healthy abroad that any traveler can afford to rely on. Health precautions really work, and the time you invest in becoming familiar with them will be amply rewarded.

Dr. Richard Dawood *devised this project and is the editor of this book. He has traveled in more than 70 countries around the world—and has survived.*

Staying healthy abroad is not a question of luck, and is much too important to be left to chance; the purpose of this book is to give you the information you need to *prevent* health problems when you travel, before they occur.

WHY PREVENTION?

Of all the hazards and infectious diseases that travelers are exposed to abroad, some are lethal, many are dangerous, and several have long-term effects upon health and well-being; some, also, may be passed on to family, friends, and contacts on the traveler's return home.

The majority of health problems in travelers, however troublesome at the time, tend to be relatively minor in their long-term implications—which is just as well, in view of the substantial numbers of travelers who experience illness abroad, and the meager attention that such problems generally receive.

A problem need not be serious, however, in order to have a devastating effect upon one's enjoyment of a trip. An undignified bout of diarrhea can be all it takes to force a major change of travel plans, mar a vacation, or interrupt a vital business deal.

Health problems in travelers are common. The risks are not decreasing, and we are all susceptible. Health care abroad is costly, travel is expensive, our leisure time is precious, and some business travelers have much at stake; if for no other reason than the most mercenary ones, prevention is a strategy for health that no traveler can afford to neglect.

PREVENTION: DEVISING A STRATEGY

Don't delegate responsibility for *your* health abroad to anyone else, however busy or preoccupied you may be with more pressing preparations for your trip; take personal charge. Business travelers are consistently at fault in this regard: they are often less well-informed about health than the average vacationer, and even when they have made efforts previously to find out about their precautions, they tend not to update their knowledge, and become complacent.

Intelligence, good health, and a general knowledge do not absolve you from the need to obtain careful advice and up-to-date information about the health risks of travel that apply to your particular circumstances and travel plans, from a reliable source. This book is intended to help you do that. Even if you are well-informed about health issues that apply to your home environment, you should not assume that this will help you overseas: many of the precautions that are necessary for travel are not logical or intuitive.

Remember that not all doctors are equally able to provide the information you need, and many will probably not provide more than a part of it unless you ask specifically about each point that concerns you. "Most physicians are remarkably ill-informed about health risks abroad and appropriate protective measures," according to one senior U.S. public health official. Two recent surveys of local health departments and specialized travel clinics in the USA found significant variation in the reliability of the advice on offer, even from supposedly knowledgeable sources. There have been at least three recent surveys of travel advice from British family physicians that have yielded similarly depressing results. Doctors are *not* the sole source of reliable health advice: nurses and other staff at immunization centers, travel clinics, and college health centers frequently have considerable experience and more time to talk to you. Listen carefully to them.

SPECIFIC PREVENTION MEASURES

Immunization offers protection from several important diseases, and should not be neglected (see pp. 498–514). An important development is the new vaccine against hepatitis A, which will soon replace the unpopular gamma-globulin injection. The vaccine against hepatitis B will probably become less expensive since being added to childhood immunization schedules; it deserves to be more widely used by travelers. The new typhoid vaccines have fewer side effects than their predecessor. And all travelers to developing countries should consider carefully whether they might benefit from protection with the new rabies vaccines. The old injected cholera vaccination is now no longer recommended, and the only remaining formal vaccination certificate requirements for travel relate to yellow fever.

Be aware of the pitfalls, however. Vaccination *regulations* are generally designed to protect countries rather than travelers, and not all individuals to whom you may turn for advice are able to make this important distinction. Regulations and *recommendations* for each country in the world are liable to change from time to time, and so should be confirmed before departure (see Appendix 8).

Immunizations don't work if they have not been given or are allowed to lapse, and their timing requires thought; not all of them offer 100 percent protection. Nor can all diseases be prevented by immunization: no traveler who has undergone even a full course of immunization should ever be allowed to assume that no further precautions will be necessary.

Prevention (prophylaxis) with drugs is an essential protective measure for travelers to malarious areas (see pp. 121–32)—malaria is by far the most dangerous infectious disease hazard most travelers are likely to come across, and is a potential killer that should never be underestimated. Drug-resistant strains of malaria are now present throughout the tropics. Chloroquine, once the most widely used preventive drug, is now seldom effective, and mefloquine (Lariam), introduced only recently, seems inevitably destined for the same fate. Although antimalarial medication is now far from infallible, it should still be taken because it reduces the likelihood and severity of disease. Drugs are not enough on their own, however, and measures to avoid mosquito bites are of the utmost importance.

Drug treatment can sometimes also be used to prevent certain diarrheal diseases, but this subject is a controversial one (see p. 25); the desired result is more likely to be achieved by careful precautions with food, water, and hygiene.

Preventing individual diseases by taking medication may seem an attractive concept, but unfortunately this is not a precaution on which travelers can rely.

GENERAL PRECAUTIONS

In most cases, each disease of concern to the traveler does not have its own, unique, specific preventive measure. There is, after all, a limit to the number of possible ways in which diseases can spread. The same approach to food hygiene provides protection against dysentery in Manila as it does against giardiasis in St. Petersburg; and insect repellents assiduously applied protect the traveler against dengue fever in the Caribbean as well as against filariasis in West Africa and unpleasant diseases in many other countries around the world.

Although detailed information about a large number of diseases appears in this book, and the list of hazards may at first glance appear frightening, the important point to realize is that prevention is not only feasible in virtually every case, but is usually not difficult and follows logical principles which relate directly to how the disease is spread. The mode of spread holds the key to prevention of each disease, but this book presents further details as well—to add interest, to provide perspective, and to give purpose to precautions that might otherwise seem obscure or not really necessary.

Because some preventive measures are common to many diseases, a degree of overlap between chapters in a book of this type is inevitable; I make no apology, for the repetition serves to emphasize their importance.

Food hygiene A recent survey of visitors to East Africa showed that only 2 percent of them were taking adequate dietary precautions. Nothing less than a process of education or reeducation in the fundamental principles of hygienic food preparation will protect travelers to most countries outside Northern Europe, North America, or Australia. Appetite is a poor guide to food safety, and food should never be assumed to be safe unless it is known to have been freshly and thoroughly cooked (heat sterilized)—in the case of meat, until no red color remains and served hot. Let this rule guide your choice from even the most tempting menu. Satisfy yourself that today's lunch is not yesterday's evening meal, reheated and rearranged. Intricate delicacies that have received much handling during preparation, and cold platters left out in the open, are highly likely to have been contaminated. Fruit and vegetables should be freshly cooked or freshly peeled.

Prawns, oysters, and other seafood feed by filtering the water around them; they are rapidly able to accumulate dangerous levels of bacteria and viruses, and only 4 percent of shellfish-growing areas in the Mediterranean now produce seafood that is fit to eat. Shellfish should be boiled vigorously for at least 10 minutes, or preferably avoided altogether. Even within the USA, public health officials estimate that the risk of gastrointestinal illnesses is 18000 percent greater from eating shellfish than from eating fish, and cholera organisms have recently been found in oysters harvested from Mobile Bay. This means that you won't always be able to eat what you want or what is on offer when you are hungry. These principles are of crucial importance to travelers, and are discussed again at length in the next chapter and elsewhere throughout the book (see also Appendix 5).

A 1988 survey of 10,000 chefs in Taiwan found that more than two-thirds had athlete's foot; most chefs smoked while cooking bare-chested over hot stoves. The local food hygiene department, with praiseworthy candor, described 90 percent of kitchens in Taiwan as "hotbeds of germs."

Expensive hotels offer no guarantee of safety from diseases of poor hygiene, and it is a grave error to assume that the food they serve is automatically safe. A recent, serious outbreak of amebic dysentery and amebic liver abscesses in a group of Italian tourists was traced to raw vegetables served on ice at a luxury hotel in Phuket. A recent survey by the British consumer travel magazine *Holiday Which?* found appalling examples of poor hygiene standards and contaminated food in hotel kitchens at popular European resorts; it concluded that a hotel's star rating bore little relation to the standard of food hygiene in its kitchen. I have myself seen waiters at a top

Paris hotel use their breath to polish plates and glasses, a particularly hazardous practice in these days of resurgent TB. If in doubt about local hygiene standards, have a look at the kitchen yourself, and check for flies; do you see any food left lying around exposed? Flies cannot discriminate between the plate of a wealthy tourist and any of their other preferred habitats. African flies carry African diseases, and you can acquire dysentery from a single fly. Do not allow luxurious surroundings to lull you into a false sense of security, and be prepared to *insist* on safe food.

Low-budget travelers are not necessarily at greater risk of illness than travelers who stick to luxury hotels. Whether you eat in a street market or anywhere else, you can rely on the same principles of food hygiene to protect you. Do you enjoy eating bread fresh from the oven, food that you have selected and watched cooking, and fresh fruit, peeled carefully yourself? (I always travel with a small spoon and a sharp knife for just this purpose.) Food like this is easy to find, is cheap, appetizing, and is almost always safe to eat.

Clean hands It is all very well to wash your hands before a meal, but if you then proceed to wipe your hands on a filthy towel that has been contaminated by others, and then touch the bathroom door handle, you are literally asking for trouble.

Water safety and purification are discussed in detail in Chapter 3 (see pp. 70–85). In most countries outside Northern Europe, North America, and Australia, water from the public drinking supply is likely to be just a very dilute solution of sewage, and should be regarded as such unless known to be safe.

Hospitality is a dangerous pitfall for the unwary. It takes diplomacy and determination to refuse food prepared (unhygienically) by someone who has clearly gone to great lengths in order to please an honored visitor. This can be an extremely delicate problem in rural areas in developing countries. My personal advice is not to relax your standards of food hygiene under any circumstances; plead illness, use any excuse, and if necessary, even permit the food to be put on your plate and toy with it, but *do not eat* food you consider to be suspect. The momentary embarrassment of offending one's host (and genuine offense is rarely taken) has to be balanced against the risk of illness that may ruin your trip or put you out of action for several days.

Insects transmit a multitude of diseases, not all of which can be prevented individually, and their bites can be a painful nuisance. With the relentless spread of drug-resistant malaria, personal protection from insects has become even more important; a notable advance is the use of bed nets impregnated with insecticide, which have proved to be over thirty times more effective than untreated nets, and in places where they have been introduced on a wide scale, the incidence of malaria has fallen considerably. Such methods are discussed in depth on pp. 182–92. Travelers to some infected areas can expect to be bitten by malaria-bearing mosquitoes at least once a day.

Sex Sex abroad has always been a risky business, but the penalties are now higher. There is a growing number of well-documented cases of HIV transmission to travelers of both sexes following heterosexual intercourse. In the USA, details of cases acquired overseas are not recorded separately, but British figures suggest that at least 450 British travelers were known to have become HIV-positive after heterosexual exposure abroad during 1992—the true figure was probably even higher, and these figures are set to rise exponentially. Estimates of HIV infection rates in many countries are of dubious accuracy, and as Dr. Peter Drotman explains elsewhere in this book, are not a reliable basis for decisions about which countries might be "safe." As far as the risks of HIV are concerned, where you go is less important than what you do when you get there.

It has been estimated that there are as many as 2 million prostitutes in Thailand alone, most of whom have had 5,000 sexual partners by the age of 19: and that one-third of male visitors to Thailand have sex with prostitutes, more than 70 percent of whom are thought to be infected with sexually transmitted diseases at any one time. In some parts of the country, at least 70 percent of prostitutes are believed to be HIV-positive. One in eleven Kenyans are now HIV-positive. An expert at an HIV conference in 1991 estimated that "every jumbo jet leaving Bangkok, Manila, Rio de Janeiro, and Algiers is carrying another ten new HIV infections."

Sun Since people from cooler climates have been taking vacations in sunny places in ever greater numbers, the incidence of skin cancer has risen significantly: the incidence of melanoma, the most serious form, is now rising in many countries by around 7 percent each year—a higher rate than for any other cancer. Skin cancers are now known to have a clear relationship not just with long-term exposure to ultraviolet light, but also with acute episodes of sunburn. (Did you know that lying in the sun can also be a significant source of extra calories? One estimate is that it adds about 300 calories per hour per hundred pounds of body weight, to your body's total energy intake.)

Exposure to ultraviolet light also causes cataract formation and retinal damage: choose good-quality sunglasses that filter out the harmful rays. A survey by Condé Nast *Traveler* has shown that some brands—especially children's—offer very little ultraviolet protection. Poor-quality sunglasses are harmful: they cause the pupil to dilate, countering the eye's natural protective response, and allowing more dangerous ultraviolet light into the eye.

The environment holds many hazards, including heat, cold, the effects of high altitude, the bites of wild animals, and accidents—the biggest hazard of all. A large part of this book is devoted to such subjects, and it is often the simplest precautions that are most important. For example, if you have children and you rent a car abroad, remember that child seats cut their risk of dying in an automobile crash by 70 percent. And if you are planning to use a moped or motorcycle, your risk of injury is at least 40 times greater than if you use a car.

Many accidents abroad relate to alcohol (at least 20 percent of drownings, for example). Remember that drinks may not come in standard measures, or even in standard strengths. Many countries have lower blood-alcohol limits for drivers, and in many countries there is also a high likelihood of being tested. Pedestrians involved in accidents are also likely to be tested. The penalties are generally high. Travel insurance policies often exclude cover for accidents, injuries, and losses that take place while under the influence of alcohol.

Remember to travel unobtrusively, be discreet with your possessions, and avoid flourishing large sums of money in poor areas: as the late Dr. Alistair Reid, an expert on hazards from wild animals, once pointed out, the greatest animal danger to travelers is man.

ILLNESS ABROAD

When prevention fails or the unavoidable occurs, coping with illness abroad and, if necessary, getting yourself or someone else home again quickly, demands resourcefulness and judgment. It helps if a doctor can be found, and knowledge of the local language is a valuable asset. Often, though, self-help is everything.

Medical treatment abroad may itself be dangerous. Publicity about AIDS has drawn attention to some of the potential hazards: screened *and* unscreened blood transfusions, nonsterile needles, syringes, and medical and dental instruments, acupuncture, and surgery may all spread HIV (see p. 429); hepatitis B, however, is much more common, and is also spread by these routes. There are numerous examples of travelers undergoing immunization in poor countries and subsequently developing hepatitis. Not all medical attention is undertaken voluntarily. Have an auto accident in Turkey, and you will almost certainly have to provide a blood sample for measurement of your blood-alcohol level; the sterility of the needle that is used will probably depend on precisely where you are unfortunate enough to have your accident.

Other hazards include drugs and vaccines that may be ineffective or dangerous; in some poor countries, where the likelihood of being bitten by a dog, and the frequency of rabies, are both high, the locally produced rabies vaccine may be almost as lethal as the disease itself. Medical skills and standards of practice also vary, and in particular, women should always make sure that a chaperon is present when they are examined. In some countries, there may be an overenthusiasm for surgical treatment, and this is undoubtedly the case in many European ski resorts; other than in a desperate emergency—a situation that is usually self-evident—repatriation is usually possible prior to any surgery.

The most usual problems, however, are inadequacy of emergency services, and scarcity or inaccessibility of skilled medical facilities. Places with reasonable facilities for local people may not necessarily be suitable for dealing with emergencies in foreigners. In Crete, for example, the annual influx of tourists swells the local population from 160,000 to 500,000. In the summer, the hospital in Heraklion has to cope with more than 10 injured tourists every day—mostly from moped accidents: not all survive the three-hour ambulance journey from the south of the island.

Adequate insurance may remove anxiety about expense, and should provide for emergency repatriation if necessary, but it is also important to have enough cash available to cover immediate costs. A general awareness of the main, likely health risks will be invaluable. Specific advice for coping with individual diseases is given in each of the chapters on the main diseases.

In my view, *all travelers to remote areas with limited medical facilities should also have a knowledge of basic first aid*—both for their own benefit, and the benefit of others—and should attend a course of instruction if necessary.

COMING HOME

The value of a post-tropical checkup is discussed in Appendix 7. All travelers should realize, however, that it is possible for symptoms of infectious diseases—especially malaria—not to appear until several weeks, or even longer, after returning home. When symptoms do appear, their significance may not be recognized immediately: roughly half of all fatal malaria cases are initially misdiagnosed as flu. The worst place to be is a country that sees few cases—the death rate for travelers with malaria is 10 times higher in Japan than in the USA, and the U.S. rate is roughly twice the UK rate. There are other pitfalls too: one vacationer died recently from appendicitis, misdiagnosed as travelers' diarrhea.

If illness does develop after a trip, make sure that your doctor understands that you have been traveling.

ATTITUDE

A positive attitude to health, and perception of one's health as a vital element in the success of a trip—rather than as an inconvenient obstacle to enjoyment—are powerful weapons indeed for any traveler.

AND FINALLY . . .

The message of this book is not that you should worry about each and every disease that is mentioned here, every time and wherever you travel; or, worse still, that you would be better off staying at home. It is simply this: by informing yourself of the nature of the hazards that travelers face and how these hazards can be overcome, you will learn healthy travel habits that will protect you wherever you go. You could, of course, learn them the hard way, as I have had to do on many of my own travels, in which case you need read no further.

2

DISEASES SPREAD MAINLY BY FOOD, DRINK, AND POOR HYGIENE

DIARRHEA AND INTESTINAL INFECTIONS

"Travel enriches the mind and loosens the bowels"—Sherwood Gorbach. Millions of travelers, all over the world, have discovered for themselves how true this statement can be. However, travelers' diarrhea is most often a preventable illness.

Dr. Herbert L. DuPont is Director of the Center for Infectious Diseases, University of Texas Medical School and School of Public Health, and has been conducting research into travelers' diarrhea for many years. He is Past President of the International Society of Travel Medicine.

Dr. Michael Barer is a medical microbiologist at the University of Newcastle upon Tyne, UK, where he teaches and conducts research on infections of the gastrointestinal tract.

If you already have diarrhea and want help, turn to *What to do if you get sick* on p. 26.

If you want quick, simple advice on how to avoid getting diarrhea in the first place, turn to *How to Prevent Diarrhea* on p. 24, and Appendix 5.

If you want to understand why these measures may or may not work, read on!

Diarrhea is among the commonest of all medical problems related to travel. All travelers, and especially those visiting tropical and semitropical developing countries, need to understand how to minimize the risk of becoming ill, and how to treat illness that does occur in order to minimize discomfort, disruption of travel plans, and more serious complications.

WHAT ARE THE RISKS?

How common is travelers' diarrhea, where does it occur most often, and what factors influence the rate of occurrence?

Any kind of travel increases the risk of developing diarrhea, and the level of risk is influenced by two main factors: your home region, and your destination.

As far as the risk of acquiring diarrhea is concerned, for travelers from industrialized countries, the world can be divided into three regions:

High risk Latin America, Africa, Southern Asia

Low risk: United States, Canada, northwestern Europe, Australia, New Zealand, and Japan

Intermediate risk: northern Mediterranean regions, China, Eastern Europe, and the former Soviet Union

When a person from a low-risk region travels to a high-risk region, the likelihood of developing a diarrheal illness is about 40 percent. When the same individual travels to an intermediate-risk area, the rate of illness is approximately 10 percent. For a traveler who goes from one low-risk region to another, the risk is between 2 and 5 percent—higher than the rate of illness in people who resist the urge to travel and just stay home. Naturally, the longer the trip, the more likely it is that illness will occur.

The 2-to-5-percent background rate of diarrhea among low-risk travelers arises from many factors, including: the stress of travel itself; the fact that many more meals are eaten at restaurants or prepared by others, with greater opportunity for contamination than when food is prepared at home; increased alcohol consumption; and the presence of poorly absorbed salts and other noninfective diarrhea-producing substances found in local, unfamiliar food and water sources.

The rate of diarrhea when a person from a high-risk region travels to either another high-risk region or to a lower-risk region is probably about the same 2-to-5-percent background rate. This reduced susceptibility, compared with that for travelers from low-risk areas, suggests that the infectious organisms that cause illness are widespread throughout the developing world.

Some of the other factors that predispose to diarrhea are listed in Table 2.1. Travelers in these categories are at additional risk, and therefore need to take much more careful precautions if they wish to avoid illness.

Most cases of travelers' diarrhea are caused by microorganisms that either damage the gut or interfere with the normal mechanisms that control water flow across the gut wall. They are transmitted in the same manner: you must actually swallow contaminated material to contract the disease.

This has two important practical consequences. First, you should identify and avoid food, drink, or anything else you might swallow that has a high risk of being contaminated. Second, you should ensure that you do not touch the food you eat, or (if you must use your fingers) that your hands are scrupulously clean and as dry as

TABLE 2.1. TRAVELERS AT INCREASED RISK OF DIARRHEA

- Travelers who are elderly, or very young
- Travelers living under conditions of reduced hygiene, in close contact with the local community
- Travelers who have little or no opportunity to select what food and drink they consume
- Travelers with an important underlying disease including: diabetes mellitus requiring insulin, heart disease requiring regular medication, chronic liver disease, and acquired immune deficiency syndrome (AIDS)
- Travelers on treatment with potent inhibitors of gastric acidity (e.g., omeprazole)

possible (if necessary, use clean paper tissues or napkins to handle food while eating); plates and cutlery should also be clean and dry.

The risk of developing diarrhea *can* be reduced considerably: travelers' diarrhea is to a major degree a preventable illness, and the necessary precautions will be considered in detail.

WHY DOES IT OCCUR, AND WHY CAN'T THE PROBLEM BE ELIMINATED?

In tropical and semitropical developing countries, the environment is heavily contaminated with microorganisms that are potentially disease-producing. Travelers from industrialized regions have typically lived their lives in a clean and uncontaminated environment, and are highly susceptible to infection in the same way that a young infant is susceptible to the organisms found in a day-care center.

In most tropical developing countries, human excreta is widely used as fertilizer (see below). General principles of personal and food hygiene are widely understood in industrialized countries, but not in developing countries, where the problems are made worse by poverty and poor education. Ignorance of correct food hygiene practices means that contaminated food is unlikely to be washed properly after purchase and during preparation; and after preparation, food will often be allowed to remain at room temperature for prolonged periods of time, which further encourages the growth of bacteria. (Room temperature in tropical countries is warmer, so safe storage times without refrigeration are much shorter.) Washing hands, keeping all kitchen surfaces clean and uncontaminated, avoiding contact between prepared and unprepared food, and eliminating flies, are basic and effective precautions that simply may not be a local priority.

Although the local water supply may be chlorinated at source, and even if it is safe most of the time, it may readily become contaminated—because of poor quality control, cross-contamination with environmental sewage following rainfall and flooding, breaks in water pipes, or because tanks and water reservoirs in houses or buildings become contaminated after filling.

Some of the factors that relate to safety of food and drink are listed in Table 2.2. The chances of acquiring an intestinal infection are also dose-related. In other words, the more you consume of a suspect food, the more likely you are to get sick. You should bear this in mind when tempted to try out any alien delicacies: the key to protection is to keep the dose (i.e., number) of infecting organisms in your food as low as possible, and below the level that will produce illness.

Travelers who prepare their own food, wash the surfaces of all fruit and vegetables carefully with clean water before consumption, eat food as soon as it is prepared or cooked, and refrigerate and store correctly any items to be eaten later, will almost certainly *not* be exposed to microorganisms capable of producing illness.

SPECIFIC FOOD HAZARDS

Some kinds of foods are safer than others. Bacteria are susceptible to heat, and if the temperature of the food or drink reaches 150°F, the item can generally be assumed to be safe to consume, and should be eaten immediately after preparation.

Bacteria also need moisture to survive, so that dry foods (e.g., bread, crackers) are safer than those that are moist (e.g., salads, sauces, buffet-style items in open dishes). Other aspects of food safety include acid content of the item (citrus is generally safe because of its citric and ascorbic acid content), and those with a high sugar content (e.g., syrups and jellies) should also be safe.

TABLE 2.2. FOOD AND DRINK: FACTORS INFLUENCING RISK OF MICROBIAL CONTAMINATION AND DIARRHEA

REDUCED RISK:

- Staying at a hotel with a history of low frequency or absent diarrhea in its other guests (though accurate information about this is often difficult to obtain)
- Eating foods you have prepared yourself, observing careful hygiene precautions including correct cleansing, handling and storage
- Eating other "safe" foods, such as those served steaming hot, citrus fruit, bread, jellies and syrups; carbonated drinks

DANGEROUS, HIGH RISK:

- Eating with local people; selecting food indiscriminately from street vendors
- Eating moist foods served at room temperature (including all buffet-style foods, sauces in open containers), fruit with its skin intact (grapes, tomatoes, strawberries)
- Drinking milk, or tap water, or brushing teeth with tap water
  Using ice not known to have been made from bottled or boiled water

The following foods can be particularly risky:

Shellfish and seafood Uncooked or poorly cooked shellfish and sea-food represent a health hazard regardless of where in the world they are consumed. In many instances this is a consequence of their mode of feeding, which involves filtration of large volumes of water, leading to accumulation of microorganisms like vibrios, *Plesio-monas, Aeromonas*, and hepatitis viruses: in many parts of the world, untreated sewage is deposited close to areas where shellfish are collected. With poor handling or storage, they may also become contaminated after harvesting, with virtually any of the bacterial or parasitic agents listed in Table 2.3. People with underlying liver disease, hemochromatosis (a disease of excess body iron stores), and AIDS are particularly susceptible to *Vibrio vulnificus* from raw oysters, and these individuals should never consume these food substances at home or abroad.

Vegetables, salads, and fruit In many of the tropical developing coun-tries, crops are grown in soil fertilized with human excreta, which assures that fruit, salads, and uncooked fresh vegetables are heavily contaminated with disease-producing microorganisms. Salads and fresh fruit are also frequently contaminated during transit, storage, or preparation. However, travelers to remoter areas who peel fruit themselves without contaminating the contents and eat the fruit immediately are at little risk of infection from this source. One almost suspects that the Almighty created bananas especially for this purpose.

Rice Freshly cooked rice is generally safe, but rice that has been left over and reheated may not be. *Bacillus cereus*, a common contam-inating organism, is able to survive the initial cooking process by producing heat-resistant spores. When left at room temperatures, these spores can produce a toxin that is not destroyed by further cooking, leading to severe vomiting and diarrhea.

Drinks Water purification is dealt with in detail in Chapter 3. How-ever, as has already been suggested in relation to salads, water contamination is not a matter that can be ignored by those who do not drink water: ice, ices, and anything else prepared locally from suspect water supplies should be considered contaminated, since freezing will kill only a fraction of any organisms present. If the local water supply is unsafe to drink, it is also unsafe to use for brushing teeth. Remember also that it is easy to swallow small quantities of water while swimming or taking a shower.

Alcohol Due caution should also be taken with alcoholic drinks, which should not be assumed to be self-sterilizing. Furthermore, excessive alcohol intake may itself cause diarrhea by an irritant action. Alcohol within a drink has a dehydrating effect, and reduces the amount of water actually available for rehydration. For these reasons, alcoholic drinks are not recommended as a source of water intake in hot countries.

Milk products Unpasteurized milk (and ice cream or yogurt made from it) should always be avoided. Diarrheal diseases are rarely contracted this way, but other diseases such as brucellosis and tuberculosis are a real problem in some regions. Listeriosis is a disease that has received much recent publicity and has also been linked to certain dairy products. As a general rule, travelers should not drink milk—not just because of the lack of pasteurization, but because of the frequent lack of refrigeration following pasteurization.

Eggs The importance of eggs as a possible source of salmonella infections is a problem in many countries where intensive farming methods are used, including the USA and the UK. There is no evidence to suggest that travelers are at greater risk of acquiring egg-associated salmonella infection, and it is possible that less intensive egg production methods that do not involve large flocks and battery conditions are less likely to produce contaminated eggs. The greatest risk is related to bulk catering where large numbers of pooled eggs are used, and large numbers of people may then be affected. Uncooked or lightly cooked eggs, and foods made with them, such as mayonnaise, sauces, mousses, milk shakes, ice cream, and sandwiches, are frequently incriminated, and in the UK several outbreaks have been linked to the Italian dessert *tiramisu,* served in restaurants. Thorough cooking kills the organisms.

Buffets People eat more buffet food when they travel: buffets are best regarded as an opportunity to present travelers with a large variety of risky foods in an attractive setting. The food looks appealing, and this is a way to try many local dishes. However, buffet foods are often the highest-risk items, and as a general rule they should be avoided. If it is absolutely essential to eat food from a buffet, and it is not possible to have something prepared freshly for

BRUCELLOSIS AND LISTERIOSIS

- Brucellosis is a bacterial disease acquired from animals. It occurs with varying but moderate frequency in most areas of the world outside Northern Europe, Australia, New Zealand, the United States, and Canada. This disease has non-specific symptoms characterized by fever, headache, profuse sweating, chills, weight loss, depression, joint pains, and generalized aching.

- For the traveler, risk of infection arises from eating unpasteurized dairy products, particularly goat cheese. Every year a number of cases are reported in recent travelers to Southern Europe, Africa, the Middle East, and South America. Most cases respond to several weeks' treatment with a combination of antibiotics. However, delay in diagnosis and initiation of appropriate therapy may lead to prolonged disability. Because the time interval between consuming the contaminated food item and onset of illness is typically a month or more, the important diagnostic clue of having eaten cheese or other unpasteurized dairy products may have been forgotten. The lengthy incubation period combined with the nonspecific symptoms of brucellosis are important factors contributing to the delays in diagnosis that often occur.

- In addition to brucellosis, a variety of other infections can be acquired from eating goat cheese in areas where pasteurization is not the norm. Bacterial infections are most common and include bovine tuberculosis, listeriosis, salmonellosis, and a variety of diarrheal agents. Listeriosis presents a particular hazard for pregnant women (see p. 446). The mother may have no symptoms, or may have a mild febrile illness; but the mother's infection may result in fetal infection. This can lead to miscarriage, stillbirth, or meningitis and septicemia in the newborn. Toxoplasmosis may also be a problem (p. 446).

                                        Dr. Arnold Kaufmann, CDC

you, the principles of food safety given in Table 2.2 and Appendix 5 should be followed closely. If there is a flame under any of the items and the food is steaming, choose food from directly over the flame: this is more likely to be at a safe temperature.

Airplane food Food served on airplanes can be a source of intestinal infection. This is not surprising considering the large number of meals prepared, the frequent flight delays that occur, and the time in the air before some meals are served. Airplane food on flights originating in tropical or semitropical developing countries are even more likely to be contaminated: follow the same precautions, or better still, don't eat it.

Cruise ships Food and water can be considered safe on most cruise ships, and the greatest risk usually arises when consuming meals on shore excursions during the cruise, which is when food precautions are particularly important. Precautions should also be followed carefully if there is any suspicion that food or water is being taken on board in a high-risk area.

FLIES

Flies live with equal happiness on excreta and on food. If you allow flies to walk on your food and then you eat it, you are asking for trouble. Flies are important vectors in the "fecal-oral" transmission of infection. Avoid buffets and cold food that have not been protected with fly screens.

HANDS

Microorganisms sticking to your hands easily contaminate food if you are careless. A conscious effort not to bring your hands up to your mouth unless they are clean is therefore worthwhile. Proper hand drying after washing is an equally important part of the cleansing process.

OTHER MODES OF TRANSMISSION

Several diarrhea-causing organisms can probably be transmitted directly from person to person or from animals. Transmission via fine droplets produced by coughing or sneezing is a possible route for the viral agents of diarrhea. Rotaviruses, the most important of these, remain largely uncontrolled worldwide and are notorious for evading even the most careful cross-infection precautions in modern hospitals.

ORGANISMS RESPONSIBLE FOR ILLNESS

The major causes of travelers' diarrhea are listed in Table 2.3. Approximately 80–85 percent of the diarrheal illnesses are caused by bacterial agents, which explains why antibacterial drugs are so effective in preventing and treating the illness. Seasonal factors sometimes influence the relative occurrence of different kinds of infecting organism, and the clinical features of a particular episode of diarrhea also give clues to its likely cause. In travelers to most parts of the developing world, enterotoxigenic *E. coli* (ETEC) is generally responsible, and is also a major cause of diarrhea in local children, in whom the illness is often life-threatening.

DIFFERENT PATTERNS OF ILLNESS: THE CLINICAL SYNDROMES

The important clinical syndromes that occur in travelers with intestinal infection are summarized in Table 2.4, along with the organisms that are usually responsible. Food-borne toxins may be found in certain foods, and often produce distinct clinical syndromes. *Staphylococcus aureus* and *Bacillus cereus* may produce a preformed enterotoxin leading to vomiting within several hours after eating a meal. A similar syndrome is caused by viral agents where vomiting is the major clinical feature. Low-grade fever commonly

TABLE 2.3. IMPORTANT CAUSATIVE AGENTS IN TRAVELERS' DIARRHEA

BACTERIA: (APPROXIMATELY 80–85 PERCENT OF CASES)
- Enterotoxigenic *Escherichia coli* (ETEC)
  40 percent in rainy summertime, 10 percent in dry wintertime

- Enteroadherent *E. coli*
  10 percent

- *Shigella*
  2–20 percent

- *Salmonella*
  4 percent

- *Aeromonas* spp or *Plesiomonas shigelloides*
  10 percent

- *Campylobacter jejuni*
  3 percent rainy summertime, 15 percent dry wintertime

VIRUSES: (10 PERCENT OF CASES)
- Norwalk and other small round viruses
- Rotavirus

PARASITIC CAUSES: (3 PERCENT OF CASES)
- *Giardia lamblia* 2 percent
- *Cryptosporidium* 1 percent
- *Entamoeba histolytica* <1 percent

MULTIPLE AGENTS: 10–15 percent of cases

NO CAUSE IDENTIFIABLE: 10–20 percent of cases

occurs in viral gastroenteritis, while fever is not commonly found in patients with an enterotoxin-related illness (an intoxication, or "food poisoning").

More than 50 percent of people with travelers' diarrhea have a nonspecific syndrome of watery diarrhea without excessive vomiting, no fever, and without passage of bloody or mucoid stools. Between 3 and 40 unformed stools are passed over a three-to-five-day period, with abdominal cramps and pain nearly always present. The cause of this syndrome can be *any* of the agents causing travelers' diarrhea. Cholera should be suspected in a person with pro-

TABLE 2.4. CLINICAL SYNDROMES ASSOCIATED WITH FOODBORNE DISEASE AND INTESTINAL INFECTIONS

VOMITING ONLY:	This is most likely to be caused by toxins produced by bacteria such as *Staphylococcus aureus* and *Bacillus cereus*: vomiting typically occurs one to five hours after eating contaminated food.
VOMITING AND DIARRHEA (GASTROENTERITIS):	This is usually due to a toxin (from *S. aureus* or *B. cereus*) or a virus (Norwalk virus or rotavirus); the incubation period and the absence or presence of fever are sometimes helpful in identifying the likely cause.
WATERY DIARRHEA:	Acute watery diarrhea, caused by any of the enteric microorganisms listed in Table 2.3, is by far the most common form of diarrheal disease in travelers. In the case of cholera, which can cause an extreme form of this syndrome, the fluid losses can be profound, with up to 60 pints per day being lost in the stools.
DYSENTERY WITH FEVER:	When fever or passage of bloody mucoid stools (dysentery) occurs, the traveler usually has an infection caused by a bacterium that invades the intestinal lining and produces inflammation. The two major causes of this syndrome in travelers are *Shigella* spp and *Campylobacter jejuni*. Other, less common causes are *Aeromonas* spp, *Vibrio parahemolyticus*, *Entamoeba histolytica*, and noninfectious inflammatory bowel disease.
PERSISTENT DIARRHEA:	When diarrhea lasts longer than two weeks it is usually due to: *Giardia*; lactose malabsorption; bacterial overgrowth syndrome; persistent infection by a bacterial agent; nonspecific injury pattern of the gut; Brainerd diarrhea
TYPHOID FEVER:	The person with typhoid will have high fever, headache, abdominal pain, and intestinal complaints that include either constipation or diarrhea.

fuse diarrhea that leads to profound loss of fluid. (Cholera is described in greater detail on p. 31.)

When fever occurs and bloody stools are passed, the traveler has dysentery, and antimicrobial therapy is necessary.

Ten percent of people with travelers' diarrhea have illness that lasts longer than one week, and 2 percent have diarrhea that lasts more than a month. In a small proportion of cases, the diarrhea will last for 2 to 12 months. In these protracted ilnesses, a different set of conditions is usually the cause (see Table 2.4), including parasites like *Giardia*); another common cause is lactose malabsorption—malabsorption of milk carbohydrate following damage to the intestinal lining and resulting loss of the intestinal enzyme, lactase, that normally breaks down lactose before absorption; and overgrowth of intestinal bacteria as a result of the sluggish movement patterns of the intestine that can also follow injury from infection.

A syndrome of chronic diarrhea occasionally occurs in travelers, in which the illness lasts many months. While the cause of this chronic disease is not known, nonspecific inflammation of the small bowel or colonic lining may be found; the intestinal lining is damaged by microorganisms and toxins, leading to malabsorption of ingested foods (sprue-like syndrome). There is also a distinct syndrome, Brainerd diarrhea, in which chronic diarrhea follows drinking raw (unpasteurized) milk or untreated water. The exact cause is not known, but the prognosis is good although diarrhea may last more than one year.

When a traveler develops typhoid fever, signs of a serious infection are usually obvious. He or she feels acutely ill with high fever, headache, and abdominal pain. The illness is usually so severe that the person is confined to bed. This situation requires prompt medical evaluation.

HOW TO PREVENT DIARRHEA

DIET RESTRICTION

Taking care about where and what you eat and drink is central to any attempt to avoid illness while traveling. Whenever possible, select a safe place to eat, or prepare food yourself. Choose safe foods (such as those identified in Table 2.2) whenever eating in a restaurant. Under extreme conditions, follow the precautions suggested in Appendix 5.

PREVENTION WITH MEDICATION ("CHEMOPROPHYLAXIS")

Most travelers *should not* take prophylactic medication. The three situations where it might be reasonable to take medication are:

- Underlying poor health (such as the medical conditions listed in Table 2.1).
- Unwillingness or inability to exercise extreme care when selecting food and drink.
- Situations where maintaining the itinerary is of extreme importance, when even a short-term illness would put the purpose of the trip at jeopardy.

Prophylaxis might also be considered for travelers on treatment with omeprazole. This approach should not be used in children.

The two prophylactic approaches that might be used include either antimicrobial agents or bismuth subsalicylate (Pepto-Bismol).

The antimicrobial agents include: trimethoprim/sulfamethoxazole (Septra, Bactrim) (160 mg./800 mg.) for trips to the interior of Mexico during rainy summertime; and for travel to Mexico at other times or for travel to other high-risk areas, norfloxacin (Noroxin) 400 mg.; ciprofloxacin (Cipro) 500 mg.; or ofloxacin (Floxin) 300 mg.; each taken once a day while traveling, to be continued for one to two days after returning home. Prophylactic antimicrobials will prevent 90 percent of the illnesses that would occur without them. This approach should not be used for travel that lasts longer than three weeks, and should be used *only* in the small minority of situations referred to above, on account of the potential side effects of the drugs and because of the difficulty of treating illnesses that may occur during prophylaxis.

Bismuth subsalicylate, taken in a dose of two tablets four times a day, with meals and at bedtime, for those with a trip lasting no more than three weeks, will prevent 65 percent of the illnesses that would occur without prophylaxis. The only side effects of this approach are harmless blackening of stools and tongue; other salicylate-containing drugs should not be taken at the same time, because this can lead to excessive salicylate blood levels.

WHAT TO DO IF YOU GET SICK

The various drugs available to treat travelers' diarrhea, and their dosages, are listed in Table 2.5.

FLUIDS AND SALTS

Even mild diarrhea may cause dehydration, and this can be exacerbated by fluid loss from sweat in a hot climate.

Oral rehydration solutions are an effective way of providing rapid replacement of lost salts and water: the carbohydrate present in these solutions speeds the active absorption of both salt and water. In adults with travelers' diarrhea, the same effect can usually be achieved simply by taking some flavored mineral water with saltine crackers. Rehydration fluids should *always* be prepared for infants.

TABLE 2.5. TREATMENT OF TRAVELERS' DIARRHEA

SYMPTOMATIC TREATMENT:
- Motility-inhibiting drugs:
  Loperamide (Imodium), Adults only: 4 mg. initially, then 2 mg. after each unformed stool, not to exceed 8 mg./day (over-the-counter dose) or 16 mg./day (prescription dose) for no more than 2 days

  Diphenoxylate (Lomotil), Adults only: 4 mg. every 6 hours as needed, for no more than 3 days
- Bismuth subsalicylate: 30 ml. (or 2 tablets) every 30 minutes for 8 doses. Repeat on day 2 if diarrhea continues.
- Attapulgite: see text

ANTIMICROBIAL TREATMENT:
- For travel to the interior of Mexico during the summer:
  Trimethoprim/sulfamethoxazole 160 mg./800 mg. once a day for 3 days
- For travel to other areas or to the interior of Mexico during other seasons:
  Norfloxacin 400 mg.; Ciprofloxacin 500 mg.; or Ofloxacin 300 mg. once a day for 3 days (these drugs should not be used in children)
- Children: 6–12 years: Trimethoprim/sulfamethoxazole 80 mg./400 mg. once a day for 3 days
  2–6 years: Trimethoprim/sulfamethoxazole 40 mg./200 mg. once a day for 3 days
  Under 2 years: Trimethoprim/sulfamethoxazole 20 mg./100 mg. once a day for 3 days
  Alternatively, erythromycin: Under 25 pounds, 250 mg./day; 25–40 pounds, 375 mg./day; 40–55 pounds, 500 mg./day; 55–80 pounds, 750 mg./day; more than 80 pounds, 1,000 mg./day in 4 divided doses for 5 days

EMPIRICAL TREATMENT OF TRAVELERS' DIARRHEA:
- With fever and/or blood (dysentery): Antimicrobial therapy alone
- No fever, no dysentery: Antimicrobial plus loperamide

Rehydration solutions may be obtained at a pharmacy as sachets containing a mixture of salts and glucose (e.g., Jianas Brothers, or WHO rehydration sachets) with instructions for use in clean water; they are sold in some form all over the world. The measures for making your own are as follows:

- 8 *level* or 4 *heaping* teaspoons of sugar (white, brown, or honey)
- + $^1/_2$ level teaspoon of salt
- added to 1 quart (approx. 1 liter) of clean water.

Rehydration is just as efficient if certain other substances are used. Substituting 10–15 teaspoons (50 grams) per quart of powdered rice instead of sugar is very effective, although the rice should be added to a small volume of boiling water before diluting it to its final volume.

Oral rehydration should be initiated early rather than late. Watch for signs of significant dehydration: a dry tongue, dark, smelly urine in small quantities, or no urine, and a weak, rapid pulse. In this situation, particularly in children, it is essential to take as much rehydration solution as possible until the urine returns to a normal appearance and volume. A simple regime for adults is to insist on a glass of oral rehydration solution for every bowel movement plus a glass every hour.

For infants and children, careful fluid replacement is necessary. As a guide, one and a half times the normal feed volume as rehydration solution plus the normal feed would be necessary. For children who are breast feeding, this should continue, with additional rehydration solution also provided.

If diarrhea is so severe that it is difficult to keep up with fluid losses, or if the affected person becomes unable to drink, *this should be treated as a medical emergency*, and the person should receive medical attention as soon as possible since intravenous rehydration may be necessary (see also pp. 457 and 521).

SYMPTOMATIC TREATMENT

There are three potentially valuable forms of symptomatic treatment: motility-inhibiting agents (that reduce intestinal movement) such as loperamide (Imodium) and diphenoxylate (Lomotil); the antisecretory drug bismuth subsalicylate (Pepto-Bismol); and intraintestinal fluid adsorbents such as attapulgite (diasorb or kaopectate).

The motility-inhibiting drugs will reduce diarrhea by 80 percent and can be useful to keep travelers on the road. These drugs should not be used in persons with fever or with dysentery (passage of bloody stools) since they can make the illness worse on these occasions. Bismuth subsalicylate will reduce diarrhea by 50 percent. *These medications should not be used in children.* Attapulgite is very safe since it is not absorbed, making it useful in children and pregnant women with travelers' diarrhea. Since most cases of travelers' diarrhea result from intestinal infection by bacterial agents, the symptomatic drugs may provide only temporary relief from symptoms, with relapse occurring after stopping the drugs.

ANTIMICROBIAL TREATMENT
Antimicrobials are sometimes necessary for curative treatment in travelers' diarrhea (Table 2.5). When patients do not have fever or dysentery, the antimicrobial can be given with loperamide to provide rapid relief of symptoms at the same time.

OTHER DIARRHEA MEDICINES
Be careful. In some countries, medication sold for prevention or treatment of diarrhea may be useless or actually harmful. For example, clioquinol (Entero-Vioform) is still a surprisingly popular remedy in some countries—despite being toxic and ineffective.

WHAT TO EAT IF YOU ARE ILL
It is important to alter the diet during a bout of diarrhea, because the intestine is injured by the infection and absorption of food is often impaired. Choose food items according to the form of the stools passed. With watery stools, only liquids such as soups and broths and easily digestible foods such as saltine crackers should be consumed. As stools assume some form and become soft, toast, potatoes, bananas, tortillas, and baked fish or chicken can be eaten. When stools become formed again, a regular diet can be followed. Milk and dairy products should be avoided during the early stages of diarrhea since lactose malabsorption (see above) may occur.

TREATING PARASITIC CAUSES OF TRAVELERS' DIARRHEA: AMEBIASIS, GIARDIASIS, AND CRYPTOSPORIDIOSIS

These parasites are important causes of intestinal infection in local inhabitants of developing countries. Amebiasis is particularly common in people living under conditions of poverty; however, it accounts for less than 1 percent of cases of travelers' diarrhea. It should be suspected when bloody diarrhea persists despite antimicrobial treatment.

Giardiasis causes about 2 percent of cases of travelers' diarrhea. Cryptosporidiosis resembles a milder form of illness than giardiasis; both should be suspected in cases where symptoms persist despite antibiotics, or when illness persists for 2 weeks or more.

Amebiasis and giardiasis are discussed in greater detail in the next chapter, and their treatment is summarized in Table 2.6. For amebiasis, two drugs are given: metronidazole (Flagyl, Protostat) and diiodohydroxyquin (also called iodoquinol; Diquinol); the latter drug treats the cysts of the organism and is necessary to prevent relapse. For giardiasis, in infants unable to take tablets, furazolidone (Furoxone) is preferred. For proven giardiasis in older children or adults, quinacrine (Atabrine) is the drug of choice, considering cost and effectiveness. When treating possible (suspected or unproven) giardiasis, metronidazole is used, since it may treat other intestinal infections. Treatment should ideally be given under medical supervision. Finally, no therapy is indicated in cryptosporidiosis.

WHEN TO SEE A PHYSICIAN

The major reasons for seeing a physician, either while traveling or on return home, include: temperature above 104°F. (40°C.); significant fever lasting longer than 48 hours; diarrhea lasting longer than four days; severe diarrhea with difficulty keeping up with fluid and salt replacement; and diarrhea with blood.

IMMUNIZATIONS

CHOLERA

There is a commercially available injectable killed cholera vaccine, but it is not very effective, and it does not confer any worthwhile benefit. Both killed and live oral cholera vaccines are being developed but the situation has been complicated by the appearance of a new strain. The problem is discussed in greater detail in the next chapter.

TYPHOID FEVER

There are three vaccines currently available. Two of them appear to be safe and effective and can be recommended: an oral living preparation, Ty 21a, that comes in capsules to be taken on alternate days for four doses; and the new Vi polysaccharide preparation, injected in a single dose, which has fewer side effects than the previous injected vaccine. All of the typhoid vaccines have roughly the same effectiveness—around 70–90 percent.

We advise travelers to developing tropical countries to have either the oral or the Vi vaccines if they are likely to live in close contact with the local community or to travel under less than ideal hygienic conditions. The vaccines are optional and are probably not necessary for travelers who will only be staying in excellent hotels and eating at the better restaurants.

FUTURE VACCINE DEVELOPMENTS

There is great interest in developing vaccines against enterotoxigenic *E. coli* (ETEC) in view of its importance in travelers and in

TABLE 2.6. AMEBIASIS, GIARDIASIS AND CRYPTOSPORIDIOSIS

Parasitic Disease	Drug	Adults	Children
Amebiasis	Metronidazole	730 mg./day In 3 divided doses/day for 10 days	35–50 mg./kilo/day
	plus		
	Diiodohydroxyquin	1950 mg./ day In 3 divided doses/day for 20 days	40 mg./kilo/day
Giardiasis	Quinacrine	300 mg./day In 3 divided doses/day for 7 days	6 mg./kilo/day
	Metronidazole	750 mg./day In 3 divided doses for 7–10 days	15 mg./kilo/day
	Furazolidone	Not given	For infants unable to take tablets: 8 mg./kilo/day in 4 divided doses for 10 days
Cryptosporidiosis	None		

children in developing countries. Because of the similarity between toxins produced by ETEC and *Vibrio cholerae*, the cause of cholera, a particularly interesting approach is the effort to develop an oral vaccine, made from the purified, nontoxic binding portion of one of the toxins that might prevent both ETEC diarrhea and cholera.

Vaccine initiatives are also being directed against many of the other agents important in diarrhea, including *Shigella*, *Campylobacter*, and rotavirus.

SUMMARY OF ADVICE FOR TRAVELERS

- Diarrheal illnesses are avoidable.
- Most travelers' diarrhea is the result of swallowing contaminated food, drink, or other material.
- The contaminating microorganisms are rendered harmless by adequate cooking.
- Food only remains safe if eaten immediately after cooking or if sealed and refrigerated without delay.
- Precautions with food are summarized in Appendix 5.
- Diarrheal episodes are usually self-limiting, get better after one to three days, and require no specific treatment.
- Replacement of water losses is the first consideration of treatment, especially with children (pp. 456–58).
- Guidelines for the place and use of antibiotics, antidiarrheal medication, and other drugs are given on pp. 25–28.

CHOLERA

An epidemic of cholera is currently spreading through South America and Africa, and a new strain is emerging in Asia. However, the risk to travelers who take reasonable hygiene precautions is extremely small. The injected cholera vaccine is discouraged by CDC and the WHO, and currently provides little or no worthwhile protection.

Dr. Ron Behrens *is Director of the Travel Clinic of the Hospital for Tropical Diseases in London, where he conducts research into ways of improving travelers' health.*

HISTORICAL BACKGROUND

The anxiety and fear associated with the name *cholera* is usually out of all proportion to the severity of the disease in its modern context. The reason is clear: during the nineteenth century, cholera was a devastating illness, causing severe dehydration and death in most of those infected. The usual source of infection was the water supply, and large numbers of people were infected and killed.

The *Vibrio cholerae* bacteria that caused classic cholera were in fact slightly different from those that cause the disease today. They produced a dramatic fluid loss, with vomiting and with several pints of watery diarrhea within hours of infection. If fluid replacement of 10–20 pints could not be provided rapidly, death would ensue.

Throughout history, cholera has always tended to occur in pandemics (worldwide epidemics) lasting decades or longer.

THE CURRENT OUTBREAKS

The outbreak currently affecting South America and West Africa is part of the seventh cholera pandemic, which started in Indonesia in 1961 and has already passed through Asia, the Middle East, Africa, southern Europe, and Japan. South America had been free of the disease for more than a century: in the Americas, more than 750,000 cases and 6,500 deaths have now been reported from 21 countries. The strain responsible has been matched with a strain originating in Bangladesh, confirming that this was the source.

The strain of cholera involved is the *El Tor 01 biotype*; it is carried by humans via trade and commercial routes. It is much less virulent than classical cholera: after infection, severe diarrhea is likely to develop in only 2–5 percent of those infected, while over 75 percent of those infected will have no symptoms at all. To put this disease in its true perspective, even during an epidemic cholera accounts for fewer than 5 percent of acute diarrheal cases in a poor community. Healthy carriers (people excreting the organism without symptoms) are an important catalyst to the spread of cholera, and remain infectious to others for more than five days after being infected.

Screening all travelers from infected areas would be highly impractical, and disease containment has never been effective in the past. Control of cholera epidemics is based on the following cardinal principles: isolate and treat patients until they are noninfectious, identify and treat their contacts, establish and enforce public hygiene measures such as protecting and treating drinking water, provide adequate sewage treatment and waste disposal, and secure uncontaminated food supplies.

An outbreak of severe cholera began in India and Bangladesh in 1992, and the cause is a non-*01* strain of organism previously known to have been harmless. It appears that this free-living bacterium has mutated and developed the capacity to cause an illness that is more like classical cholera. This strain is able to live freely in the environment; adults and children in the affected regions have no immunity to it, despite previous exposure to other strains, and no vaccine protects against it. It therefore poses a much bigger threat to travelers and the communities from which they travel.

Within twelve months of the first report, the organism had spread to Thailand, and the disease will undoubtedly spread rapidly to other countries and continents. The first case in an American traveler was reported in June 1993. It is likely that we are seeing the start of the eighth worldwide cholera pandemic from this non-*01* strain.

LEGISLATION AND CONTROL

In an effort to control the spread of cholera across international boundaries through travel, mandatory cholera vaccination was introduced in 1969 by the World Health Organization. The intentions and scope of these regulations have on many occasions been over-interpreted and misapplied: measures such as placing aircraft passengers in quarantine, disinfecting mail, and prohibiting importation of canned foodstuffs have been enforced at various times.

Control measures consisted mainly of checking immunization of travelers at borders, and reporting cases of cholera that did occur. Despite intensive surveillance, however, most countries could not prevent the spread of cholera across their borders—which was often carried by illegal immigrants via small, unsupervised ports.

International requirements for cholera immunization have had little impact on worldwide cholera spread and were formally abandoned in 1973. WHO stopped publishing cholera vaccination certificates in 1989. WHO, along with other organizations such as the Centers for Disease Control and Prevention, does not now recommend cholera immunization for any traveler, and states that immunization certificates should *not* be required.

CHOLERA VACCINATION

The original cholera vaccine has been found to protect only half of recipients, for a limited period of only 8 to 12 weeks. Serious reactions to the cholera vaccine have been reported when it is combined with the typhoid vaccine, but are rare; a more important drawback is the false sense of security that it engenders.

One reason for the continuing demand for vaccination is the lingering anxiety that border health officials might insist on cholera certification as a condition of entry. This appears to occur despite the ostensible absence of international requirements. Vaccination at the border carries added risks if sterile equipment is not used, with obvious concerns about transmission of hepatitis B and HIV. Until WHO requirements on cholera immunization are fully enforced, it is very difficult to give firm advice on cholera vaccination. If it can be obtained, local information on what border officials are demanding may help you decide whether or not to have a cholera shot; if not, the alternatives are to take along an exemption certificate or a letter from your physician stating that vaccination is medically inadvisable for you, or to travel without and argue your case.

HOW IT IS SPREAD

The bacteria that cause the disease survive mainly in estuarine waters and semisaline coastal lagoons; it has been suggested that certain kinds of algae act as an environmental reservoir.

Cholera is spread by contamination of food and water by feces or raw sewage. Shellfish and seafood have been a major source of infection in South America, where *ceviche*—a dish that contains marinated uncooked fish—is a delicacy in many countries. Unwashed vegetables irrigated with contaminated water or untreated sewage are also a source.

As with all diarrheal illnesses, the likelihood of infection depends on the weakest link in the food and water hygiene chain. Where the water supply is chlorinated and remains uncontaminated the risk of

During the current South American outbreak, one traveler brought a cooked crab home to New Jersey in his suitcase, after a visit to Ecuador, and served it up in a salad to his friends. Four of them developed cholera.

On St. Valentine's Day 1992, an Aerolíneas Argentinas Boeing 747 flight between Buenos Aires and Los Angeles made a stop in Lima. Five of the passengers suffered diarrhea, and 75 passengers were later found to have developed cholera as the result of a contaminated seafood salad served on board; one person died. This episode created a major diplomatic incident between Argentina and Peru, who view cholera as more of a political problem than a medical issue. During 1992, CDC recorded 102 cases in the USA—more than in any year since it began collecting data in 1961.

cholera is very low. A recent investigation in Peru revealed that many people with cholera had been drinking unboiled water, stored in containers. This is a common practice: water is stored in large containers, left uncovered, and scooped out as required. This carries a high risk of contamination, and when the water is used for making ice, cleaning vegetables, or brewing homemade alcoholic beverages, the risk of infection is carried over to those products. People who drank the homemade brews were at highest risk.

THE ILLNESS

Diarrhea caused by the *El Tor* strain is a mild illness, unlike the more profuse diarrhea associated with classic cholera. Its onset is quite sudden, but in no way can it be differentiated from most other causes of travelers' diarrhea. Vomiting is frequent and is thought to reflect dehydration; it improves as fluid replacement progresses.

Hospital treatment is not normally necessary unless sufficient oral fluid intake proves difficult, and intravenous rehydration is required. The illness lasts between three and five days and leaves no disability when properly treated.

Disease caused by the new non-*01* strain is more like classical cholera, and much more severe. Prompt rehydration is vital, and medical attention should be sought immediately.

TREATMENT

Oral antibiotics such as tetracycline can reduce the length of infection and reduce fluid loss, if taken early in the illness.

The diarrhea of cholera is no different from other types of travelers' diarrhea, and its treatment with plenty of oral rehydration solution is the simplest and most effective measure (see p. 26). Since fluid loss is the most important complication of severe cholera, the development of effective oral rehydration therapy has to a large extent disarmed the disease, reducing the death rate from over 80 percent to less than 1 percent.

Scientific research has established that the intestine absorbs salt and water most rapidly and efficiently in the presence of a carbohydrate such as sugar or glucose. Rehydration fluids take advantage of this effect, and generally consist of glucose (or sucrose), salt, and water (the sugar can be replaced by a number of other carbohydrates such as powdered rice, potato, or wheat—the effect in the presence of salt is the same).

CHOLERA AND THE TRAVELER

Cholera is a disease associated with urban squalor and extreme poverty, and an absence of the most basic hygiene facilities and education—conditions typical of the *barrios* of Latin American cities. It is exceptional for travelers to use water supplies or food from such areas, and the risk of cholera in travelers is incredibly remote.

In the 20 years before the current outbreaks, only 10 cases of cholera were reported in travelers from the USA, though an estimated 6 million travelers had visited cholera endemic areas. The majority of these victims had been vaccinated against cholera. The number of cases in travelers from the USA has now increased considerably, however. The risk of contracting symptomatic cholera appears to be around one in 500,000 travelers, and the illness is likely to be similar to travelers' diarrhea.

VACCINES FOR THE FUTURE

New vaccines against cholera and other diarrheal diseases are under development. Several are now being tested in countries where cholera is endemic, where the impact of the vaccines is most likely to be seen. Using genetic manipulation techniques, scientists have created cholera organisms that are "sheep in wolf's clothing"; one type uses killed bacteria, while another uses live organisms. What is unusual about these vaccines is that they are swallowed, so that immunity occurs in the intestine—at the natural site of infection. Protection against cholera with these new vaccines appears to be around 60–70 percent for adults—a great improvement on the current injected vaccine.

To enhance the effect, a further maneuver is the use of a neutralized cholera toxin to stimulate the intestine to produce antibodies to the toxin produced in natural infection. This two-pronged approach ensures immunity to both the organism and its toxin.

These oral vaccines may also protect against other forms of diarrhea caused by *Escherichia coli*, the bacteria responsible for most of travelers' diarrhea; this effect could be of considerable benefit to tropical travelers in the future.

Most of the new vaccines were developed before the recent outbreaks of non-*01* cholera became a problem, and are not likely to be effective: further research will be necessary.

SUMMARY OF ADVICE FOR TRAVELERS

- The current South American outbreak is a serious hazard to the local communities that are affected, but the risk to individual travelers is extremely small, and should not deter anyone from visiting the affected regions.
- Cholera is spread by contaminated food and water; hygiene precautions are the most reliable way of avoiding risk.
- There are no official vaccination certificate requirements for travel to any country.
- The injected cholera vaccine is not recommended by CDC or the WHO and is not considered to provide worthwhile protection.

INTESTINAL PARASITES

Travelers to rural areas in the tropics are at greatest risk from parasitic intestinal infections. All travelers should choose their food with care, because complications of intestinal parasites are occasionally serious.

Dr. David Haddock was a Senior Lecturer in Tropical Medicine at the Liverpool School of Tropical Medicine, U.K. He also worked for long periods in Tanzania, Ghana, Nigeria, and Saudi Arabia, and was a WHO consultant in Ghana and the Sudan.

Dr. George Wyatt *is a Senior Lecturer in Tropical Medicine at the Liverpool School of Tropical Medicine.*

Most people who live in developing countries harbor one or more varieties of intestinal parasite, and travelers to those countries are at risk of infection. "Host" and parasite usually coexist in reasonable harmony, and most often no serious condition results from the relationship. In a few cases, however, serious illness and even death may occur unless treatment is given.

Intestinal parasite infestations usually follow swallowing infective forms of the parasite (eggs or larvae) in food or water contaminated with human or animal feces containing excreted parasites. The frequency and severity of infection with intestinal parasites is therefore highest in areas with low standards of hygiene, poor sewage disposal, and unsatisfactory water supplies. Flies are abundant in such areas and are able to carry infective parasites on their feet directly from feces to food. Some types of intestinal worm cause infection when their larvae penetrate the skin (bare feet especially), when the skin comes into contact with soil contaminated with feces. Tapeworm infections follow eating infected meat or fish that has not been thoroughly cooked.

INTESTINAL PARASITES AND THE TRAVELER

Travelers usually have to rely on food prepared by others, and it is difficult to influence other people's standard of food hygiene or preparation. Even seemingly high-class hotels and restaurants may be sources of infection. Water supplies are often contaminated, and should be regarded with suspicion. In many countries intestinal infections with bacteria, viruses, and parasites are the commonest health hazards to visitors; such infections are difficult to avoid completely, but sensible precautions greatly diminish the risks.

As mentioned in the previous sections and on pp. 71–77, all drinking water should be boiled or sterilized; cold drinks or ices should not be bought from street vendors. Raw salads and vegetables are notorious sources of parasitic infections, and are usually best avoided completely. Meat should be thoroughly cooked until all trace of red color is lost. Fruit should be peeled carefully. In addition to such general precautions, the possibility of infection by parasitic skin penetration makes it unsafe to walk around without shoes in many tropical areas.

TYPES OF INTESTINAL PARASITE

Parasites of the intestinal tract fall into two groups—the *protozoa* and the *metazoa* (worms).

The protozoa are microscopic, single-celled creatures which multiply by simple cell division to produce more adult parasites within the intestine. As in the case of infection with bacteria, an initially light infection can rapidly build up to a heavy one. The protozoa include *amebae* and *giardia*.

The second group of parasites, the metazoa, or worms, are complex multicellular animals which may be as small as a fraction of an inch or, in the case of tapeworms, up to several feet long. Generally, intestinal worms excrete eggs in the feces but cannot reproduce adult worms inside the body. Their eggs have to undergo development outside the body, often in the soil.

The severity of human infection often depends upon the number of adult worms in the intestine, and light infections are often relatively harmless. The number of adult worms depends upon the number of infective forms that have been swallowed, or that have penetrated the skin. Worms can damage the lining of the intestine, or suck blood from the lining, causing anemia. They can also cause mechanical disturbances in the gut, or can migrate into the side-alleys of the intestine.

Unlike many bacterial and viral infections, parasitic infections do not lead to reliable immunity from further infection with the same parasite. So repeated infection is common, and chronic infection is also a problem because the worms may survive for several years—indeed a beef tapeworm may survive in the intestines for twenty-five years.

SOME PROTOZOAL INFECTIONS OF THE INTESTINE

AMEBIC DYSENTERY (AMEBIASIS)

This infection is caused by an ameba called *Entamoeba histolytica*. This single-celled creature secretes enzymes to digest particles of food in the intestine and then absorbs the products by engulfing them. The ameba usually lives in the large intestine and is about five times the size of a red blood cell. Sometimes amebae invade the intestinal wall by digesting the tissues and so causing dysentery, or they may be carried to the liver or other organs and cause abscesses. Different strains of amebae vary in their capacity to cause disease: some are harmless but may be very difficult to differentiate from the harmful strains.

Amebae living in the cavity or on the surface of the intestine cause no symptoms, but as they are passed out in the feces they round up and secrete a thick protective wall to form resistant infective cysts. In the absence of proper hygiene, food or water may be contaminated by these cysts, and the amebae re-form when the cysts reach the large intestine of another person.

Amebae that invade the wall of the large intestine cause ulceration and bleeding. The patient suffers from a slowly developing and often recurrent dysentery with blood and slimy mucus in the feces. Dysentery may persist or recur for months and may occasionally lead on to perforation of the intestine, and peritonitis. Amebic liver abscesses sometimes occur in people who already have dysentery; more often, however, there are no intestinal symptoms, just severe pain over the liver and high fever. These abscesses are very dangerous and require urgent treatment.

Amebiasis is a frequent infection in travelers or expatriates resident in the tropics and infection may be present in up to 20 percent of local residents. Most of these people have no symptoms, but they pass cysts in their feces and are therefore potentially infective to others. Once a person is infected, carriage of amebae may last for months or many years, and it is possible to develop disease many years after initial exposure so that even asymptomatic expatriate carriers usually need treatment.

Intestinal infection with *E. histolytica* is readily detected if stool specimens are examined by a competent technician, although amebae may not be found in every stool. Effective drug treatment is available, usually with metronidazole (Flagyl, Protostat), but since many other conditions may simulate amebiasis, laboratory confirmation before treatment is always advisable.

GIARDIASIS
The cause of giardiasis is a tiny one-celled parasite called *Giardia lamblia*, which is about three times the size of a red blood cell. It

lives in the small intestine and may damage the lining. *Giardia* occurs in Europe and North America, but infection is much more common in countries with a low standard of hygiene. As with *E. histolytica* resistant infective cysts are passed in the stools and infection is acquired by swallowing these cysts in contaminated water or food.

Some infected individuals have no symptoms, but excrete infective cysts in their feces for weeks or months. Others have moderate diarrhea, often with passage of excess gas and a distended abdomen; this may persist for several weeks though rarely for longer than six months (see also pp. 28–29). A very small proportion of those infected have severe diarrhea with fatty stools and marked weight loss, weakness, and anemia. This is due to a reduced ability to absorb food from the intestine (malabsorption).

Giardiasis is the commonest cause of diarrhea persisting for weeks after return home. The diagnosis is made by microscopic examination of stool specimens and treatment with metronidazole or other drugs is usually highly effective.

SOME WORM INFECTIONS OF THE INTESTINE

HOOKWORM INFECTION (ANKYLOSTOMIASIS)

About 600 million people around the world are infected with hookworms. These worms live in the small intestine, and attach themselves to its lining by means of teeth or cutting plates. The worms suck blood from their hosts.

Each worm causes a blood loss of 0.03–0.1 ml. of blood daily. There may be 100 or more worms in the intestine, and chronic blood loss eventually leads to anemia, particularly if iron intake in the diet is also low.

Hookworm eggs are passed in the feces, and if soil conditions are warm and moist, infective larvae take about a week to hatch and can survive for several weeks. The larvae can penetrate intact skin, sometimes producing an itchy rash, and find their way to the lungs through the bloodstream. They undergo further development in the lungs for several days, causing a cough, before migrating through the air passages and the esophagus to the small intestine, where they mature to form half-inch-long adults, which may survive for up to nine years.

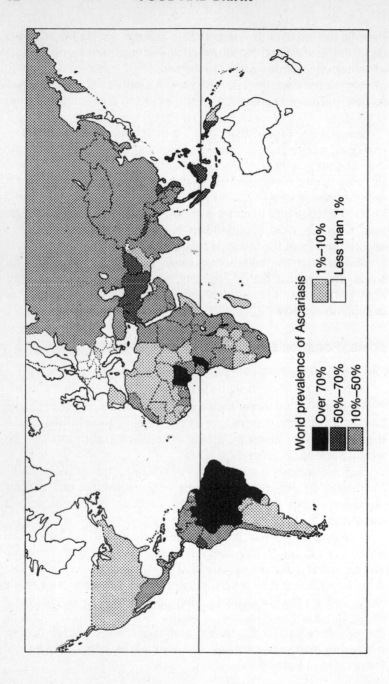

World prevalence of Ascariasis

Over 70%

50%–70%

10%–50%

1%–10%

Less than 1%

Barefooted farmers working in tropical areas are particularly liable to heavy infection, and severe anemia due to hookworm infection can cause cardiac failure and death.

Visitors to rural areas in the tropics may acquire light infections, especially if they wander around with bare feet.

Diagnosis and treatment Diagnosis is made by microscopic examination of the stools and identifying hookworm eggs. The anemia is treated with iron preparations and the worms are eliminated with drugs such as mebendazole (Vermox).

Creeping eruption Certain hookworm larvae, which normally parasitize dogs, are able to penetrate human skin but are unable to mature further. These larvae wander around aimlessly under the skin for several months. In the course of their migration, the worms produce an intensely itchy, red, moving, worm-shaped trail. (See also pp. 107 and 365.)

This condition is called creeping eruption and causes considerable irritation; secondary infection with bacteria may occur as a result of scratching. The rash is usually on the feet or legs, and cure is obtained by treatment with thiabendazole (Mintezol) tablets or ointment.

Creeping eruption is not uncommon in places where beaches are contaminated with dog feces; it occurs in North, Central, and South America, the Caribbean, Africa, and Asia.

STRONGYLOIDES STERCORALIS (STRONGYLOIDIASIS)

Strongyloides is common in many tropical areas. Like hookworm, larvae of *Strongyloides* are excreted in feces, develop in the soil, and cause infection by penetrating the skin.

The larvae reach the small intestine in the same way, mature and reside in its lining. Infection is often harmless, but sometimes causes intestinal ulceration with abdominal pain, diarrhea, and failure to absorb certain nutrients. However, the larvae are also able to mature in the intestine and penetrate the lining of the intestine or the skin around the anus, perpetuating the infection. Infection may last for a lifetime. Larvae wandering beneath the skin may produce a creep-

Map 2.1. World distribution of ascariasis. Percentage figures refer to the proportion of the local population affected. (Reproduced, with modifications, by kind permission of the Editor, *Parasitology Today.*) The prevalence of ascariasis varies considerably *within* countries.

ing eruption on the trunk (see also larva currens, p. 108). If someone with strongyloidiasis is given steroid or other medication that suppresses immunity, the infection can rapidly become generalized and cause death. This has happened occasionally in patients who have been immunosuppressed for transplant surgery.

Diagnosis is made by finding larvae in the feces, or by serological blood tests, and treatment is with albendazole.

ROUNDWORM INFECTIONS (ASCARIASIS)

About 1 billion people in the world and perhaps one third of the inhabitants of tropical Africa are thought to harbor the common roundworm *Ascaris lumbricoides*. Roundworms are large, stout, whitish worms 5–11 inches long and about 0.4 inches in diameter. Infection is acquired by swallowing infective eggs, often on vegetables. Eggs are passed in the feces of infected persons, especially children, and need to mature in suitable soil before they become infective.

Heavy infections with roundworms in local children can cause serious disease ranging from abdominal colic and distension to nutritional disturbance and even blockage of the small intestine by a tangled mass of worms. Infection with a few worms in an expatriate rarely causes trouble but they should always be expelled because very occasionally they can enter a bile duct or other orifice and cause disease.

The diagnosis is made by finding the eggs on microscopy of the feces. A number of drugs are available for treatment; one such is mebendazole (Vermox).

THE BEEF TAPEWORM

The beef tapeworm *Taenia saginata* is long and ribbon-like, about half-an-inch broad and up to several yards in length. Each worm has hundreds of segments, each of which is a hermaphrodite creature. *Taenia saginata* resides in the small intestine, attached to the intestinal lining by suckers at its head. It usually causes surprisingly little disturbance to its host, who may be unaware of its presence until segments are discovered in the feces, or even wriggle out of the anus. Some patients suffer from recurrent abdominal pains.

When detached segments or eggs from human feces contaminate pastures, cattle become infected. The worms do not reach their adult state in cattle, but form cysts in their muscles—a quarter to a half-inch in diameter. People become infected when they eat inadequately cooked beef containing cysts. The swallowed cysts develop into adult worms in the small intestine.

Infection is widespread in many parts of the Middle East, Africa, and South America; Ethiopia has a particularly high prevalence. Diagnosis is made by examining stools for segments and eggs. Treatment is with niclosamide (Niclocide) tablets.

Prevention depends on proper disposal of sewage, meat inspection, and *thorough cooking of meat.* In some countries (such as Francc), raw or lightly cooked meat is regarded as a delicacy and is a source of tapeworm infection.

In the Far East, lightly cooked or raw fish is consumed widely and is a source of infection with certain parasites infecting the liver and the gut, such as *Clonorchis sinensis* (the Chinese liver fluke).

THE PORK TAPEWORM

Infection with the pork tapeworm *Taenia solium* is acquired by consumption of infected pork. Unfortunately, as is not the case with beef tapeworms, infection can also be acquired directly from swallowing the tapeworm's eggs. Furthermore it is possible for eggs to be regurgitated from the small intestine into the stomach if there is a tapeworm present.

On exposure to stomach contents, these eggs become infective. Larvae that develop from the eggs spread throughout the body and form cysts in the muscles and brain—a condition called cysticercosis. Cysticercosis may cause epilepsy, cerebral degeneration, and even death.

Taenia solium infection needs to be diagnosed and treated with some urgency, because cysticercosis is a hazard both to the infected individual and to others who may become infected by contamination with his or her feces. An outbreak occurred recently within an Orthodox Jewish community in New York, and its probable source was infection in a housekeeper from Mexico.

The infection is treated with niclosamide or other drugs, with special precautions to avoid cysticercosis. There are also drugs, including praziquantel, that are effective against cysticercosis. Prevention involves awareness of the problem and avoidance of undercooked pork.

HYDATID CYSTS

Hydatid cysts are caused by *Echinococcus granulosus*: the adult form of this parasite is a small tapeworm that lives in the intestines of dogs. Its eggs are infective to man, sheep, goats, camels, and horses, and are passed in dogs' feces. Larvae develop from any eggs that are eaten, and these form slowly growing larval cysts in the tissues. Dogs become infected when they eat organs of sheep or other animals that contain these larval cysts. Humans usually become infected by stroking dogs: eggs from the fur adhere to the fingers, and are subsequently swallowed.

In humans, larval cysts form most often in the liver, but the lungs, brain, bones, and other tissues may also be affected. The cysts grow very slowly but behave like expanding tumors that may not become obvious for five to ten years after infection. Surgical excision is necessary, and is sometimes difficult. Drug treatment is being developed but is still unreliable. Prevention depends upon avoiding contact with dogs in endemic areas, proper disposal of animal carcasses, deworming dogs, and food hygiene.

OTHER PARASITIC WORMS

A form of meningitis is caused by the larvae of the parasitic worm *Angiostrongylus cantonensis*. The disease occurs in Southeast Asia and the Pacific, and occasionally leads to serious complications such as blindness or paralysis. The disease is spread by eating undercooked snails or slugs. Escargots prepared by the traditional French methods, at high temperature, are safe.

SUMMARY OF ADVICE FOR TRAVELERS

- Travelers to rural, tropical areas are at greatest risk from intestinal parasites. Most parasitic infections are not life-threatening, but they may occasionally be very dangerous. Symptoms of infection may not appear for months or even years after leaving an endemic area. Most infestations can be avoided by commonsense precautions—so follow this book's advice on food and water hygiene, wear shoes, and avoid handling dogs.

- At the moment no drugs or vaccines are available for preventing these infections, but effective treatment exists for most of them if it is given sufficiently early. Travelers who have spent prolonged periods abroad or who have lived in close contact with local communities should have an examination on return home to detect possible hidden infection.

POLIOMYELITIS

Polio remains a problem in many countries with poor hygiene, and is a serious hazard to travelers who have not been immunized.

Dr. George Wyatt is a Senior Lecturer in Tropical Medicine at the Liverpool School of Tropical Medicine.

Poliomyelitis, or polio, was once widely known as "infantile paralysis" because it caused paralysis chiefly in young children. As hygiene improved in many parts of the world, infection became more common later in life, when its effects tend to be more serious; in Europe, major epidemics of polio caused death and severe disability in young adults during the 1940s and 1950s.

With the introduction and widespread use of polio vaccines polio has now been largely eliminated from developed countries, and the WHO has set the year 2000 as a target for its eradication (see p. 547). In the Americas, the number of cases fell from 800 in 1985 to just 9 cases in 1991; there were no cases in 1992. However, it remains common in developing countries elsewhere, and is especially common in young children; in many areas up to 1 percent of schoolchildren may be lame from previous polio.

INFECTION

Polio is caused by a virus, which is spread from person to person either in mucus from the nose and throat, or by contamination of food or drink with infected feces. There are three varieties of polio virus. After infection a person may become a "carrier," and continue to excrete the virus in the feces for many weeks.

Once the virus has traveled to the motor nerve cells in the spinal cord and brain, it damages these cells and causes paralysis of the muscles they control.

Poliomyelitis occurs in two phases—an initial nonspecific illness of fever, headache, muscle pains, and perhaps a stiff neck, followed after a short interval by a return of muscle pains and the rapid development of paralysis over the next 24 hours. The paralysis may be limited to a single limb or may spread rapidly to involve much of the body. Very severe polio is sometimes fatal because the muscles used in breathing or swallowing are affected. In those who survive, recovery of muscle power takes place over the next few months, but some permanent disability often remains.

Fortunately most young children infected with the polio virus escape with little or no damage, although a few are left with a wasted paralyzed limb. Infection in adults all too often produces severe paralysis.

POLIO AND THE TRAVELER

Polio is a serious hazard for nonimmunized travelers in developing countries, and many tragedies have occurred, resulting in death or permanent paralysis. Polio virus still circulates constantly in areas with poor levels of hygiene and low immunization rates in local inhabitants.

Most travelers will have received a full primary course of immunization in childhood, but some may have missed immunization and older people in particular may never have been offered the vaccine. Because so little polio virus has been circulating in the last twenty years, unvaccinated persons should never assume that they are *naturally* immune whatever their age.

IMMUNIZATION

There are two types of polio vaccine (see pp. 505–6). The type most often used is a modified live virus vaccine given by mouth as drops or on a sugar lump. There is also a killed vaccine given by injection, which is also highly effective and is preferred for travelers who are pregnant or who have a depressed immune system because of disease or drugs (such as high doses of corticosteroids).

People who have never been immunized or who have no record of immunization should receive three doses of polio vaccine, preferably at monthly intervals before they travel. People who have been fully immunized at any time in the past need only a single booster dose of polio vaccine every ten years if they intend to travel.

Oral polio vaccine is both highly effective and very safe. There is, however, an extremely small risk of the vaccine virus causing paralysis in unvaccinated close contacts of the person being immunized, especially if these people are immunosuppressed. This is why it is usual for all members of the same household who have not been immunized before to be offered immunization at the same time.

While there are theoretical objections to immunization with two live virus vaccines at the same time, I have never heard of anyone coming to any harm from being immunized against polio and yellow fever together. This theoretical objection should not stop people from receiving both vaccines on the same day if there is not sufficient time for the usual three-week interval between vaccines. Normal immune globulin for protection against viral hepatitis may also contain antibodies against polio, so it is therefore usually given last, shortly before travel and at least three weeks after the last dose of oral polio vaccine (see pp. 505–6); if there is insufficient time, however, polio and immune globulin may be given together.

SUMMARY OF ADVICE FOR TRAVELERS

• Full immunization against polio is essential for anyone traveling to a developing country and advisable for those traveling anywhere outside Northern Europe and the Americas. Although good general hygiene may somewhat reduce the risk of catching polio, it is unreliable and cannot replace immunization.

VIRAL HEPATITIS

Hepatitis is common in travelers to areas outside North America, Northern Europe, and Australia, and may result in an unpleasant prolonged illness. All travelers should understand how the different types of hepatitis are spread.
Professor Arie J. Zuckerman *is Dean and Director of the WHO Collaborating Center for Reference and Research on Viral Diseases, Royal Free Hospital School of Medicine, London.*

Viral hepatitis is common throughout the world and is a major public health problem. At least six different viruses are capable of causing the infection, and the illnesses associated with each (which are all very similar) are as follows:

1. Hepatitis A, also known in the past as infectious hepatitis or epidemic jaundice;

2. Hepatitis B, also known in the past as serum hepatitis;

3. Hepatitis C;

4. Hepatitis D (Delta hepatitis);

5. Hepatitis E;

6. Non-A, non-B hepatitis, which is caused by several different viruses (although, by definition, not by the viruses responsible for hepatitis A and B).

The viruses responsible for hepatitis A, B, C, D, and E have been "characterized," i.e., a great deal is known about their size, structure, and biology. Sensitive laboratory tests are available for detecting components of the viruses (viral antigens), and antibodies against them, in the blood or tissues of people who have been infected with these viruses—and hence a diagnosis of infection can be made with precision.

The viruses responsible for some forms of non-A, non-B hepatitis have not, on the other hand, been fully characterized, and specific laboratory tests are not available for detecting them. The diagnosis of non-A, non-B hepatitis is thus made (as the name implies) in cases of hepatitis where hepatitis A, B, C, D, and E, and other viruses known to cause liver damage have been excluded.

THE ILLNESS

The illness in all forms of hepatitis is similar, and results from acute inflammation of the liver. It is frequently heralded by symptoms such as fever, chills, headache, fatigue, generalized weakness, and aches and pains. A few days later, there is often loss of appetite, nausea, vomiting, right upper abdominal pain or tenderness, followed closely by dark urine, light-colored feces, and jaundice of the skin or the sclerae (outer coating of the eyeballs). Many infections, particularly in children, are without specific symptoms or without jaundice. In others, jaundice may be severe and prolonged; complete liver failure may occur, and the patient may lapse into a coma.

HEPATITIS A

Hepatitis A is common in all parts of the world, but the exact incidence is difficult to estimate because of the high proportion of nonsymptomatic cases and infections without jaundice. Surveys of antibody to hepatitis A have shown that while the prevalence of hepatitis A in industrialized countries (particularly North America, northern Europe, and Australia) is decreasing, the infection is virtually universal in most other regions, particularly in countries with warm climates.

Only one form of hepatitis A has been identified, and the antibody that develops against it persists for many years, frequently providing lifelong immunity.

HOW IT IS SPREAD

Hepatitis A virus is spread by the fecal-oral route, usually by person-to-person contact, particularly in conditions of poor sanitation and overcrowding. Outbreaks result most frequently from fecal contamination of drinking water and food (although waterborne transmission is less often a factor in industrialized countries, or where the piped water supply has been adequately treated and chlorinated).

Food-borne outbreaks, which have become more important and frequent in developed countries, may be due to the shedding of the virus in the feces of infected food handlers during the incubation period of the illness: the source of the outbreak can often be traced to cooking. Raw or inadequately cooked shellfish cultivated in sewage-contaminated tidal or coastal water, and raw vegetables grown in soil fertilized with untreated human feces and excreta, are associated with a high risk of infection with hepatitis A virus. Hepatitis A infection is frequently contracted by travelers from areas of low to areas of high prevalence. Hepatitis A virus is very rarely transmitted by blood transfusion or by inoculation.

The incubation period of the virus is between three and five weeks, with an average of 28 days.

AGE INCIDENCE AND SEASONAL PATTERNS

All age groups are susceptible. The highest incidence is observed in children of school age, but in North America and in many countries in Northern Europe most cases occur in adults, frequently after travel abroad. In temperate zones the characteristic seasonal trend is for an increase in incidence in the autumn and early winter months, falling progressively to a minimum in midsummer, but recently this seasonal trend has been lost in some countries. In many tropical countries, the peak of reported infection tends to occur during the rainy season with low incidence in the dry months.

CONSEQUENCES OF INFECTION
The illness caused by hepatitis A is described above. Although the disease has a low mortality, patients may be incapacitated for many weeks. There is no evidence of persistence of infection with hepatitis A virus nor of progression to chronic liver disease.

CONTROL
Control of the infection is difficult. Since fecal shedding of the virus and therefore infectivity is at its highest during the incubation period, strict isolation of cases is not a useful measure. Spread of infection is reduced by simple hygienic measures and the sanitary disposal of excreta.

HEPATITIS A AND THE TRAVELER
Protection against hepatitis A is strongly recommended for travelers who are not already immune (this can be checked with a blood test), and who are traveling to endemic areas.

Normal human immune globulin (sometimes also called gamma globulin) contains the hepatitis A antibody and will prevent or lessen the severity of the illness, while not always preventing excretion of the virus or the development of asymptomatic hepatitis. Immune globulin injections may be required every four to six months for people at risk. Immune globulin for intramuscular administration prepared by cold ethanol fractionation according to the Cohn method is safe and without any risk of transmitting blood-borne infections including HIV (the virus causing AIDS). This is the method of preparation used by all reputable manufacturers in the USA and other industrialized countries. In such circumstances a 16 percent solution of immune globulin in a dose of 2 i.u. hepatitis A antibody per kilogram of body weight may be given intramuscularly before exposure to the virus or early during the incubation period.

New vaccines against hepatitis A have recently been developed; they have been licensed in Australia and Europe and are shortly expected to be licensed in the USA. Clinical trials have shown that they provide effective immunity lasting several years. Such vaccines represent a major step forward for travelers, eliminating the need for repeated doses of immune globulin. Among their many advan- tages, they are also less painful.

Other preventive measures include strict personal hygiene, avoid- ing raw or inadequately cooked shellfish, avoiding raw vegetables, and not drinking untreated water or unpasteurized milk.

HEPATITIS B

Like hepatitis A, hepatitis B occurs throughout the world. Its con- tinued survival is ensured by the large number of individuals who are carriers of the virus, estimated to be at least 300 million world- wide. Hepatitis B can be spread either from carriers or from people with inapparent infection, or during the incubation period, illness, or early convalescence.

A person is defined as a carrier if hepatitis B surface antigen—a marker of the virus—persists in his circulation for more than six months following infection. A person may be a lifelong carrier and remain apparently healthy, although variable degrees of liver dam- age can occur.

The prevalence of hepatitis B carriers varies from one region of the world to another. In North America, Northern Europe, and Australia, 0.1 percent of the population are carriers (at least among blood donors); in Central and Eastern Europe up to 5 percent; in Southern Europe, countries bordering the Mediterranean, and parts of Central and South America, a higher frequency; and in parts of Africa, Asia, and the Pacific area, 20 percent or more of the appar- ently healthy population may be carriers.

The incidence of hepatitis B tends to be higher among adults living in urban communities and among those living in poor con- ditions. The infection may become established in closed institutions such as institutions for the mentally handicapped.

Certain groups of people—recipients of unscreened blood trans- fusions and blood products, health care and laboratory personnel, staff in institutions for the mentally handicapped, male homosexu- als, prostitutes, and abusers of injectable drugs and narcotics—are at considerably increased risk of contracting hepatitis B. Travelers or expatriates belonging to any of these groups are at higher risk in countries where the carrier rate is high.

HOW IT IS SPREAD

Transmission of the infection may result from accidental inoculation with minute amounts of blood which may occur during medical, surgical, or dental procedures; during immunization with inadequately sterilized syringes and needles; sharing of needles during intravenous drug abuse; during tattooing, ear piercing, and nose piercing; during acupuncture, during laboratory accidents, and accidental inoculation with razors and similar objects that have been contaminated with blood.

However, hepatitis B is not spread exclusively by blood or blood products. Hepatitis B surface antigen has been found in other body fluids such as saliva, menstrual and vaginal discharges, and seminal fluid, and these have been implicated as vehicles of transmission of the infection. In certain defined circumstances the virus may be infective by mouth, and there is much evidence for the transmission of hepatitis B by sexual contact. The sexually promiscuous, particularly male homosexuals, are at high risk.

In the tropics and in warm climates, additional factors may be important for the transmission of hepatitis B. These include traditional tattooing and scarification, bloodletting, ritual circumcision, and repeated biting by bloodsucking insects. Results of investigations into the role that biting insects play in the spread of hepatitis B are conflicting. Hepatitis B surface antigen has been detected in several species of mosquito and in bedbugs that have either been trapped in the wild or fed experimentally on infected blood, but no convincing evidence of multiplication of the virus in insects has been obtained. Mechanical transmission of the infection via an insect's biting parts is a theoretical possibility, but appears to be rare.

Hepatitis B also tends to occur within family groups, although the precise mechanism of intrafamilial spread is not known.

Transmission of hepatitis B virus from carrier mothers to their babies can occur around the time of birth and appears to be an important factor in determining the prevalence of the infection in some regions, particularly in China and Southeast Asia.

The incubation period is about 60–180 days.

THE CARRIER STATE

Progression to the carrier state is more common in males, more likely to follow infections acquired in childhood than in adult life, and more likely to occur in people with natural or acquired immune deficiencies. The carrier state becomes established in approximately 5–10 percent of infected adults. In countries where hepatitis B infection is common the highest prevalence of surface antigen is found in children aged four to eight, with steadily declining rates among older age groups.

There is an urgent need to define the mechanisms that lead to the carrier state and to introduce methods of interruption of transmission. This is a complex and vexed issue, with considerable personal, social, and economic implications.

CONSEQUENCES OF INFECTION

The symptoms and manifestations of hepatitis B are similar to those of the other types of viral hepatitis. However, the picture is complicated by the carrier state and by chronic liver disease, which may follow the infection. Chronic liver disease may be severe and may progress to primary liver cancer. In many parts of the world primary liver cancer is one of the commonest human cancers, particularly in men.

PREVENTION AND CONTROL

Immunization against hepatitis B can be carried out in two ways.

Passive immunization, using hepatitis B immune globulin (hepatitis B gammaglobulin) which contains antibody against hepatitis B. This is not used for prevention in travelers, but can be used as a protective measure after accidental exposure, such as when blood or other material containing hepatitis B surface antigen is inoculated, swallowed, or splashed in the eyes. Two doses administered thirty days apart are required: the first dose should preferably be administered within 48 hours, but not later than seven days following exposure. A course of active immunization should be started at the same time.

Active immunization, using a vaccine that contains hepatitis B antigen and "primes" the body's immune system to produce its own antibodies. The new hepatitis B vaccines have been developed using recombinant DNA technology (genetic engineering): they are safe and effective.

Among the high-risk groups who might benefit from the vaccine are homosexual men, drug addicts, prostitutes, people who require multiple transfusions, people with immune deficiencies or malignant disease, and health-care personnel. Immunization should also be considered by nonimmune persons living in areas where the prevalence of hepatitis B infection is high. Strategies for immunization against hepatitis B are under review, and hepatitis B has recently been added to the childhood immunization schedule.

The currently available vaccines are expensive, costing around $150 for a course of immunization ($70 for children). Vaccination of travelers is advisable if (1) they belong to a high-risk group; (2) they will remain in an endemic area for longer than about six months; (3) they will reside in rural areas or engage in sporting or other activities that carry an increased risk of accidents, injury, or occupational exposure to blood; (4) they are likely to need medical treatment abroad—such as kidney dialysis or blood transfusion.

HEPATITIS B AND THE TRAVELER

Travelers should take commonsense precautions to reduce the risk of hepatitis B. They should employ great caution in any intimate or sexual contact (particularly male homosexual contact) with possible hepatitis B carriers; they should where possible avoid any procedure involving penetration of the skin, for example, tattooing, ear piercing, any sort of injections, blood transfusions, and many medical, surgical, and dental procedures carried out under dubious sanitary conditions.

The delta virus is a defective infectious agent that can only infect actively in the presence of hepatitis B. The infection is common in parts of Southern Europe, the Middle East, parts of tropical Africa, and in parts of South America. The virus is spread in the same way as hepatitis B and precautions against it are identical. Immunization against hepatitis B will also protect against Delta hepatitis.

HEPATITIS C

The hepatitis C virus, which is considered to be responsible for the majority of cases of non-A, non-B hepatitis, was identified by molecular biology techniques in 1989. Although in general the illness is mild and often without jaundice, severe hepatitis does occur and in many patients the infection is followed by a persistent carrier state. Chronic liver damage may occur in as many as 50 percent of patients, and there is preliminary evidence of an association between hepatitis C virus and primary liver cancer in some parts of the world.

The virus is transmitted by blood and blood products. Surprisingly, blood transfusion accounts for only a small proportion of cases in industrialized countries, although between 0.01 and 2 percent of volunteer blood donors are carriers of hepatitis C virus. There is a very high prevalence of infection among intravenous narcotic drug abusers. Preliminary evidence indicates transmission by the sexual route and during childbirth, but the route of infection has not been determined in as many as 50 percent of cases.

Vaccines against hepatitis C are being developed. Methods of prevention are at present identical to those that apply to hepatitis B.

There is also considerable evidence for the existence of other non-A, non-B, and non-C hepatitis viruses.

NON-A, NON-B HEPATITIS

Improved laboratory diagnosis of hepatitis A, B, and C has enabled a previously unrecognized form of hepatitis, unrelated to either type A, B, or C, to be identified. It is referred to as non-A, non-B hepatitis, and it is now known to be the most common form of hepatitis occurring after a blood transfusion and the administration of blood-clotting factors in some countries. It has been found in every country in which it has been sought, has some features in common with hepatitis B, and has been detected in patients on dialysis and among drug addicts. In several countries a significant number of cases are not associated with transfusion, and such sporadic cases have been found to account for up to 15–20 percent of all adult patients with viral hepatitis.

In general, the illness is mild, often without jaundice or other symptoms. However, there is evidence that the infection may be followed by the development of a persistent carrier state: chronic hepatitis may occur in as many as 40–50 percent of patients after infection associated with blood transfusion or treatment by renal dialysis. About 10 percent of patients with the sporadic form of the infection may progress to chronic liver damage.

There are no known methods of preventing non-A, non-B hepatitis (beyond the precautions applicable to hepatitis B).

HEPATITIS E

An epidemic illness similar to that caused by hepatitis A and commonly transmitted by contaminated water has been observed in India, Myanmar, the southeastern part of the former Soviet Union, parts of the Middle East, East Africa, North Africa, and parts of West Africa, and in Mexico. The virus responsible for this type of hepatitis has now been identified and characterized as hepatitis E. There is evidence that this virus is prevalent in many nonindustrialized countries and where a safe piped water supply is not available.

It should be noted that although infection does not lead to chronic liver damage, it is extremely serious during pregnancy, causing a high mortality. The severity of the illness during pregnancy dictates an urgent need for a vaccine.

Methods of prevention include strict personal hygiene, not drinking untreated water, and not eating raw or inadequately cooked shellfish and raw vegetables. Immune globulin is not considered to afford any protection.

TREATMENT OF VIRAL HEPATITIS

No specific treatment is available for any of the types of viral hepatitis. A number of antiviral substances are under study for the management of chronic liver disease associated with hepatitis B. Bed rest is required during the acute phase. A low-fat diet is usually preferred during the acute phase of the disease. Alcohol should not be consumed for six months after recovery.

Women using oral contraceptives (the Pill or progestogen-only Pill) can carry on with this contraceptive method during convalescence and recovery from hepatitis.

Evacuation of a patient with acute hepatitis is not usually necessary unless serious complications develop, when special facilities may be required.

THE DIFFERENT TYPES OF HEPATITIS VIRUS

The five hepatitis viruses, A, B, C, D, and E, are distinct infectious agents and infection with one virus does not confer immunity against another infection with a different virus. Similarly, vaccination against hepatitis A or hepatitis B does not protect

SUMMARY OF ADVICE FOR TRAVELERS

- Hepatitis A and the enteric form of non-A, non-B hepatitis are a risk to travelers in areas of the world where hygienic and sanitary conditions are poor. Protection with immune globulin, or where it is available, hepatitis A vaccine, should be considered for nonimmune travelers anywhere outside the USA, Canada, Northern Europe, Australia, and New Zealand. Strict personal hygiene, avoidance of untreated water and raw or inadequately cooked food, particularly raw vegetables, shellfish, and milk, can help prevent infection. Similar precautions apply to hepatitis E.

- Hepatitis B is a risk to certain groups of people in industrialized countries, notably health-care personnel and male homosexuals. The risk increases in developing countries, where there are generally more carriers. Caution should be observed with regard to intimate or sexual contact with inhabitants of these countries. Active immunization with hepatitis B vaccine is advisable for health-care personnel, members of other risk categories working in the subtropics or tropics, and long-term travelers to endemic areas.

- Penetration of the skin by any object that may have come in contact with someone else's blood or other body fluids—as in tattooing, ear piercing, sharing of razors, acupuncture, needle sharing by drug abusers, and any medical, dental, or surgical procedure, including blood transfusion and donation under dubious hygienic conditions—should be avoided.

- Hepatitis C is transmitted in the same manner as hepatitis B, and in some parts of the world is particularly associated with narcotic drug addiction.

- Non-A, non-B hepatitis is principally a risk of blood transfusion. No preventive immunization is available, and avoidance is by measures similar to those advised for hepatitis B and C.

- Travelers who develop a general malaise and symptoms such as right upper abdominal pain, jaundice, and dark-colored urine either abroad or after their return should suspect viral hepatitis, and should seek medical advice immediately.

against another hepatitis virus. The only exception is immunization against hepatitis B which will afford protection against infection with the defective interfering delta virus (hepatitis D). It should be emphasized that the hepatitis viruses are common in all countries.

The highest-risk areas for hepatitis A include Central and Eastern Europe, the Mediterranean countries, the Middle East, developing countries in Africa, Asia, and Central and South America.

The highest-risk areas for hepatitis B include Southeast Asia, the

People's Republic of China, the Pacific islands, sub-Saharan Africa, and a number of countries in Central Asia and South America. Note that in certain population groups the rates of infection are very high, especially among homosexual men, prostitutes, and drug addicts.

POISONS AND CONTAMINANTS IN FOOD

Certain foods need to be treated with caution while abroad: in tropical countries, fish and shellfish can pose a particular hazard.

Dr. Elizabeth Driver is a medical consultant in a law firm in London. She has worked as a toxicologist at the Medical Research Council and in the Tropical Metabolism Research Unit in Jamaica.

One of the most enjoyable aspects of visiting a foreign country is the opportunity to sample the local cuisine—and provided such food is carefully prepared and cooked, this usually carries little risk.

Unfortunately, some foreign delicacies or even staple foodstuffs contain contaminants and biological toxins in their raw or uncooked form, and although local culinary methods have usually evolved for dealing with such contaminants prior to consumption, cases of poisoning still occasionally occur. This risk of poisoning is in addition to the hazards of food-borne infection considered elsewhere in this section.

Travelers should therefore know which foods carry a significant danger, and either avoid them completely or exercise extreme caution. The foods themselves range from cassava, eaten as a staple throughout the tropics, to "fugu" or puffer fish, considered a delicacy in Japan and much of the Indo-Pacific.

TYPES OF POISONING

The variety of potential food contaminants and toxins is vast and their effects range from the trivial and inconvenient to the frankly dramatic. In general, however, poisoning can be classified into "acute" and "chronic" varieties. *Acute* poisoning is more or less immediate in onset and may follow consumption of a single portion of contaminated food. *Chronic* poisoning is a long-term process which generally follows repeated consumption of small amounts of a toxic substance over an extended period—so it is unlikely to appear in travelers on a short trip.

ACUTE POISONING

Acute poisoning may be produced by foods of either plant or animal origin.

PLANT TOXINS

In places where potentially poisonous plant material is part of the local diet, methods of preparation have evolved that minimize the risk. Travelers should be wary of preparing unusual foods for themselves, but may be reasonably confident, except in times of drought or famine, that food prepared by local people will be innocuous. Poisoning is much more likely to result from eating wild berries or fungi. The two most toxic flowering plants are the castor bean (*Ricinus communis*) and the rosary pea (*Abrus precatorius*). The latter is sometimes encountered in bead necklaces, usually of African origin, and should be confined to this decorative use. If seeds with broken coats are swallowed, persistent diarrhea, often with bloody mucus, begins after a latent period of up to three days. Death may result. Many mushrooms are toxic, but generally produce gastrointestinal symptoms, sweating, or headache, which will resolve spontaneously after a few hours of discomfort. A few mushrooms have an alcohol-sensitizing effect, while others induce hallucinations. Only *Amanita phalloides* and similar types are likely to be fatal.

Cassava (manioc) is a shrub that produces starchy tubers rather like yams or sweet potatoes, and also protein-rich leaves that can be used as a green vegetable. Because it is drought and pest resistant and will grow on poor soil, it is a major staple crop in tropical countries. It originates from South America but is now the major energy supply for 20–40 percent of the population of sub-Saharan Africa.

Cassava roots and leaves contain natural chemicals that break down to release cyanide. The bitter varieties, which are grown in large quantities because of their drought resistance and higher yields, contain more of these toxic chemicals and must be processed before consumption, whereas the sweet varieties can be eaten fresh. Consequently, processing methods such as soaking in water, grating and fermenting the mash in sacks or prolonged sun-drying of the roots have been developed to remove the toxins. Consumption of the unprocessed roots can result in acute cyanide poisoning.

The acute effects of eating improperly prepared cassava are abdominal pain and vomiting, progressing to mental confusion and to a variety of neurological problems. In Tanzania the neurological disorder is called *"Konzo,"* which literally means *"weak legs."* Konzo is caused by abrupt, symmetrical, and permanent damage to parts of the spinal cord which can lead to difficulties in walking, talking, and vision. In other parts of Africa, blindness is recognized as being related to eating manioc. Deafness and loss of sensation are also features of the so-called *tropical ataxic neuropathy.* In parts of rural Nigeria, where the staple food is cassava, the prevalence of this syndrome can be as high as 80 per 1000.

Lathyrism is a disease very similar to Konzo and is characterized by the same acute onset of permanent selective damage to parts of the spinal cord. It also occurs in epidemics during acute food shortages. Lathyrism is caused by high consumption of the drought-resistant chickling pea (*Lathyrus sativus*).

Ackee Travelers to Jamaica or Nigeria may be introduced to the delights of the fruit of *Blighia sapida*, known as the *ackee* in Jamaica and *isin* in Nigeria.

In Jamaica, this strange fruit is served up with bacon or salt-fish as a kind of scrambled-egg look-alike. Problems arise if the fruit is eaten unripe or has been improperly prepared, as it contains a potent toxin that rapidly lowers the blood sugar level. The victim succumbs rapidly to vomiting, followed by convulsions, coma, and death in the majority of cases. This is more likely to occur in the already malnourished, but the unripe fruit can be lethal to anyone. Correct preparation involves boiling the fruit and then discarding the water.

Cycads Various species of cycad grow throughout the tropical areas of the Far East including southern Japan, southern China, the Philippines, Indonesia, the East Indies, and northern Australia. Both the seeds and stems of several species of cycad are used for food, but degenerative diseases may result from eating them.

Amyotrophic lateral sclerosis (ALS) is a progressive fatal disorder of adults resulting from degeneration of cells in the brain and spinal cord. It is particularly common among the indigenous (Chamorro) population of the islands of Guam and Rota, where a clinical variant of Parkinson-like dementia (PD) is also seen. Recently, it has been shown that this disorder is associated with eating the highly toxic seeds of the false sago palm (*Cycas circinalis L.*). During the Japanese occupation of Guam from 1941 to 1944, when rice was hard to obtain, cycad seed represented a major source of food for the indigenous residents of Guam. Cycad flour, used to make tortillas, atole (a drink), and soup, is prepared from the endosperm of ripe (green-brown) seeds. This is removed from the seed integument and halved, sliced, or crushed, then soaked in fresh water to remove unidentified acutely poisonous substances. This is then dried in the sun and ground to form a flour. Cycad flour products are now favored by middle-aged and elderly traditional Chamorros living in rural communities. In addition, the fresh seed integument is chewed to relieve thirst. Improperly washed *Cycas* seed has caused acute seizures in humans but ALS and PD are the result of more prolonged ingestion.

The condition is ultimately fatal. It rarely occurs outside the Chamorro population, but one ex-marine who stayed in Guam after World War II developed ALS and a second was diagnosed as having Alzheimer's disease. ALS-PD also occurs in other Western Pacific islands and in the Kii Peninsula of Japan.

ANIMAL TOXINS

Animal toxins fall into two categories. First, a normal constituent of the animal or one of its organs may be toxic. For example Eskimos have always known of the toxicity of polar bear liver, which contains immensely high levels of vitamin A. Second, the animal itself may be contaminated with toxins.

The vast majority of poisonings are the result of eating fish or other forms of seafood. There are approximately 1,200 marine species known to be poisonous or venomous. They are found throughout the world but only pose a medical or socioeconomic hazard in a few areas.

Puffer fish The puffer fish—known as "fugu" in Japan—is a kind of culinary Russian Roulette. It is said to be sufficiently delicious to warrant the considerable risk attached to its consumption. Japanese chefs have to be specially licensed to carry out the delicate operation of removing the roe, liver, and skin which contain the lethal *tetrodotoxin*, but every year several deaths occur from eating fugu. About 40 percent of those who develop significant signs and symptoms die. Death is said to be preceded by a tingling sensation of the lips. Recent studies have indicated that tetrodotoxin is more widespread than was first thought: it has also been identified in crabs.

Paralytic shellfish poisoning Rather less dramatic in onset, but no less unpleasant, is the poisoning caused by eating fish, or more often shellfish, that have ingested plankton containing *saxitoxin*. In some areas of the world, such as the Caribbean, dinoflagellate protozoa may be present in such large numbers that the sea looks red and the amount of saxitoxin in the flesh of fish or shellfish will be correspondingly high. Fishermen in areas that are commonly affected know not to harvest the fish when there is a "red tide." Symptoms of poisoning are slowing of the heart rate even to the point of heart failure, and muscle paralysis. Mild poisoning may result from ingesting just 1 mg. of the toxin, which could be found in a single clam. Without treatment 4 mg. of the toxin would be fatal.

MOLLUSC-ASSOCIATED INTOXICATIONS

The ability of mussels, clams, and oysters to concentrate toxins from water and pass them on to humans makes them particularly dangerous. This can occur equally in cold climates: in December 1987 over 250 Canadians were poisoned when they ate mussels which had been raised in river estuaries in Prince Edward Island in Eastern Canada. Nineteen were hospitalized, of whom 12 required intensive care because of seizures, coma, profuse respiratory secretions, or unstable blood pressure, and 3 died. Many had prolonged neurological abnormalities including memory loss, disorientation, and confusion which had not resolved 24 months after the incident. The mussels were found to contain domoic acid, a neuroexcitatory amino acid derived from a planktonic diatom which the mussels had concentrated. In Canada steps have been taken to prevent the recurrence of shellfish poisoning due to domoic acid: they are tested for the presence of the toxin before commercial distribution.

Ciguatera is the most common food-borne illness worldwide due to a chemical toxin. Ciguatera is a circumtropical variety of food poisoning caused by eating a wide variety of coral reef fish that have accumulated *ciguatoxin* via the marine food chain. The term *ciguatera* was derived from a name used in the eighteenth century in the Spanish Antilles for intoxication brought about by ingestion of the cigua or turban shell. Ciguatera was recorded in the West Indies in the fifteenth century and noted in the Pacific as early as 1606, when Spanish explorers suffered from ciguatera in the New Hebrides.

Ciguatera can occur anywhere around the world in a belt from 35° north to 35° south. It is particularly common in the tropical Pacific and the Caribbean and it is also reported in Florida. Outbreaks of ciguatera occur sporadically: the problem may suddenly appear in any one location after years of absence and is not signaled by any visible change in the sea.

Ciguatoxic fish are species that feed on algae or detritus around tropical reefs, especially the surgeon fish, parrot fish, and larger reef carnivores and omnivores that prey on these, such as reef sharks, moray eels, snappers, some inshore tunas, groupers, and barracuda. In Florida, the sale of barracuda is banned. The toxin accumulates in the flesh, skin, and viscera of the fish but since the toxins are much more concentrated in the viscera than in the flesh, it is advisable to avoid eating the brain, spinal cord, intestines, gonads, and liver of all species of reef fish.

Symptoms appear between one and six hours after eating the fish and are very varied, ranging from mild gastroenteritis to death. Several different toxins are almost certainly involved and symptoms depend on the relative amounts of each of these toxins. In New Caledonia the common name for ciguatera is *"la gratte"* or "the itch." In Samoa the typical course for ciguatera is gastroenteritis followed by general weakness, followed by "pins and needles" lasting three weeks or longer. Neurological symptoms can persist for months or even years. In French Polynesia, the gastrointestinal symptoms seem to be more common in victims who have eaten herbivorous fish such as the surgeon fish *"maito,"* whereas cardiovascular and other disorders prevail in cases caused by toxic carnivores such as snappers and groupers. In the Gambier Islands the parrot fish causes most of the ciguatera intoxications: symptoms begin like the typical ciguatera syndrome but are followed by a staggering walk, loss of balance, and tremor, lasting a month or more.

Ciguatera is occasionally fatal. In acute cases death may be caused by respiratory failure due to paralysis of the respiratory muscles but may also result from the severe dehydration caused by the vomiting and diarrhea.

Recently, it has been shown that ciguatoxin may be present in the semen of men affected with ciguatera and may be capable of producing symptoms in both males and females during sexual intercourse. Two male visitors to the Bahamas developed ciguatera after eating grouper. Five days later both men had sexual intercourse and reported painful ejaculation with severe, prolonged urethritis following sex. The wives, who had not eaten any of the fish, had no symptoms until engaging in intercourse: both then reported pain immediately following ejaculation, and vaginal burning and stinging that persisted for two or three weeks.

Scombroid poisoning Some fish of the mackerel or tuna varieties may be the cause of poisoning if they are inadequately refrigerated and preserved. Cooking does not destroy the toxin. A toxic substance, originally thought to be histamine, is formed by the action of enzymes on the muscle of the dead fish. Recent research suggests that another toxin, *saurine*, is also formed. This causes nausea, vomiting, diarrhea, and epigastric pain. The face of the victim becomes flushed and burning and there may be numbness, thirst, and generalized urticaria. Fortunately all these signs and symptoms, which arise within about two hours of the meal, subside within 12–16 hours. No treatment is required. It is said that the flesh of affected fish tastes rather peppery. This type of poisoning may occur anywhere in the world.

CHRONIC POISONING

The long-term effects of food toxins are of rather less importance to travelers than acute poisons, but travelers should none the less be aware of the dangers of certain molds and metals.

MYCOTOXINS
Mycotoxins, the toxins produced by molds, have been implicated in several diseases both in tropical and in temperate climates. Moldy foods are more commonly consumed during times of famine. Many of their effects are chronic but acute poisoning may also occur.

Acute mildewed sugarcane poisoning has been reported in China: there were 217 outbreaks of the poisoning between 1972 and 1989, affecting 884 patients and causing 88 deaths. The poison is characterized by a sudden onset of gastrointestinal symptoms followed by toxic encephalopathy. Most of the victims were children who had eaten mildewed sugarcane harvested in late October and stored during the winter. The outbreaks of poisoning usually occur between January and March, mainly in the northern part of China.

Mold-contaminated food may be consumed directly by man, or by domestic animals reared for food—pigs, for example—which are capable of accumulating toxins in their flesh. Balkan nephropathy, a strange and serious disease of the kidneys confined to areas of the former Yugoslavia, Romania, and Bulgaria, was first recognized thirty years ago. Only recently has it been linked to consumption of a mold that grows on maize.

Aflatoxin is the toxin of *Aspergillus flavus*, which grows on peanuts and other crops, including pistachios, almonds, walnuts, pecans, brazil nuts, oil seeds (cottonseed and copra), and grains (corn, grain sorghum, and millet). In tropical regions aflatoxin can be produced in unrefrigerated prepared foods. Contamination may occur in the field, especially during times of drought and other stresses that allow insect damage and predispose the plant to mold attack, and may also occur due to inadequate storage conditions.

The toxin is highly carcinogenic and consumption of moldy peanuts explains the high incidence of liver cancer in some parts of Africa—particularly West Africa. This has serious economic implications for many of the countries involved. Aflatoxin metabolites are sometimes present in the milk of dairy cows that have consumed contaminated feed.

Eating moldy cornmeal may be one of the factors involved in the high incidence of cancer of the esophagus found in areas of China. Excessive consumption of pickles and preserved foods containing nitrites may also be contributing factors.

Poor nutritional status, particularly combined with deficiency of vitamins A and C, probably increases susceptibility to mycotoxins. The well-nourished traveler may be at rather less risk than the indigenous population, but would still be well advised to avoid moldy foods.

Trichothecenes These mycotoxins are produced by a number of commonly occurring molds and occur most often in moldy cereal grains. There have been many reported cases of trichothecene toxicity in farm animals and a few in humans. Disruption of agriculture during World War II resulted in millet, wheat, and barley being over-wintered in the fields in Siberia. Consumption of these grains led to an outbreak of vomiting, skin inflammation, diarrhea, and multiple hemorrhages in inhabitants of the area around Orenburg in Siberia. The exposure was fatal to over 10 percent of the individuals who consumed the moldy grain.

METALS

Various metals can be toxic. Lead from cooking pots is found in high levels in home-brewed beers in various parts of Africa, and can lead to chronic poisoning. Mercury present in seed dressing has caused poisoning in starving peasants in Iraq, forced by hunger to eat the grain intended for planting.

CANCER AND PLANTS

In developed countries concern has focused on the potential of food additives to cause cancer and it is often forgotten that naturally occurring constituents of plants can be much more potent carcinogens. These hazards are not unique to the traveler but may become significant if a particularly monotonous diet is consumed. For example, basil, mushrooms, celery, and lettuce all contain high levels of chemicals that are known to cause cancer when fed to experimental animals.

Safrole is a known carcinogen present in many plants eaten in various parts of the world. Oil of sassafras, which was used in "natural" sarsaparilla root beer in the USA, is about 75 percent safrole. Black pepper contains small amounts of safrole and large amounts of the related compound piperine.

Hydrazines are found in many mushrooms including the most commonly grown commercial mushroom (*Agaricus bisporus*): they cause lung tumors in mice.

Fucoumarins are potent light-activated carcinogens and are present in high levels in celery, parsnips, figs, and parsley. The level in celery can increase about a hundredfold if the plant is bruised or diseased.

Pyrrolizidines are known to cause liver and lung damage and tumors in animals and man. They are found particularly in herb teas such as comfrey tea and in the bush teas brewed in parts of the Caribbean.

Fortunately, many plants also contain substances that protect against the development of cancer including vitamin E, beta carotene, ascorbic acid, and selenium. Both at home and abroad it is advisable to eat a balanced, mixed diet and to avoid excessive consumption of any single food.

RADIATION

Years after the accident at Chernobyl, farmers in villages in Byelorus are still being instructed not to consume the crops or milk they produce. Replacements are supposed to be delivered weekly by the government. The combination of the national food shortage and political upheavals means that this does not happen and the locally produced foods are often consumed, some reaching regional markets that cannot all be policed properly. Another bizarre government policy is to distribute modestly contaminated foods to distant regions, while bringing food from these regions to the contamination zone. Travelers would be well advised to avoid foods that are obviously locally produced, such as mushrooms, fruit, and vegetables.

SUMMARY OF ADVICE FOR TRAVELERS

- Food toxins and contaminants are so diverse that there are no really hard-and-fast rules for the traveler to follow. Generally, where food is known to be hazardous—such as with cassava or puffer fish—traditional local methods of preparation have evolved to minimize the risk. Most such traditions have a basis in fact, and are best observed.
- Obviously decayed or moldy foods, either plant or animal, are likely to cause toxic effects.
- Problems are more likely to arise in areas of drought and famine.

3 WATER

SAFE WATER

Careful choice or treatment of water—whether for drinking, washing, preparing food, or swimming in—is one of the most important health precautions a traveler can take.

Dr. Hemda Garelick is a Research Fellow at the London School of Hygiene and Tropical Medicine.

Water is essential for our survival: according to our size, activity, culture, health status, climate, and choice of clothing, we require between four and ten pints of water (two and five liters) every day.

In the developed world, the availability of safe water in more or less unlimited quantities is taken for granted. This does not apply in the developing world: in many countries, easy access to a safe water supply—and that does not necessarily mean a piped water supply—is available to only about 70-80 percent of the urban population and to about 40 percent of the rural population. Figures for access to sanitary facilities are even worse, so it is hardly surprising that water-related diseases remain a major problem in the developing world and that travelers to such countries are at risk.

WATER AND DISEASE

Water-related infections can be divided into four groups, according to how they are transmitted:

1. Those spread by drinking contaminated water;
2. Those spread through lack of hygiene and sanitary facilities (lack of water);
3. Those spread through *direct* contact with contaminated water (e.g., swimming) or *indirect* contact (e.g., eating fish that carry infection from contaminated water);
4. Those spread through bites of insects that need water in order to breed (see particularly malaria, pp. 121–32);

In the first two categories, the infections of greatest importance to the traveler are those transmitted by the fecal-oral route, that is from one person's feces to another person's mouth.

These include diarrheal diseases, dysenteries, typhoid, poliomyelitis, hepatitis A, and worm infections, discussed in earlier chapters.

In the third category, diseases transmitted through direct or indirect contact with water include schistosomiasis (see pp. 94–99), Guinea worm, fish tapeworms, and liver flukes.

Chemical contamination (unless gross) is likely to affect travelers far less than the local population, because the harmful effects tend to be cumulative and related to duration of exposure. In contrast, biological contamination (e.g., pathogenic microorganisms) has a more acute effect on travelers than on local people who may have acquired partial or full immunity to locally prevalent infections.

WATER AND THE TRAVELER

Contamination of water supplies is usually due to poor sanitation close to water sources, sewage disposal into the sources themselves, leakage of sewage into distribution systems, or contamination with industrial or farm waste. Even if a piped water supply is safe at its source, it is not always safe by the time it reaches the faucet. *Intermittent* water supplies should be regarded with particular suspicion.

Travelers on short trips to areas with water supplies of uncertain quality should avoid drinking water from the faucet or untreated water from any other source. It is best to keep to hot drinks, bottled or canned drinks of well-known brand names—international standards of water treatment are usually followed at bottling plants. Carbonated drinks are acidic, and slightly safer. Make sure that all bottles are opened in your presence, and that their rims are clean and dry.

Boiling is always a good way of treating water. Some hotels supply boiled water on request and this can be used for drinking, or for brushing teeth. Portable boiling elements that can boil small quantities of water are useful when the right voltage of electricity is available. Refuse politely any cold drink from an unknown source.

Ice is only as safe as the water from which it is made, and should not be put in drinks unless it is known to be safe. Drinks can be cooled by placing them on ice rather than adding ice to them.

Alcohol may be a medical disinfectant, but should not be relied upon to sterilize water. Ethanol is most effective at a concentration of 50–70 percent; below 20 percent, its bactericidal action is negligible. Spirits labeled 95 proof contain only about 47 percent alcohol. Beware of methylated alcohol, which is very poisonous and should never be added to drinking water.

If no other safe water supply can be obtained, water from the faucet that is too hot to touch can be left to cool and is generally safe to drink.

Anyone planning a trip to remote areas, or intending to live in countries where drinking water is not readily available, should know about the various possible methods for making water safe.

WATER TREATMENT

The choice of processes used in a public water treatment plant depends on the physical, chemical, and microbiological characteristics of the water, but the main steps generally necessary are these:

1. The removal of suspended solids by precipitation, sedimentation, or filtration;
2. Disinfection—usually by chlorination—to inactivate and kill the possible pathogens (disease-causing infective agents).

Treating small quantities of water is based on similar principles but is rather easier, and a wider range of processes is possible.

Begin by choosing the purest possible source. This is likely to be water from the local piped supply, well water, spring water, or collected rainwater, all of which are preferable to surface water— e.g., rivers, streams, or pond water—which tends to be polluted. Rainwater can be collected from roofs, which should be clean and made of tiles or sheeting, not of lead or thatch.

BOILING

Boiling is the most effective way of sterilizing water. It kills all infective agents including amebic cysts, which are resistant to chlorine.

This treatment is not affected by the turbidity or the chemical characteristics of the water. The only limitation of boiling is that it is not always practical and is generally suitable only for small quantities. The water should be boiled vigorously for five minutes (this is sufficient even at high altitude).

Boiling tends to make water taste flat, because it reduces the amount of dissolved gases. To improve the taste, drinking water should be allowed to cool in a covered, partially filled container for a few hours, in the same container in which it has been boiled.

FILTRATION

Filtration is a process that should be used when boiling is not practicable. It is either an initial step or can produce safe water in a single step when the right equipment is used.

Removal of suspended solids In order to make disinfection (with chlorine or iodine) as effective as possible, suspended solids and organic matter must be removed. Organic matter interferes with the process of chemical disinfection, and pathogens adsorbed to suspended solids are less susceptible to disinfection.

Filtration through a closely woven cloth is adequate, and filtration bags such as the Millbank bag are available commercially. These can take from about one to six gallons and are not expensive ($10–$20, depending on size). However, it is important to remember that although the water may look clear it has not yet been made safe, and requires further treatment.

Removal of pathogens Ceramic filter "candles" of a very fine pore size (which can be as fine as 0.5 micron [0.00002 inch], the finer the better) are available commercially, and some units can be attached to piped water supplies. They remove most pathogens found in water (bacteria, amebic cysts, and some viruses). Some of the filters are impregnated with silver, which acts as a limited bactericide.

Manufacturers' instructions on the operation and maintenance of filters should be followed. Filters should be examined regularly for cracks and leaks. They should be cleaned by scrubbing, and boiled (unless impregnated with silver) when clogged and at weekly intervals.

Disposable paper cartridge filters are also available. They should be kept wet when in use, or the paper filter may shrink or crack.

Most carbon filters are not recommended for making water safe. They are normally used to improve the taste of clean water. They remove organic matter, dissolved chlorine, and pathogens by a mechanism of adsorption, not by mechanical straining. When over-loaded they can shed the adsorbed material, and unless it is impregnated with silver, bacteria may even grow on the filter. The efficiency of the filter over a period of time will depend on the organic load of the water: travelers may find it difficult to determine when the filter is exhausted. Some ceramic filter candles have the option of adding activated carbon to improve the taste. It is important to ensure that any such combined filter does not rely on the carbon for removal of pathogens. Only in cases of high chemical contamination will addition of activated carbon to the filter be advantageous to health.

Filtered water should always be boiled or disinfected before being given to babies and small children.

There are a great many convenient-looking purification devices on the market based on filtration, and they are often recommended to travelers. The manufacturers frequently make extravagant claims about the effectiveness and safety of their products without producing any objective and convincing evidence to support their claims—such as precise details of how and by whom microbiological tests were performed. Without this evidence, such gadgets must always be regarded with suspicion, however useful they may seem. The safest purification methods remain boiling and chemical disinfection.

CHEMICAL DISINFECTION
Chemical disinfection is recommended when boiling or fine-pore filtration is not possible, or when extra safety is required.

Choosing a water filter or purifier

Keeping to bottled or boiled water is the best option for most travelers, but there are many situations—such as hiking or trekking through tropical jungle or desert terrain—where it is simply not practicable. There are limits to how much water can be carried, and boiling takes time, effort, and fuel.

As an alternative to chemical purification, a large number of water filters and purification devices have appeared on the market; they seem attractive, but claims are sometimes made for them that are difficult to assess. Here are the most important points to watch for.

Water filters for travel should be dependable, be easily maintained, and give some strong indication of when their useful life has ended. Nothing lasts a lifetime, so be wary of units that are claimed to be able to cope with thousands of gallons. While it may be true that thousands of gallons can be run through, the number that will be treated effectively may be a different matter. Using a commonly recognized technique of "methylene blue" dye extraction, testing has shown that for most activated carbon filters, "breakthrough" usually occurs after less than about 50 gallons.

Don't be misled by the terms used in manufacturers' literature. A "filter" removes suspended solids by mechanical straining; *further purification is almost always required*. However, a "purifier" both filters and sterilizes, giving safe drinking water with no need for further treatment. Product literature sometimes makes much play of a filter unit being "bacteriostatic"—particularly in relation to activated carbon units. This merely means that bacterial growth is inhibited, NOT that bacteria are actually killed. Only a "bactericide" will do this. Manufacturers' literature does not always give results of virus removal tests, even when a unit may be quite effective. Such tests may require a high degree of skill to perform, and can be expensive.

Bear in mind that no uniform, objective, agreed standards exist for such devices, and that external safeguards on quality control are generally lacking. Look therefore for test data from a good university department or endorsement by reputable independent organizations.

In practice, the most common problems with filters are that they tend to clog easily and that they may lose their effectiveness by cracking or becoming damaged without the user being aware of what has happened. Don't forget that filtration alone is not enough to make water safe to drink.

(**Andreas King,** Assistant Editor, *Water & Waste Treatment Journal,* London.)

Chlorine This is the most widely used water disinfectant. It kills living organisms by inactivating biologically active compounds. However, it also reacts with any other organic matter that may be present in the water, and this reduces the amount of chlorine available to kill pathogens. Pathogens adsorbed to suspended solids may also be protected from disinfection. Water should thus be filtered before disinfection (see above).

Chlorine is an effective disinfectant against bacteria and some viruses, although less effective against amebic cysts. The amount of chlorine needed for inactivation of amebic cysts is 10 times that needed for inactivation of bacteria.

Iodine This works in a similar way to chlorine and is thought to be a more effective disinfectant, especially against amebic cysts.

Both chlorine-based and iodine-based disinfection tablets are available commercially. When these are used, it is important to follow manufacturers' instructions carefully, and to make sure that water to be treated is clear.

Liquid chlorine laundry bleach and first aid tincture of iodine can also be used. The exact constituents and concentration of the solutions should be determined before use. Liquid chlorine laundry bleach usually contains 4–6 percent available chlorine, and one to two drops (one drop = 0.05 ml.) of such a solution (or alternatively four to eight drops of a 1 percent solution) should be added to each quart or liter of water. Tincture of iodine usually contains 2 percent iodine, and four drops of the solution should be added to one quart or liter of water.

In both cases, the treated water should be allowed to stand for 20–30 minutes before use, although very cold water should be allowed to stand longer (a few hours if possible).

The use of iodine in this way is *not* thought to be harmful, though regular long-term use should probably be avoided on theoretical grounds; likewise, use in pregnancy has not been associated with harmful effects, but is probably also best avoided on theoretical grounds; anyone with a thyroid problem should consult a physician first.

STORAGE OF TREATED WATER

Treated water should be stored in conditions that will prevent recontamination, and preferably in the same container in which it has been treated. If this is impractical, make sure that storage containers are either sterile or disinfected. They should always be covered, and should ideally have a tap at the bottom or a narrow opening, thus minimizing the risk of contamination when drawing off the treated water. Store water in a cool place, away from children.

SANITATION AND HYGIENE

Sanitary facilities should be kept as far away as possible from water and food. Hands must always be washed before handling food and drink. Personal hygiene should be maintained at the highest standard possible.

FOOD HYGIENE

Food—especially fresh food obtained locally in areas where sanitary conditions are poor—should always be regarded as contaminated.

Fruit and vegetables should be washed thoroughly in clean soapy water and then rinsed with treated water. Rinsing alone is not enough—sterilizing chemicals in treated water will not kill pathogens on fruit and vegetables because contact time is not long enough.

Soaking in chlorine (e.g., using tablets or liquid chlorine bleach) or iodine—the concentration of either should be roughly three times that normally used for drinking-water purification—is usually also effective, though the contact time necessary depends on how badly contaminated the food is.

Soaking in potassium permanganate, traditionally recommended for this purpose, is less reliable; permanganate has few medical uses these days.

Dipping in boiling water is a simple and effective alternative.

Avoid eating any raw vegetables or cold food prepared by others—especially in restaurants and hotels, and especially salads. (If you really must eat a salad that looks unsafe, plenty of lemon juice or strong vinegar in the dressing will slightly reduce the risk.)

Seafood, fish, and meat should always be well cooked, and unpasteurized milk should be boiled or avoided.

SWIMMING

From the point of view of infection, swimming in the sea is usually safe, unless it is close to sewage outfalls or highly populated areas with no proper sanitary facilities. Swimming in fresh surface water is not advised, especially in areas where schistosomiasis (bilharzia) (see pp. 94–99) and Guinea worm are found.

MANUFACTURERS AND SUPPLIERS: WATER PURIFICATION PRODUCTS

TETRAGLYCINE HYPERIODIDE
TABLETS
Wisconsin Pharmacal Co. (Potable Aqua iodination tablets)
6769 North Industrial Rd.
Milwaukee, WI 53223
Tel. (414) 677-4121

FILTRATION BAGS (MILLBANK)
Johnson-Progress Ltd
Carpenters Rd.
Stratford, London E15 2DS, UK.
Tel. (081) 534-7431
Fax (081) 519-8768;
accepts mail orders

FILTRATION UNITS, PUMPS, AND PURIFICATION UNITS
First Need Filters: General Ecology Inc.
151 Sheree Blvd.
Lionville, PA 19341
Tel. (215) 363-7900
(800) 441-8166

Katadyn Filters: Katadyn USA Inc.
12219 St. James Rd.
Potomac, MD 20854
Tel. (301) 251-0570
(also supplies industrial and ultra-violet purification units)

Performance Filters (NA), Inc.
2940 Portsmouth Ave.
Cincinnati, OH 45208
Tel. (513) 271-2600

Timberline Filters, Inc.
Box 12007
Boulder, CO 80303
Tel. (303) 440-8779

Basic Designs, Inc.
Box 2507
Santa Rosa, CA 95405
Tel. (707) 575-1220

Pur filters: Recovery Engineering, Inc.
2229 Edgewood Ave. South
Minneapolis, MN 55426
Tel. (800) 845-7873

MSR
Box 24547-0
Seattle, WA 98124
Tel. (206) 624-7048

DISTILLATION
TapWorks distiller: Ecowater Consumer Products
Box 64420
Saint Paul, MN 55164
Tel. (612) 739-5330

SPECIALIST RETAIL OUTLETS
Most of the above products can be obtained from camping and sporting goods stores, such as Eastern Mountain Sports, Paragon, Herman's.

ALGAL BLOOMS

Pollution of sea water, lakes, and rivers with fertilizers, sewage, and organic material has caused sudden increases in the growth of microscopic plants or algae—algal blooms. The phenomenon is on the increase, with recent dramatic blooms along the Adriatic and elsewhere. The algae can be toxic or merely a slimy nuisance, interfering with swimming, windsurfing, and other watersports. This chapter explains the background to the problem.

Dr. Robin Philipp is a Senior Lecturer in Public Health Medicine and Occupational Medicine, and the Director of the WHO Collaborating Center for Environmental Health Promotion and Ecology, both at the University of Bristol, UK. He has a particular interest in the health risks associated with water.

INTRODUCTION

Blue-green algae (BGA) are microscopic plants found in fresh and brackish waters. They have some characteristics of bacteria and are therefore described as photosynthetic bacteria, also called cyanobacteria. They are particularly common in lowland, nutrient-laden waters in the warm, sunny summer months. Mountain reservoirs generally have low numbers, except where contributory water sources drain forested areas on which phosphate or nitrogenous fertilizers have been used.

Some free-floating algae contain gas bubbles that regulate buoyancy in response to the light intensity. Normally this keeps them away from the surface, but in windy conditions that mix the water, the cells may become too buoyant and rise rapidly to the surface if the wind subsides abruptly. They accumulate downwind and at the water's edge to form scums that look like blue-green paint or jelly. In high density within the water, they can also form a visible blue-green bloom; they may also be colored purple or red. They are an increasing problem due to nutrient enrichment of natural waters, agricultural fertilizer runoff, domestic and industrial effluents, and possibly global warming. Scums and blooms can also encourage other bacterial growth and colonization by insects.

TOXINS

Toxins produced by some BGA have caused deaths in agricultural livestock, pets, wild animals, and fish. Toxicity can fluctuate daily in that BGA can be toxic one day and not the next. Blooms can also appear one day, disappear suddenly, and reappear at any time. The toxins are of three main types—those that affect the nervous system, those that damage the liver, and those that irritate the skin.

HARMFUL EFFECTS ON WILDLIFE AND MAN

Deaths have occurred in animals venturing into thick concentrations of algae to bathe and drink the water, or licking scum and deposits off their fur when coming ashore. Inhalation of aerosols containing desiccated algal material can also occur. No deaths have been reported in humans, although harmful effects of BGA on human health have been widely reported, most commonly in developed countries with hot climates such as Australia and parts of the USA, but also from the UK, Canada, China, Scandinavia, the Baltic States, the former USSR, South Africa, Zimbabwe, India, New Zealand, Israel, Venezuela, and Argentina.

In humans, ingestion of toxic algae or body immersion in scum-containing water has been associated with dizziness, headaches, muscle cramps, runny nose, sore eyes, hay fever, asthma, pneumonia, nausea, vomiting, gastroenteritis, and liver damage, and skin contact has been associated with burning, itching, and inflammation of the skin, eyes, and lips, sore throat, and dizziness. Recent outbreaks of gastroenteritis affecting travelers to Nepal have been attributed to BGA-like organisms, and these are currently under investigation.

THE MAIN EXPOSURE SITUATIONS AND ASSOCIATED RISKS

DRINKING WATER
BGA can give a "musty," "geranium," or "vegetable" taste and odor to drinking water. Dense blooms of blue-green algae in drinking water reservoirs have occasionally resulted in inflammation of the liver and gastroenteritis in people who have been drinking affected water.

EATING CONTAMINATED FISH OR MEAT

Some BGA toxins can accumulate in freshwater shellfish such as the swan mussel (*Anadonta cygnea*). BGA toxins can also accumulate in some fish organs, particularly the liver. In the 1920s and 1930s, for example, outbreaks of a condition called Haff disease were common around the Baltic Coast and were linked with eating fish, in particular, fish liver from fresh waters affected by algal blooms: the livers were regarded as a delicacy if tasting of musty blue-green-algal-type flavor compounds. Haff disease was occasionally fatal, and was characterized by muscular pain, vomiting, respiratory distress, and the passage of brownish-black urine. Elsewhere, there do not seem to have been any such outbreaks, even when freshwater algal blooms have been prominent. There is no evidence at present that algal toxins can affect the flesh of fish. Fish are therefore considered safe to eat provided they are properly gutted and cleaned. The flesh of animals which have been drinking water that is affected by an algal bloom is also safe to eat.

CONTACT WITH SEAWATER ALGAE AND EATING SHELLFISH

Seawater algal blooms are caused by increased nutrient loads and low oxygen levels in the water. They cause "red algal tides" and mucilage formation. Mucilage is an amorphous, messy, viscous substance suspended in the water. It can be deposited on beaches.

The commonest toxic algae to be found in marine waters are called dinoflagellates (they are single-celled, motile algae). Their toxins are mainly a problem when they become concentrated by fish and shellfish that are subsequently eaten by humans. Toxic marine dinoflagellates can cause several illnesses.

Paralytic shellfish poisoning (PSP) occurs in several parts of the world. It begins with numbness and tingling around the mouth and in the hands and fingers within 5–30 minutes of eating affected shellfish, followed by numbness and weakness of the arms and legs. Usually the illness is mild and self-limiting, but in severe cases when large amounts of toxin have been eaten, paralysis of the diaphragm leads to respiratory failure, which may be fatal. There is no evidence that PSP can be caused by skin exposure, drinking seawater, or from inhaling seawater droplets.

Algae associated with *diarrheic shellfish poisoning* (DSP) are *Dinophysis* and *Prorocentrum* (okadaic acid). The symptoms and signs of DSP are mainly diarrhea, nausea, vomiting, abdominal pain, and chills coming on within 30 minutes to 12 hours of eating shell-fish.

Neurotoxic shellfish poisoning (NSP) resembles PSP, but is non-fatal and paralysis does not occur. So far, blooms causing it have only been reported in the Gulf of Mexico. Sea spray containing the same algae (*Ptychodiscus brevis*) or their toxins cause an irritant aerosol that leads to inflammation of the eyes and nose, with cough and tingling lips; with windy conditions, the effects can be observed up to a few miles inland.

Amnesic shellfish poisoning is a rare illness first recognized in 1987 when a mysterious outbreak in Canada was traced to a bloom of the diatom *Nitzschia pungens*. (Diatoms are unicellular plankton with a silicified cell wall, and are widely distributed.) The illness was associated with a shellfish toxin (domoic acid) which had become concentrated in mussels. Severe headache, vomiting, abdominal cramps, and diarrhea were followed by confusion, memory loss, disorientation, and coma. *Nitzschia pungens* is widely distributed in the coastal waters of the Atlantic, Pacific, and Indian oceans.

Ciguatera and *puffer-fish poisoning* resemble PSP, and the term *pelagic paralysis* has been proposed to cover all three because their neurotoxins are believed to act in the same way. Ciguatera is mainly a hazard in Pacific and Caribbean waters: the dinoflagellates involved are benthic (found at the bottom of an ocean) and therefore probably not related to blooms. It is, however, the most common form of fish poisoning and the most frequently reported food-borne disease of a chemical nature in southeast Florida and Hawaii. Puffer-fish poisoning is still a public health hazard in Japan. Both types of poisoning may occur in Europe from imported fish.

Marine cyanophyte dermatitis is a severe contact dermatitis known as swimmers' itch or seaweed dermatitis. It may occur after swimming or handling fishing nets in seas containing blooms of the filamentous marine cyanophyte *Lynbya majuscula*. Two of the toxic agents are known to be potent tumor-producing compounds. So far, outbreaks have only been reported from Japan and Hawaii. A toxic dermatitis known as Dogger Bank itch or weed rash also occurs in European trawler fishermen from the handling of trawl nets. It is caused by moss animals called sea chervils found in the North Sea, and not by algae.

Skin irritation in bathers can also be caused by jellyfish fragments or by small crustacea in the bloom which become trapped inside bathing suits. The bloom may also dry on the skin after bathing and irritate or sensitize it if it is not washed off. Hay fever or asthma may also be provoked by bloom material drying on the shore, becoming airborne, and affecting sunbathers and others exposed to onshore winds.

HINTS FOR PERSONAL HEALTH

The risk of harmful effects from different patterns of exposure to BGA is not fully understood. Unfortunately, the potential toxicity of a bloom or scum cannot be determined by its appearance, odor, texture, or any other simple feature. If treated with reasonable care, there is little hazard to human health: although algal scums and blooms are not always harmful, it is sensible to regard them as such. The following points will help minimize possible risks associated with drinking water and recreational exposures.

DRINKING WATER

Standard water treatment does not remove algal toxins from water. The toxins are heat stable and unlikely to be destroyed by boiling. There is also no evidence that water-purification tablets either destroy the toxins or encourage their release from algal cells. Although an extremely uncommon and temporary phenomenon, any drinking-water supply that is obviously discolored blue-green should be avoided. Nevertheless, there is little present evidence of particular risks from public supplies.

Shellfish are best avoided if there is doubt about the purity of the waters they came from.

In rural or wilderness areas where raw water is consumed, take the following precautions to reduce the risk of exposure.

- Where possible, take drinking water from flowing rather than still water.

- In still water, scums and decaying cells accumulate downwind on the surface, and are more likely to be associated with the release of toxins. Water should therefore be taken away from any visible scum, out from the water's edge, from below the surface, and on the windward side of a lake or reservoir.

- Brownish, peaty upland waters are less likely to be contaminated with BGA than lowland nutrient-enriched waters.

- If drinking water has been taken in the presence of a scum or algal bloom, the water should be filtered to remove particles of algal material.

- Affected water is generally safe for irrigation, but if in doubt, avoid eating leafy vegetables, or at least wash them carefully in clean, treated water.

FRESHWATER RECREATIONAL ACTIVITIES

Studies have not yet identified any particular illnesses that could be linked to BGA exposure through recreation. As a precaution, though, the following guidance is recommended.

- If the water is clear there is little danger of ill-effects as a result of recreational contact.

- Toxins are more concentrated where there are visible algal scums. These areas should always be avoided. Direct contact with a visible scum, or swallowing appreciable amounts, are associated with the highest chances of a health risk.

- On a lee shore and windy day, algae and scum can be found at some distance from the water's edge—avoid these areas.

- If sailing, windsurfing, or undertaking any other activity likely to involve accidental water immersion in the presence of scums or algal blooms, wear clothing that is close-fitting at the wrists and neck, and also boots and sailing suits that fit into the boot tops.

- Spend as little time as possible in shallow water launching and recovering boats; launching and recovery should be undertaken in areas away from thick aggregations of algae or scum.

- After coming ashore, hose, shower, or wash yourself down to remove any scum or algae.

- All clothing and bathing suits should be washed and thoroughly dried after any contact with scums or blooms. Do not store wet clothes.

- During sailing or boating activities when scums or blooms are present, keep capsize drills to a minimum, ensure rescue boats are on hand to take crews out of the water as soon as possible, and wash boats and wet gear down immediately on coming ashore. Races should be staged away from affected areas.

- When fishing, keep away from algal scums and clean your hands after handling fish or fishing tackle.
- If any health effects are experienced subsequently, whatever the nature of the exposure, seek prompt medical attention.

SEAWATER BATHING

- As far as exposure to algae is concerned, seawater is generally safe to bathe in provided there is no red algal tide or mucilage, and the water is not otherwise obviously polluted.
- Avoid floating clumps of seaweed or aggregations along the shoreline.
- On the beach, do not sit downwind of any bloom material drying on the shore which could form an aerosol and be inhaled.
- If available, use beach showers after bathing, and rinse bathing suits thoroughly in fresh water to remove salt, crustaceans, algae, or jellyfish fragments that can cause skin irritation.

4 DISEASES OF "CONTACT"

TUBERCULOSIS

After decades of consistently declining incidence, an unprecedented resurgence of tuberculosis (TB) is occurring in the United States and in some European countries. TB is also on the increase in many developing countries, largely because of the spread of human immunodeficiency virus (HIV) infection. Compared to HIV seronegative persons, HIV seropositive individuals are at greatly increased risk of developing active tuberculous disease if they are also infected with the bacterium that causes TB.

Dr. Sonia B. Richards *is an infectious disease specialist currently working for the Centers for Disease Control and Prevention as a medical epidemiologist.*

Dr. C. Robert Horsburgh Jr. *is a medical epidemiologist, also at the Centers for Disease Control and Prevention, who conducts research on the relationship between TB and HIV infection.*

As a traveler, you need to be concerned about TB if your itinerary includes travel to areas with a high prevalence of TB. TB is found most commonly in the tropics, particularly in Southeast Asia and sub-Saharan Africa. It is also quite common in the Middle East and Latin America. Travelers who need to be particularly concerned include those who 1) work with sick people, as in a hospital or refugee camp, 2) live in close quarters with foreign-country nationals, or 3) stay abroad for several months.

SOURCES OF INFECTION

Tuberculosis is caused by the tubercle bacillus, *Mycobacterium tuberculosis.* The disease principally affects the lungs, although virtually any organ can be involved. It is almost always spread by the airborne route. Individuals with pulmonary disease harbor numerous tubercle bacilli in their sputum. Upon coughing or sneezing, they produce a fine mist of sputum particles that dries quickly, leaving a cloud of tiny "droplet nuclei." These can remain suspended in the air and, if inhaled, are small enough to carry bacilli into the uppermost portions of the lungs, where they cause a primary focus of infection.

Prolonged exposure to an infectious environment is usually required for transmission to occur and brief contact is usually of little risk. Thus, household contacts and health-care workers caring for patients with TB are at risk of getting the disease; however, casual contact as in a bus or in a marketplace poses minimal risk.

TB can also be contracted by drinking unpasteurized milk from cows that are infected with *Mycobacterium bovis,* in which case the bacilli enter the body through the tonsils and lymph glands of the neck. Although infection from ingestion of contaminated milk was once commonplace, it is now distinctly unusual in industrialized countries. Elsewhere in the world, such infection can be avoided simply by boiling milk and avoiding unpasteurized milk products.

One does not contract TB from contact with objects. Special housekeeping measures for dishes and bedclothes are therefore not necessary for the prevention of TB.

TUBERCULOUS INFECTION VS. DISEASE

TB does not always cause serious illness and in most individuals the primary focus heals without overt signs of disease. In the first few weeks following infection with the tubercle bacillus, there is no evidence of infection. Tissue hypersensitivity develops within 2–10 weeks and is manifested by a reactive TB skin test. (The skin test should be performed using the Mantoux technique [i.e., intradermal injection of 5 units of tuberculin] rather than Tine or other multiple puncture tests that are less useful.) Persons who have a positive TB skin test but no signs or symptoms of the disease are said to have "tuberculous infection," but not the disease. Once a person is infected, the TB skin test will usually remain positive for many years, perhaps even for a lifetime.

Some persons with tuberculous infection will later develop active tuberculous disease. For those who progress to overt disease, the time interval between initial tuberculous infection and the onset of disease may vary from several weeks to many years. Immunologically normal adults who have been infected are estimated to have a 10 percent chance of progressing to active TB during their lifetime. This risk is distinctly higher in young children, in whom tuberculosis is more likely to develop as an immediate complication of the primary infection. Certain medical conditions which weaken the immune system increase the likelihood that an infected person will develop symptoms of active TB. These conditions include: HIV infection, diabetes mellitus, silicosis, cancer, cancer chemotherapy, immunosuppressive therapy, intestinal bypass surgery, severe kidney disease, and malnutrition.

TB AND HIV

Infection with HIV has emerged as the single most important co-existent medical problem for those infected with tubercle bacilli. Whether HIV-infected persons are at greater risk of acquiring tuberculous infection is unclear; however, once infection has been established, they are clearly more likely to progress to active disease. Since TB often occurs at an early stage of immunodeficiency, the HIV-infected traveler need not have been diagnosed with AIDS or be seriously ill to be at increased risk of developing active tuberculous disease.

SYMPTOMS

The most characteristic symptom of pulmonary TB is a cough which lasts several weeks or longer and produces sputum which may occasionally be blood-tinged. Other nonspecific symptoms include fever, weight loss, loss of appetite, fatigue, and night sweats.

IMMUNIZATION

Immunization against TB is performed with a live, attenuated vaccine derived from *Mycobacterium bovis*, a bacterium related to the tubercle bacillus, and is commonly known as Bacille Calmette-Guérin (BCG) after the French scientists who first introduced it. The vaccine, which is applied intradermally, produces a small ulcer that heals within three months, leaving a permanent scar. In the United States, it is accepted that BCG protects children against miliary TB (a bloodborne form of TB) and against tuberculous meningitis; however, its efficacy in preventing other forms of TB in children or adult TB has been widely variable in several scientific studies and remains the subject of debate. For these reasons, a BCG vaccination program is not routinely offered to the entire population in the United States.

The general population in the United States is at low risk for acquiring tuberculous infection and it is believed that the prevention of TB is most reliably accomplished by periodic Mantoux skin testing of those at higher risk, followed by administration of preventive therapy for those whose skin test reactions convert from negative to positive. However, BCG vaccination may contribute to TB control in selected population groups and is recommended by the American Committee on Immunization Practices for: 1) uninfected children who are at high risk for continuous or repeated exposure to persons with infectious TB who remain untreated, 2) uninfected children who are continuously exposed to drug-resistant TB, or 3) uninfected children who are members of groups without regular access to health care.

The World Health Organization recommends BCG immunization as soon after birth as possible, and in many developing countries it is given in the first year of life. In the UK, BCG is offered to children 12–14 years of age if they have a negative Mantoux skin test and are therefore not already immune to TB. Conversion of the Mantoux test to positive and development of immunity are thought to occur about 6 weeks after immunization. BCG vaccine is not recommended for adults with HIV infection because of possible adverse effects, but the World Health Organization does recommend BCG for infants in developing countries regardless of HIV-infection status.

TREATMENT

Treatment with antituberculous drugs is usually quite effective to cure TB. However, several months of medication are required because tubercle bacilli multiply much more slowly than other bacteria and a correspondingly longer period of contact with the drugs is needed to kill them. Previous regimens lasted 9–18 months; however, it is now generally accepted that 6 months of treatment is effective for most persons. The standard regimen in the United States consists of isoniazid (INH), rifampin (RIF), and pyrazinamide (PZA) for 2 months, followed by INH and RIF for an additional 4 months. Persons with TB who are HIV seropositive usually can be treated successfully with the standard regimen, provided the duration is prolonged to 9 months. Some strains of TB are resistant to these antibiotics, necessitating individualized regimens.

INH PROPHYLAXIS

For those persons who acquire tuberculous infection (a positive Mantoux test but no evidence of active TB), preventative therapy with INH is administered for 6–12 months for those under age 35. Beyond this age, the toxic effect of INH on the liver is significant enough to preclude its routine use unless infection with TB is known to have occurred within the previous 2 years or the individual has a coexisting disease such as HIV infection (or other medical condition mentioned previously) that weakens the immune system and increases the risk of developing active TB.

SUMMARY OF ADVICE FOR TRAVELERS

- No special precautions are required for those traveling within Europe or North America.

- HIV-infected travelers should be aware that they are at increased risk of becoming ill from TB and should avoid traveling to areas where TB is common.

- Persons traveling or living in areas where there is an increased risk of exposure to TB should ensure that their milk is boiled or pasteurized and that their butter is made from pasteurized milk. Yogurt and cheese are not thought to pose a risk since the souring of the milk during the manufacturing process probably kills tubercle bacilli.

- In an area where TB is common, any family with a foreign national in its employ should try to ensure that the employee undergoes TB skin testing at the time of hire and be evaluated for active TB if the skin test is positive.

- If an employee develops a cough lasting longer than two weeks, he or she should receive a chest X-ray and sputum examination. In the event that the employee is diagnosed with active TB, the entire family should undergo TB skin testing.

- Travelers who are likely to be exposed to TB should consider undergoing a TB skin test prior to commencing travel and have the test repeated 6 or more weeks after returning.

- Travelers who believe that they have had a significant exposure to TB should see their physician for an examination and a TB skin test even if they feel well and have no symptoms.

- If a previously negative TB skin test converts to positive, an evaluation should be carried out by a physician and consideration given to preventative antituberculous therapy.

TETANUS

All travelers should be immunized against tetanus, because the risks are widespread and correct treatment following injury may be difficult to obtain overseas.

Dr. David Haddock *was a Senior Lecturer in Tropical Medicine at the Liverpool School of Tropical Medicine. He also worked for long periods in Tanzania, Ghana, Nigeria, and Saudi Arabia, and was a WHO consultant in Ghana and the Sudan.*

Dr. George Wyatt is a Senior Lecturer in Tropical Medicine at the Liverpool School of Tropical Medicine.

Tetanus is a leading cause of death in many developing countries, particularly in hot, moist tropical areas. Probably 500,000 people die each year from tetanus, though 90 percent of these are newborn infants—who are at special risk owing to unhygienic methods of cutting and dressing the umbilical cord after birth, with contamination and infection.

Sixty years ago, tetanus used to be common in the USA and Europe, but immunization and good medical care have greatly reduced its incidence. Globally, it is an important disease because it is common, often fatal, and although difficult to treat, is easily prevented.

HOW INFECTION OCCURS AND HOW DISEASE IS SPREAD

Tetanus is caused by infection of wounds with a bacterium called *Clostridium tetani*, which damages the nervous system and muscles with a powerful toxin. The toxin causes forceful, continuous muscle contraction and severe spasm, often leading to death from respiratory problems and exhaustion. As little as 0.1 mg. of toxin may be fatal to an adult and the fatality rate from tetanus is about 40–50 percent in the absence of highly specialized treatment. The first sign of disease is often spasm of the jaw muscles—which is why the disease is often called "lockjaw." The muscle spasm interferes with swallowing.

Clostridium tetani lives in the intestinal tracts of man and animals, where it does not cause disease; but the bacteria produce spores, which are passed in the feces and contaminate the environment. Spores of *Cl. tetani* persist for years in soil and dust, and are resistant to heat, drying, chemicals, and sunlight; steam heat under pressure (autoclaving) at 240°F. (115°C.) for five minutes is necessary to destroy them.

Most outdoor environments are contaminated with tetanus spores, particularly in agricultural areas where animal manure is used.

Tetanus bacilli can develop from the spores and produce toxin in the absence of oxygen, and they multiply in deep, dirty wounds

WOUNDS AND INJURIES ASSOCIATED WITH TETANUS

- Deep, dirty wounds
- Compound fractures (fractures with broken overlying skin)
- Bites from animals and humans
- Nonsterile injections
- Operations
- Tattooing, ear piercing, and traditional circumcision
- Chronic ulcers and ear infections
- The uterus following childbirth, miscarriage, or abortion
- Infected umbilical cords in the newborn
- The symptoms of tetanus usually begin 7–14 days after injury.

containing foreign material and in dead tissue, where surrounding oxygen levels are very low. Many different kinds of injury favor multiplication of tetanus bacilli, and some are listed above, *although in about 30 percent of cases the injury is probably a small puncture wound, too small to attract attention.*

Many wounds causing tetanus occur on the feet or legs. Walking around with bare feet is inadvisable because of the tetanus hazard, and also because of the dangers of skin-penetrating worm larvae (p. 43) and jigger fleas (p. 174).

PREVENTION

The best method of prevention is by immunization with tetanus toxoid in infancy, with booster doses every 10 years (although immunity probably lasts for longer than this). Those who suffer an injury may require a further dose, especially if it has been longer than five years since their last immunization.

Injured persons who have not been immunized previously or are unsure of their immunization status need to be given ready-made tetanus antibodies in the form of human tetanus immune globulin (HTIG) in one arm and tetanus toxoid in the other. If HTIG is not available antitetanus serum (ATS) produced in horses can be used, but there is an increased risk of allergic reactions particularly if the person has been exposed to horse serum before. Another important preventive measure is the proper cleaning of wounds with removal of any dead tissue. Professional treatment of dirty or deep wounds should be obtained if possible. First-aid treatment includes washing the wound with clean water and soap or weak detergents soon after the injury. Strong antiseptics may damage the tissues and should be avoided. Antibiotics cannot be relied upon to prevent tetanus by themselves.

Travelers should make every effort to ensure that they receive protection against tetanus after any serious injury—this protection may not be offered routinely in some areas.

SUMMARY OF ADVICE FOR TRAVELERS

- Tetanus is rare in travelers taking a conventional vacation, but is a greater hazard for those going on safari, trekking, hiking, climbing, or exploring.

- All travelers should check that they have received a primary immunization course against tetanus and that they have had a booster injection within the last 10 years. Many older people may not have received primary immunization.

- Primary immunization against tetanus is obtained by three injections of tetanus toxoid. In children (under seven years old) this is given as part of the DPT series. After this age, it is normally given as Td (tetanus-diphtheria toxoid), with intervals of 4–8 weeks between the first and second doses and 6–12 months between the second and third doses. After this, immunity is maintained by booster doses of toxoid every 10 years, or sooner if there is an injury. Too frequent injections of toxoid should be avoided as allergic reactions may occur. It is safe to have tetanus toxoid injections at the same time as other immunizations.

SCHISTOSOMIASIS (BILHARZIA)

Schistosomiasis is an unpleasant disease spread by contact with fresh water. Travelers are at risk in most tropical areas.

Dr. Clinton Manson-Bahr taught and practiced in Africa and the Western Pacific for 23 years. He is a descendant of Sir Patrick Manson, the founder of modern Tropical Medicine, and is the editor of Manson's Tropical Diseases.

Schistosomiasis, or bilharzia as it is also called, is found throughout the tropics and subtropics. It is a grave problem in countries where it is common, because although not a "killer" disease in the usual sense, it gnaws insidiously at the general health of entire populations. The geographical distribution of the disease is shown in Map 4.1.

At least 200 million people around the world are afflicted, and this figure is rising rapidly; ironically, the dams, irrigation schemes, and agricultural projects so necessary for the fight against world poverty and hunger themselves create conditions in which the disease thrives. Schistosomiasis is a special problem in young children; it hinders development and reduces life expectancy. It remains a problem in China despite an attempt at eradication that involved the entire nation.

HOW INFECTION IS SPREAD

Schistosomiasis is an infection with one of three kinds of worm, called *Schistosoma haematobium* (urinary schistosomiasis), *Schistosoma mansoni* (intestinal schistosomiasis), and *Schistosoma japonicum* (Far Eastern schistosomiasis).

The fully grown worms live in the veins of the urinary bladder (*S. haematobium*), or the wall of the intestine (*S. mansoni* and *S. japonicum*). The worms produce large numbers of eggs, which leave the body through the lining of the bladder or intestines. On contact with fresh water, larvae hatch from the eggs and infect certain varieties of snail in which they develop further, and multiply. More larvae are produced (called *cercariae*), which swim freely in fresh water, and actively seek out and penetrate the skin of a human host.

After burrowing through the skin, the young worms find their way (by an unknown route via the lungs) to veins of the bowel or bladder once again. The adult worms lay eggs for the rest of their lives, which may be as long as 15 years. So many eggs and larvae are produced that a single infected person passing eggs daily can infect a whole river if the appropriate snails abound.

Water is necessary for drinking and washing, and in rural communities around the world, daily exposure to infection is inevitable from an early age. In the Nile valley, East Africa (especially the coastal regions), West Africa (especially the savannah), along the Euphrates and the Tigris rivers in the Middle East, and in parts of Brazil, the majority of the population may be infected from child-

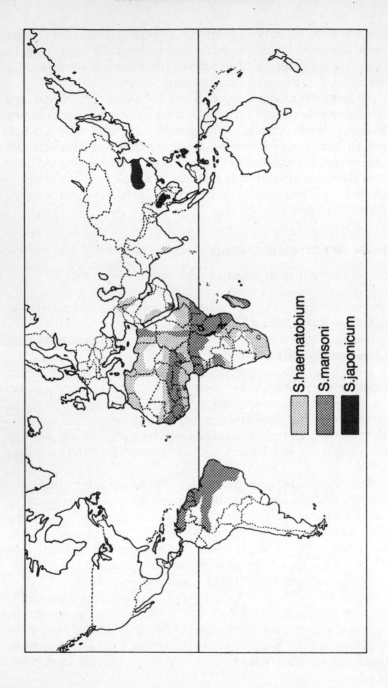

S.haematobium

S.mansoni

S.japonicum

hood. Almost all children of school age pass large numbers of eggs in the urine or stool daily, and children are mainly responsible for the spread of infection. Later in life some immunity builds up so that the worst effects of infection may be avoided.

Most of the harmful effects of the disease are due to the eggs; these cause bleeding, ulceration, and the formation of small tumors as they penetrate the wall of the intestine and bladder. Long-term effects include severe liver damage (the eggs cause liver fibrosis), kidney failure, and cancer of the bladder.

DISEASE IN TRAVELERS

Expatriates and travelers with no previous exposure to schistosomiasis may become seriously ill in the early stages of an infection, though it is unusual for them to suffer in the same way as local people who are exposed to the disease over a long period.

A few hours after contact with infected water, there is tingling of the skin and sometimes a slight rash where the larvae enter the body (cercarial dermatitis).

These symptoms subside, but weeks later, once the worms begin producing eggs, a high fever may develop. This may be severe, and may be confused with typhoid or malaria. An increased number of white blood cells (especially of a type called *eosinophils*) appear in the blood, which may give a clue to the true diagnosis, although not many doctors outside the tropics are aware of this. Travelers should always tell their doctor if they think there is a possibility that they may have been exposed to infection.

This fever, sometimes called "Katayama fever," does not always occur, and symptoms may be no more than a general feeling of lassitude and ill health. Once the infection becomes established, abdominal pain and blood in the urine or feces are common.

TREATMENT

A new drug is now available for treatment of all forms of schistosomiasis, and is very effective. Praziquantel tablets are given, usually as a single dose, and side effects are rare.

Map 4.1 Geographical distribution of schistosomiasis (bilharzia). The disease occurs in 74 countries. Travelers requiring specific, localized information may wish to consult the WHO Atlas listed under "Further Reading."

TRAVELERS AT RISK

Travelers to all countries shown on Map 4.1 (p. 96) may be in danger of infection. Especially at risk are those who swim in streams, rivers, or lakes, or who take part in watersports such as waterskiing and windsurfing in freshwater areas; watersports are particularly dangerous because they may involve exposure to surface water over a large area. Activities such as snipe and duck shooting and cross-country walking safaris where streams have to be crossed are also hazardous.

Some areas are especially risky: the Nile valley, Lake Victoria, Lake Malawi, the Tigris and Euphrates river systems, and artificial lakes such as Lake Kariba in Zimbabwe and Lake Volta in Ghana, which are both notorious. Even small collections of water far from human habitation can give rise to serious infections since baboons can harbor *S. mansoni*, the commonest cause of Katayama fever.

PERSONAL PROTECTION

No vaccine is available and none is foreseen in the near future.

Never assume fresh water to be free from bilharzia in an endemic area. Infection can occur on contact with infected water from streams, rivers, and lakes. Even deep water, far offshore, cannot be regarded as safe, and it is dangerous to swim from boats in infected lakes. Salt water and brackish water are safe from schistosomiasis, however, and so is heavily polluted water.

Since the larvae die quickly on removal from water and cannot survive drying, quick drying of exposed skin and clothing does offer some protection. Rubber boots and wetsuits are protective also, but must be dried quickly in the sun after use. Water that has been chlorinated or stored in a snail-free environment for 48 hours is safe, since any cercariae present will have died off.

Swimming pools that are snail-free are safe, but care must be taken that any water entering the pool has been treated. Neglected swimming pools can rapidly become colonized with snails. Dams are especially dangerous and invariably become infected within 10 years of construction.

CHECKUP ON RETURN HOME (SEE APPENDIX 7)

A checkup should involve examination of the urine and feces for the presence of eggs. Remember that eggs take 30–40 days to be produced following initial infection, so tests made earlier than this

IF CONTACT WITH WATER CANNOT BE AVOIDED, ALWAYS OBSERVE THE FOLLOWING PRECAUTIONS

- Do not cross streams at points where there is much human contact, such as village river crossings; always cross upstream of a village.
- Wear long pants and sleeves and dry out immediately in the sun after contact.
- Wear waterproof footwear when possible.
- The risk is greatest during the hottest, sunniest part of the day, and close to aquatic vegetation.
- Always take particular care to avoid contact with water in the tropics and remember the risks of baboon-contaminated water. Resist the temptation to strip off and swim after a long hot hike.

will be negative. Samples should be taken at least 40 days after the last possible exposure. Modern egg concentration methods should always be asked for specifically.

A white-blood-cell count is advisable for the presence of eosinophilia and there is now also a specific and highly accurate blood test (ELISA) for schistosomiasis.

SWIMMERS' ITCH

Swimmers' itch is an intensified variety of cercarial dermatitis caused by schistosome larvae which die in the skin and do not develop further. This condition can occur in temperate as well as in tropical countries—recent outbreaks have occurred in the USA. There have also been reports of cases occurring in salt water, affecting swimmers in Long Island Sound. Some hours after exposure to the water an itching sensation develops on the exposed skin surfaces, followed by a rash composed of small red intensely irritant papules which fade after 24 hours. No further symptoms occur and no harm results. Antihistamines (pp. 527–28) are all that is necessary for treatment.

DIPHTHERIA

Diphtheria is a potentially serious infection, rarely seen in western countries these days, but still an important hazard to travelers who have not been immunized. All travelers should be protected.

Dr. Clinton Manson-Bahr *taught and practiced in Africa and the Western Pacific for 23 years. He is a descendant of Sir Patrick Manson, the founder of modern Tropical Medicine, and is the editor of Manson's* Tropical Diseases.

Diphtheria is caused by a bacillus which in many people lives quite harmlessly in the throat or on the skin without causing disease. People who harbor the bacillus in this way are known as "carriers"; they are unaffected either because they have been immunized against diphtheria or because they have previously come in contact with the bacillus and have acquired immunity.

Problems arise only when the bacillus spreads from a carrier to a nonimmune or susceptible individual. Throat infection with the bacillus may then result in the formation of a thick white membrane which swells and obstructs breathing, possibly causing suffocation.

On the skin, the bacillus can cause an ulcer known as "Veldt sore." This is seen most commonly in dry, semi-desert regions where washing facilities are scarce. More important, however, the bacillus produces a powerful toxin that may damage the nervous system, causing paralysis of the limbs or swallowing mechanism; the toxin can also affect the heart.

Penicillin is effective against the diphtheria bacillus, and an antitoxin is available to neutralize the toxin.

Infection is spread by direct skin contact with contaminated dust or by inhalation of infective droplets produced when a carrier coughs. Diphtheria of the skin can be prevented by daily washing, and by keeping the skin clean and dry.

PATTERNS OF DISEASE AND IMMUNITY

Over the past decade, the incidence of diphtheria in the USA has been between one and three cases each year. The very low incidence of diphtheria in developed countries is due to the safe and reliable vaccine, which is widely available and offered to all infants routinely.

Doctors working in developing countries have also reported a steady decline in serious disease, but for a different reason: diphtheria infection of the skin is now known to be widespread in hot, humid climates and this effectively immunizes the local population against the more dangerous forms of the disease.

More recently, however, severe disease has reappeared in tropical countries with an improving standard of hygiene—more frequent washing has meant a decline in the number of skin infections and therefore a fall in the number of people acquiring "natural" immunity.

DIPHTHERIA AND THE TRAVELER

There has also been a major resurgence of the disease in the former Soviet Union, with several thousand cases occurring since 1991, largely the result of a collapse in public immunization programs. Tourists have been affected and an elderly Belgian visitor died recently from diphtheria.

Travelers, especially to the tropics, are potentially at risk from all forms of diphtheria unless they have been adequately immunized. There have been at least five recent cases of skin infection with diphtheria in travelers, including a severe case in a nineteen-year-old Australian visitor to Bali. As a result of various vaccine scares, especially during the mid-1970s, many young adults may have no protection.

All travelers who are in doubt about their immune status or who have not been adequately immunized should have the necessary additional doses of vaccine.

Diphtheria is readily treatable if treatment is sought promptly when symptoms appear, but prevention is much easier, and clearly preferable. Most people have been adequately protected, but many travelers are still at risk and should take advantage of the protection that the vaccine offers.

MENINGITIS

Meningitis is of little risk to travelers, even for those traveling through the "meningitis belt" in Africa. Anyone who has had the spleen removed should take particular precautions.

Dr. Christopher Ellis *is a Consultant Physician in the Department of Communicable and Tropical Diseases, East Birmingham Hospital, U.K., and spent part of his career working in Nigeria.*

The term *meningitis* means infection of the membrane lining the brain and spinal cord. Many different types of bacteria and viruses can cause meningitis; in general untreated bacterial infections can rapidly be fatal, whereas if a virus is responsible, the infection always subsides without treatment.

Whatever the cause, the patient suffers severe headache and neck stiffness which prevents bending the head forward, and usually prefers to remain in darkness because light is painful to the eyes.

VIRAL MENINGITIS

All travelers should ensure that they are immune to one particular form of meningitis: that caused by the polio virus (see pp. 47–49). In polio, a form of meningitis usually precedes the paralysis. However, provided the traveler has been immunized as a child, with a booster when necessary before traveling to areas where the disease is still rife, there is no risk whatsoever from this infection.

Other forms of viral meningitis are also more common in areas with inadequate sanitation, since most of the causative viruses are carried from person to person by contaminated food and water. In practice, however, infections are usually not serious, and travelers are seldom affected by anything more than a severe headache in conjunction with a bout of stomach trouble.

MENINGOCOCCAL MENINGITIS

Meningitis caused by one species of bacterium, the meningococcus, is a particular hazard to travelers because it may occur in epidemics arising apparently out of the blue. Epidemics are especially likely to occur where people are crowded together, and infection is acquired by inhaling bacteria in tiny droplets of mucus coughed or sneezed into the air—either by someone suffering from the disease, or more often by a healthy "carrier." Exposure to cigarette smoke is said to increase the risk. Between epidemics the bacterium survives in the throats of a tiny proportion of the population and only occasionally produces an isolated case of meningitis.

Even in hot countries the onset of cooler weather leads to people crowding together more than usual, so that "winter" in such countries is often associated with a sharp increase in the number of (healthy) carriers, and sometimes with an outbreak of disease.

SYMPTOMS AND TREATMENT

Meningococcal infection often causes a scattered blotchy rash which may precede the usual features of meningitis by a few hours. The disease may be rapidly fatal, death occurring within a few hours of the patient's first feeling unwell, so treatment should be started immediately the diagnosis is made or strongly suspected.

Strictly speaking, the diagnosis can be proved only by growing the meningococcus from the fluid that circulates around the brain and spinal cord (the *cerebrospinal* fluid); but in practice, a physician should be able to make the diagnosis with a fair degree of certainty when faced with a patient who has a fever and the characteristic rash, and with even more certainty if the features of meningitis are present. Naturally, if an epidemic was in progress a physician would be particularly inclined to treat a patient, even if no means of proving the diagnosis was available.

Ideally, treatment consists of large doses of penicillin injected intravenously, but where this is impossible, Penicillin G should be given intramuscularly in a dose of 2 mega units, 1 mega unit into each buttock. One mega unit should be repeated every eight hours till the temperature is normal. In people allergic to penicillin, chloramphenicol is an alternative and a single intramuscular dose of this antibiotic has produced complete cures. The same may well be true of a single dose of penicillin given intramuscularly, but if more is available, then it should be given as described.

THE MENINGITIS BELT

The meningitis belt is a semidesert region known as the Sahel which extends across Africa just to the south of the Sahara desert (between latitudes 10° and 15° north).

Outbreaks of meningococcal meningitis occur regularly in this region with the onset of cooler weather. Every 15 years or so epidemics occur on a large scale with great loss of life. Sudan, Ethiopia, and Chad have had recent outbreaks. The meningitis season coincides with winter in the USA and Europe, and ends with the start of the rains. It therefore coincides with the best time for overland crossing of the Sahara.

PREVENTION

A vaccine is now available that protects against the epidemic strains of meningococcal meningitis most likely to infect travelers. A single dose protects for about three years. Trekkers and overlanders visiting the African meningitis belt in the dry season, or spending several weeks in Nepal, should be protected. Pilgrims to the Holy Places in Saudi Arabia must be vaccinated.

SUMMARY OF ADVICE FOR TRAVELERS

- The risk to visitors to any area where an epidemic of meningococcal meningitis is in progress is small, but someone intending to live in close contact with the local population during an epidemic should be immunized beforehand with meningococcal vaccine—see p. 510.

- Travelers who have had the spleen surgically removed (e.g., after trauma to the abdomen) *should be immunized even if only passing through* the meningitis belt, as their chances of developing meningitis are much increased. They are also at increased risk of malaria, a fact that is not widely realized.

- People who have been in close contact with sufferers from meningococcal infection may be protected from infection by taking antibiotics by mouth for four days after contact, but I would emphasize that the vast majority of people in close contact with sufferers do not come down with meningitis even if they take no precautions of any kind.

LEGIONNAIRES' DISEASE

Although reports of outbreaks of legionnaires' disease occasionally receive publicity, the risks to travelers are in fact very small.

Dr. Christopher Bartlett *has been involved in research on legionnaires' disease and related infections since 1977, and has investigated many outbreaks. He is a member of the WHO Working Group on Legionnaires' Disease.*

Legionnaires' disease is a newly recognized disease, so named after a dramatic outbreak of respiratory illness among delegates attending an American Legion convention in Philadelphia in 1976. Despite exhaustive investigation the cause remained a mystery for nearly six months, until eventually a small bacterium now called *Legionella pneumophila* was shown to be responsible. Subsequent studies showed that the disease was not in fact new, and cases dating back to 1947 have now been identified in retrospect.

The bacterium had escaped recognition because it did not grow on the conventional nutrients used to culture microorganisms in diagnostic laboratories. *Legionella pneumophila* is found naturally in mud, lakes, rivers, and streams. Surveys have shown that it commonly colonizes domestic hot- and cold-water systems and cooling towers used for air-conditioning and industrial purposes.

WHAT IS LEGIONNAIRES' DISEASE?

The principal feature of legionnaires' disease is pneumonia, with fever and cough and often shortness of breath and chest pain as the main symptoms. Diarrhea or vomiting may also occur in the first few days, and confusion often develops at this stage; a small proportion of victims also develop difficulties with speech and balance.

Legionnaires' disease occurs both sporadically and in outbreaks, and it is the latter that have received the most attention in the media. Although legionnaires' disease is often described as a "killer" disease, in reality the proportion of fatalities is similar to that seen in many other types of pneumonia.

The infection does not appear to be spread from person to person but is acquired from environmental sources. The investigation of outbreaks has shown that hot-water systems in public buildings are an important source of infection and, less commonly, the fine water mist generated by cooling towers has also been implicated. Inadequately treated whirlpools, hot tubs, and spas have also been shown to serve as occasional sources of legionella infections. There has been one outbreak from a misting device in a store. The infection is acquired by the inhalation of fine water droplets carrying *Legionella pneumophila*. Drinking water containing bacteria is unlikely to cause the infection. Most people are probably in contact with low concentrations of the bacterium quite frequently at home, at work, and elsewhere, but only rarely does this exposure lead to infection.

The diagnosis of legionnaires' disease is not straightforward, because although it is not too difficult to establish that an individual has pneumonia, identification of *Legionella pneumophila* as the cause (rather than any of the other organisms which might be responsible) presents technical problems. Special nutrient media for

SUMMARY OF ADVICE FOR TRAVELERS

- Immunization is not available, but most people are probably not susceptible to *Legionella pneumophila*. The infection is readily treatable if the diagnosis is considered by the attending doctor, so if you should develop a chest infection it would be worth mentioning any recent travel to your physician.

growing *Legionella pneumophila* from clinical specimens have been developed only recently and are not yet widely in use in diagnostic laboratories. Furthermore, the organism may be present only in very low concentrations in the patient's sputum, and consequently may be difficult to detect.

The diagnosis can be confirmed by a blood test to detect the specific antibody produced by the patient to combat the infection. With this method, however, it is not possible to make the diagnosis at an early stage of the illness, because at least a week may elapse before measurable levels of antibody appear in the bloodstream.

Several antibiotics, principally erythromycin and rifampicin, have been shown to be effective in treating the infection. Many doctors now include one such antibiotic in the early treatment of any undiagnosed primary pneumonia to take account of the possibility of legionnaires' disease.

LEGIONNAIRES' DISEASE AND THE TRAVELER

Only about 3 percent of all primary pneumonias are due to *Legionella pneumophila* and the majority of these are *not* associated with travel overseas.

During the 10-year period 1981 to 1990, 742 cases of legionnaires' disease were identified among British travelers overseas—a very low frequency considering the many millions who went abroad during that period. Outbreaks have occurred among guests staying at several hotels in the UK and abroad.

There have certainly been cases at many popular European resorts. Investigations into outbreaks related to travel have revealed that hotels' water systems have been the source of infection in most cases, and have shown that, fortunately, growth of *Legionella pneumophila* can be controlled by continuous chlorination of the water or by raising the circulating hot water temperatures to above 122°F. (50°C.).

Many cases among British travelers have been associated with visits to the Mediterranean region, but this, to a large extent, reflects the popularity of the region as a vacation destination.

CREEPING ERUPTION (LARVA MIGRANS AND LARVA CURRENS)

These rather alarming skin problems are caused by skin contact with soil or beaches contaminated with feces. Treatment is easy and effective.

Dr. Clinton Manson-Bahr taught and practiced in Africa and the Western Pacific for 23 years. He is a descendant of Sir Patrick Manson, the founder of modern Tropical Medicine, and is the editor of Manson's Tropical Diseases.

LARVA MIGRANS

Hookworm larvae from dogs, cats, and various other animals occasionally burrow into human skin. Although they are unable to develop further in humans, they are still a nuisance because they migrate aimlessly under the skin, exciting an unpleasant skin reaction and causing slowly moving, itchy red lines. The red lines may sometimes be accompanied by considerable blistering, but any intensely irritant area—especially on the feet—should be suspected.

Larva migrans is contracted by walking in bare feet on sand or soil contaminated by dog or cat feces. Sandy beaches, *above* the high-water mark, are often contaminated: the beaches of West, East, and South Africa as well as Malaysia, Sri Lanka, and Thailand are all areas where this infection is common. It also occurs in the USA (especially the Atlantic and Gulf coasts), South America, and the Caribbean. *Sand below the high-water line is safe*; take great care on beaches obviously fouled by dogs.

Areas underneath houses raised on stilts are also dangerous. Treatment is easy and very satisfactory. The drug used is thiabendazole (Mintezol), which can be taken by mouth or applied to the skin as an ointment (the ointment has to be prepared specially by a pharmacist from thiabendazole tablets: 0.5g. thiabendazole crushed and mixed with 10 g. petroleum jelly—this has fewer side effects than oral treatment). Cooling the skin with ethyl chloride also kills the larvae.

PREVENTION

Larva migrans can be prevented by wearing shoes or sandals at all times and by preventing children (who are most often affected) from running around barefoot on the beach. Use a beach mat or beach towel when sunbathing, and choose your beach carefully.

LARVA CURRENS

Larva currens is a similar condition to larva migrans, but is caused by the human worm *Strongyloides*. The eggs of this worm hatch in the bowel, and larvae are passed out of the feces. However, the larvae sometimes penetrate the skin of the anus, causing a reinfection. This results in an irritating rash round the buttocks, extending up the back. The rash is composed of irritant red lines and weals which move quite quickly and may vanish within a few hours, appearing and disappearing repeatedly over a period of many years. (Many ex-prisoners from World War II who were held in the Far East still suffer more than 40 years after infection.)

The infection is picked up from moist soil in villages and rural areas in Thailand, Malaysia, and Vietnam. Treatment with thiabendazole (Mintezol) is effective even after more than 40 years.

There are also animal forms of *Strongyloides* which are especially common on mounds in tropical swamps. The worms move around under the skin, causing lesions similar to those of larva migrans.

PREVENTION

Avoid contact with moist soil under houses and wear shoes at all times. Do not sit on the ground with wet bathing suits or clothes since this will attract infective larvae. Avoid mounds in swamps, especially those fouled with feces.

SUMMARY OF ADVICE FOR TRAVELERS

• Walking around barefoot on soil or sandy beaches above the high-water line is risky in many parts of the world—as the editor of this book has now discovered twice to his own cost, in Florida and in the Caribbean!

HANSEN'S DISEASE (LEPROSY)

This disease poses a negligible hazard to travelers, though in some situations people may worry unduly about the risks.

Dr. Stanley Browne was a leprologist of international reputation. Past President of the Royal Society of Tropical Medicine, he advised on Hansen's disease in 68 countries.

Vacationers and business travelers alike may well harbor important misconceptions about Hansen's disease (formerly known as leprosy, and now often simply abbreviated to HD). Half-remembered stories from the Bible and from films like *Ben-Hur*, pictures of horrible deformities and the specter of frightful contagion—these are the sum total of most people's "knowledge."

How then do you react to rumors: HD in Spain, in Malta, in Italy? It can't be true . . . but it is. On visiting these countries, you will most probably never see a case; and even if you do, you probably won't recognize it.

If your travels take your farther afield, say to Lagos or Madras, you may be accosted by beggars holding out their deformed and ulcerating hands. So this is HD. You shudder and turn away quickly, embarrassed and perhaps a little frightened. Will you catch HD? You are half-reassured by a dimly remembered phrase about "prolonged and close contact" being necessary for infection to occur.

But what is HD? How much HD is there in countries advertised in glossy, inviting travel brochures? What risk is there to the traveler, and are there any special precautions you should take?

WHAT IS HD?

HANSEN'S BACILLUS AND ITS EFFECTS

HD is caused by a tiny bacillus that can survive only in human tissues. It prefers to live in the skin and lining of the nose. It multiplies very slowly. The only symptoms of an early infection may be a nonitching rash and perhaps an occasional bloodstained discharge from the nose.

The potential seriousness of the disease derives not from the rash (which may disappear spontaneously), but from Hansen's bacilli accumulating in the main nerves of the limbs and face. Dead bacilli inside nerves provoke inflammation which eventually destroys the nerve fibers, resulting in muscle paralysis and loss of feeling in hands and feet. This can lead to repeated injury—from handling objects that most people would find too hot to touch, or from walking carelessly over rough ground—resulting ultimately in scarring, ulceration, and deformity. The disease does *not* cause fingers and toes to drop off.

HOW INFECTION IS SPREAD

Hansen's bacilli are spread in small droplets of nasal discharge from some patients with early, untreated HD—who may look and feel healthy, with only slight signs in the skin and nose.

The disease is *not* particularly contagious or infectious, and chance contact is unlikely to lead to infection: most people exposed to living Hansen's bacilli have some degree of built-in resistance to the disease, and will never develop signs of infection. Very few medical workers in daily contact with HD patients ever catch HD; they take no precautions beyond washing their hands, and perhaps wearing a face mask when examining patients' noses.

Ulceration of the hands and feet is *not* a sign of infectivity. Most beggars with overt signs of HD are *not* contagious.

GEOGRAPHICAL OCCURRENCE

HD is present in most countries, although the proportion of the population affected varies widely. As many as 15 million people were previously thought to be affected worldwide, though 5.5 million is now thought to be a more accurate estimate: most of them live within the medico-geographical tropics. In Europe, most HD sufferers live in southern countries—Portugal, Spain, Italy, Greece, Turkey, the southern Commonwealth of Independent States (formerly the USSR), and the Mediterranean islands. There is a small number of cases—around 140—each year in the USA, mostly in the South and in Hawaii.

The HD problem worldwide is now improving. Modern drugs kill 99.8 percent of HD bacteria within a few days of the first dose, and there has been much recent progress in developing more effective treatment regimens.

SUMMARY OF ADVICE FOR TRAVELERS

- At present no vaccine is available to protect travelers from HD, and no preventive medicine is necessary.

- Due to the low infectivity of the disease, and most people's inbuilt resistance, the chances of a traveler's catching HD *are virtually nil*—the only precaution necessary might be to avoid being sneezed at. HD is a much less frightening disease than you may have imagined.

ANTHRAX

Although anthrax is most uncommon in travelers, certain handicrafts may be contaminated and should be avoided.

Dr. Arnold F. Kaufmann *is Chief of Bacterial Zoonoses Activity, Centers for Disease Control and Prevention, Atlanta, Georgia, USA, and specializes in public health control of anthrax and other infections acquired from animals.*

Anthrax is a lethal bacterial disease of livestock that is occasionally transmitted to humans. A disease of considerable historic significance, anthrax occurs or has occurred in virtually every country of the world. It is currently only a minor public health problem, even in developing countries, due to the wide use of animal anthrax vaccines. Lapses in local control programs, however, can have serious consequences such as the recent epidemic of almost 10,000 human cases in Zimbabwe. The most frequent victims of this disease are persons closely associated with raising livestock or working in industries processing animal bones, hair, and hides.

HOW IT IS SPREAD

Anthrax is caused by *Bacillus anthracis*, a bacterium normally present in various types of soil. The anthrax bacillus has a cyclic pattern of replication, growing rapidly when environmental conditions are optimal and then forming spores to survive adverse periods. These spores are resistant to disinfectants and can remain viable for many

SUMMARY OF ADVICE FOR TRAVELERS

* Although cutaneous anthrax may cause severe illness, the disease is only weakly contagious and presents little risk to the average traveler. Only one travel-associated case has occurred in a U.S. citizen in the past 40 years. This patient acquired her infection from a goatskin handicraft purchased in Haiti.

* Subsequent studies revealed that Haitian handicrafts incorporating dried or poorly tanned goatskins were commonly contaminated with anthrax spores. As a result, rugs, drums, and other handicrafts containing goatskin with attached hair (the spores are found in the hair) are not permitted to be brought into the USA. Another case, not in a traveler, was traced to a coarse goat-hair yarn produced in Pakistan.

* Travelers should not buy any item made of coarse goat hair or goatskin with attached hair in any poor country.

* General commonsense precautions of eating only well-cooked meat and avoiding unnecessary handling of dead animals also apply. Otherwise, no special precautions or immunizations are necessary.

years. Animals become infected by grazing on soils where the anthrax bacillus is in its active growth phase.

Human anthrax results not from contact with the soil but from handling the tissues of infected animals.

When an animal dies of anthrax, the important control measure is either to bury or to burn the carcass. Poverty or failure to recognize the cause of death, however, frequently leads animal owners in developing countries to salvage anything of value. The meat may be eaten, and by-products such as bones, skin, and hair sold or used. Anthrax spore contamination of these by-products, which may be made into handicrafts or exported for industrial processing, can become a hazard to people far away.

FORMS OF ANTHRAX

Human anthrax has three forms, namely cutaneous (skin), gastrointestinal, and inhalation forms, and these directly reflect the route of the infection.

Cutaneous anthrax, the most common, results when the anthrax bacillus is introduced beneath the skin, e.g., by a puncture, abrasion, or through a preexisting break in the skin while handling contaminated materials. A red, raised area develops at the site of the infection—rather like an insect bite—and characteristically progresses to a large blister, finally becoming an ulcer covered with a dark scab. This form of the disease is diagnosed easily and can be treated effectively with common antibiotics such as penicillin and tetracycline.

Gastrointestinal anthrax results from eating raw or undercooked meat from infected animals, and causes severe abdominal symptoms.

Inhalation anthrax is almost exclusively an occupational respiratory disease, associated with industrial processing of goat hair from western Asia. These two forms of the disease are difficult to diagnose and are often fatal; however, both are so rare as to be a negligible risk.

VIRAL HEMORRHAGIC FEVERS

Lassa fever and other viral hemorrhagic fevers periodically hit the headlines, but in fact the risk to travelers is extremely small.

Dr. Susan Fisher-Hoch is a medical epidemiologist in the National Center for Infectious Diseases, Centers for Disease Control and Prevention, Atlanta.

Viral hemorrhagic fevers (VHFs) are found on every continent except Australia and North America, and are caused by viruses of rodents, ticks, or mosquitoes; details of some of them are summarized in Table 4.1. They occur mostly in rural areas, so that infection is usually confined to the more adventurous travelers, or those involved in medical care, agricultural, mining, or other projects. It is important to remember that infections in nonresidents of endemic areas are very rare: most fevers in short-term visitors are due to common diseases, and most of these, like typhoid or malaria, are eminently treatable.

Hemorrhagic fevers are diseases of poverty, and most sufferers are local people who have poor housing conditions and little or no access to medical care. Four VHFs, Lassa fever, Marburg and Ebola viruses, and Congo-Crimean Hemorrhagic Fever (CCHF), have been shown to spread from person to person, especially in hospitals with poor hygiene conditions or where needles or other equipment

are reused. Indeed it was the high mortality in early hospital outbreaks that led to their fearsome reputation as "killer" diseases.

However, we now know that there are many mild or asymptomatic cases of these fevers, and that infection can be avoided by
simple, basic hygiene precautions. Effective treatment is now available for some VHFs.

LASSA FEVER

GEOGRAPHICAL OCCURRENCE
Lassa fever is found in West Africa, from southern Senegal to
the Cameroon, principally in Guinea, Sierra Leone, Liberia, and
Nigeria, but presumably also in other West African countries where
data have not yet been collected. It is by far the most important
VHF transmissible from human to human because of the very large
numbers of cases that occur each year in West Africa.

HOW INFECTION IS SPREAD
Humans are infected from the urine of a local rodent, *Mastomys
natalensis*—the multimammate rat—which is larger than a mouse
but smaller than the common rat. It infests village homes throughout Africa, though only in West Africa does it appear to carry Lassa
virus. The disease is most common in secondary bush, though it is
also found in savannah areas. Along the coast and in the dry hin-
terland Lassa fever is uncommon. The rat is nocturnal, and feeds
on unprotected food and refuse in the house, on which it may
deposit the virus. Infection can be prevented, therefore, by enclosing
all food in rat-proof containers, and ridding the house of rats.

THE ILLNESS
The disease has an incubation period of one to two weeks, and
the illness lasts about two weeks. During the first week, fever,
headache, and other general symptoms develop slowly, and make
the illness very difficult to diagnose. Many people then recover, and
may not know they have been infected; others develop further symptoms, such as vomiting, diarrhea, and in severe cases, bleeding and
collapse.

The disease can be treated successfully with intravenous ribavirin, if it is started as soon as possible after onset of symptoms. Any

persons who know that they may have been exposed to Lassa fever either from contact with rodents or patients, and who then develop a fever, should therefore make sure they receive expert medical treatment as quickly as possible.

The risk to women during the last three months of pregnancy is very high. The baby is usually lost, and the mother may also die, especially if she is being looked after in a hospital where standards of supportive care are poor. Children, on the other hand, appear to have milder infections. Recovery in survivors is usually complete except for the risk of deafness, which is quite common following Lassa fever.

Person-to-person spread is from contact with blood and body fluids. Lassa fever is not spread by the respiratory route, so entering a patient's room carries no risk. It can be spread, however, by sexual contact while the patient is sick or just recovering. Avoiding intimate contact with blood or other fluids from people with fevers is

TABLE 4.1. VIRAL HEMORRHAGIC FEVERS

	Virus	Geo-graphic distribution	Host /Vector	Estimated incubation period (days)	Estimated untreated mortality (percent)
Lassa fever	Arenavirus	West Africa	rodent	7–22	17
Junín	Arenavirus	Argentina	rodent	7–14	17
Machupo	Arenavirus	Bolivia	rodent	7–14	15
Guanarito etc.	Arenavirus	Venezuela /Brazil	rodent*	?	60
CCHF	Bunyavirus	Africa/Asia	tick /small mammal	2–9	15–30
Ebola	Filovirus	Africa (?Asia)	? monkey	3–10	?0–90
Marburg	Filovirus	Africa?	monkey	2–21	20–30
Rift Valley Fever	Bunyavirus	Africa	mosquito /mammals	3–6	?0-50
Dengue fever	Flavivirus	Africa/Asia	mosquito /human	5–8	0
Yellow Fever	Flavivirus	Africa /S.America	mosquito /primates	3–7	10–50
HFRS	Hantavirus	Northern Hemisphere	rodent	10–35	2–10

*Probably similar to Junín and Lassa, but insufficient data currently available.

therefore the most important method of avoiding infection in hospitals and clinics.

Despite this knowledge, there continue to be devastating outbreaks and deaths in hospitals in endemic areas, as the result of failure to employ careful disinfection techniques and measures to prevent blood-to-blood contact, or where surgical facilities are very primitive. In contrast, more than 1,500 Lassa fever patients have been cared for in one rural hospital in Sierra Leone without any cross-infection, simply on the basis of disinfection measures using chlorine solutions, and gloves that are disinfected, washed, and reused. There is no risk of infection from recovered persons.

INTERNATIONAL SPREAD

The rural areas where the disease is endemic are within reach of international airports, and the incubation period is long enough to allow ample time for displacement of infected persons by modern transportation before illness appears; cases have been imported into Europe and North America.

Since 1970 there have been two documented importations of Lassa fever to the United States, one of whom died. There have been about ten cases imported to the United Kingdom, and one each to Canada, Australia, the Netherlands, Israel, and Japan, none of whom died. Unfortunately, the patient who died in the United States in 1989 visited four emergency rooms before he saw anyone who was aware that he had recently returned from Nigeria, or who knew anything about Lassa fever.

It is therefore essential for travelers to make sure their physicians have all details of travel and possible exposure to viruses, and that Lassa fever should be considered as a possible diagnosis. Simple infectious-disease precautions for the care of patients in regular isolation rooms are recommended, using gloves, gowns and masks and strict disinfection.* Patient isolators (bubbles) are no longer considered necessary or desirable.

PROSPECTS FOR A VACCINE

Though an experimental vaccine has been developed and successfully tested in animals, there are currently no plans for devel-

---

*Further details of procedures and advice on care and treatment can be found in the CDC publication: *Morbidity and Mortality Weekly Report,* 1988, Volume 37, Supplement 3.

opment of human vaccines, mainly because of the high cost involved.

SOUTH AMERICAN HEMORRHAGIC FEVERS

At least three, possibly four, hemorrhagic fevers are recognized in South America: Junín in Argentina, Machupo in Bolivia, and Guanarito in Venezuela. These are caused by rodent viruses related to Lassa virus, which they resemble closely. Outbreaks are very focal, and have only ever involved farmers and local people in clearly defined areas. There is no person-to-person spread, and no cases have ever been recorded in travelers.

Treatment with immune plasma and possibly ribavirin is recommended for Junín virus infection. A vaccine for human use is currently undergoing evaluation in Argentina.

MARBURG AND EBOLA VIRUSES

Marburg and Ebola viruses are related to each other. They are extremely rare, and their reservoir in nature is not known, though in some instances monkeys may be involved.

Marburg disease was first recognized in 1967, when there were 32 cases and 7 deaths in laboratory personnel working with African green monkeys recently imported to Germany from Uganda—hence the popular name "Green Monkey Disease."

In 1976 simultaneous outbreaks of a lethal hemorrhagic fever, Ebola, occurred among humans in Zaire and Sudan, and another in 1979 in Sudan. These outbreaks were again associated with needle sharing in remote clinics and hospitals. There have been no more cases or outbreaks since 1979, and Ebola virus seems to have disappeared for the present.

Small outbreaks and single cases of Marburg disease continue to occur in East, Central, and southern Africa. Two were in visitors to a single cave in Kenya, and one was a hitchhiker in Zimbabwe. Cases are extremely rare, however, and the source has never been found. In 1989 monkeys infected with a virus related to Ebola were imported into the United States, and many of them became sick and died. The source of this virus has also not been found, but it has become clear that this Asian strain is not able to cause severe disease in humans.

THE ILLNESS

Both Ebola and Marburg disease have an incubation period of less than one week, and have a very sudden, violent onset with rapid deterioration, bleeding, and shock. No imported cases have ever been seen outside Africa. Unfortunately, there is currently no specific treatment. Recovery, in survivors, is complete.

CONGO-CRIMEAN HEMORRHAGIC FEVER (CCHF)

CCHF is widely distributed throughout Africa, parts of southern and eastern Europe, and the Middle East and Asia. Human cases are rare, but are associated with close contact with animal blood or infected humans, or with tick bites. Thus animal herders in dry areas, farmers, slaughterhouse workers, butchers, and people sleeping or working on tick-infested ground may be infected. Hospital outbreaks have been associated with high mortality, but were again associated with unhygienic practices, including mouth-to-mouth resuscitation. Good nursing techniques and care with blood and needles is sufficient to prevent transmission.

THE ILLNESS

CCHF has a very short incubation period, as little as three days, and a very sudden onset with violent headaches, fevers, and body pains. Patients may then bleed, and a small number may die. With good hospital care and with ribavirin, however, most will survive, and recover rapidly and completely.

Prevention is best assured by avoiding ticks and intimate contact with blood from animals or infected people.

HEMORRHAGIC FEVER WITH RENAL SYNDROME

This infection is very common in parts of Asia, particularly China, where it results in thousands of infections each year, with major economic impact. It is seasonal, mostly in the early summer and fall. It is caused by a family of viruses of small field rodents, voles and rats, which excrete it in the urine. There are rural and urban forms, depending on the host rodent. It is present, however, throughout the former Soviet Union and most of Europe, so it is not strictly a disease of exotic places. This is the same disease as Korean Hemorrhagic Fever, which affected 3,000 United Nations

Troops during the war there in the 1950s, and is closely related to an old disease in Scandinavia, called nephropathia epidemica. Recently a new virus causing severe disease has been described in rural parts of the former Yugoslavia.

THE ILLNESS

The clinical picture is slightly different from the other VHFs, in that the incubation period may be two or three weeks and the onset is slow. Some patients may experience brief kidney failure and a very few bleed and may die, but most make a complete recovery. Treatment with ribavirin may be effective, but must be started early in disease.

PREVENTION

Avoidance of contact with rodent urine is the most important preventive measure. HFRS is a disease of poverty, though paradoxically, the recently increased rural prosperity in China has allowed expansion of rodent populations, and big epidemics of HFRS disease are being seen. Person-to-person spread has not been reported. Vaccines are currently under development in China and in the United States.

YELLOW FEVER, DENGUE, AND RIFT VALLEY FEVER

The viruses that cause these hemorrhagic fevers are spread by mosquitoes. Yellow fever and dengue are discussed in greater detail on pp. 132–39. Yellow fever is the oldest and one of the most severe of the hemorrhagic fevers, but there is a safe and effective vaccine; there is no vaccine for dengue, but in most adults the disease is self-limiting and seldom serious.

Rift Valley Fever is mainly a veterinarian problem, though there have been two large human outbreaks in Egypt and in Mauritania. The disease is usually mild, but occasional severe cases do occur. There is an animal vaccine, but no special recommendations for protection of humans, beyond protection from mosquito bites.

CONCLUSION

Viral hemorrhagic fevers are not viruses of humans. Though the illnesses may be dramatic, there is an excellent chance of survival with good medical care. In fact they are far less insidious and less lethal than HIV infection, which they resemble in their capacity for blood transmission, especially within hospitals. As with HIV, with some basic knowledge it is normally possible to avoid infection. As is not the case with HIV, recovery is complete within a month or two of infection, and fully effective treatment may be available.

Human infection is an accident for the virus as well as the individual, and with care, can be avoided.

Medical staff who are planning to care for or be in contact with patients in areas endemic for VHFs may be at special risk. They should seek additional, thorough briefing about the fevers they may encounter in the areas they are planning to visit, and ensure they understand the symptoms of the diseases and appropriate protective measures and therapy. Veterinary personnel should also obtain relevant detailed information on areas they may visit.

5

DISEASES SPREAD BY INSECTS

MALARIA

Malaria is one of the most important disease hazards facing travelers to tropical countries. Drug-resistant malaria continues to spread at an alarming rate, complicating the identification of effective drug regimens. Travelers can protect themselves by taking antimalarial

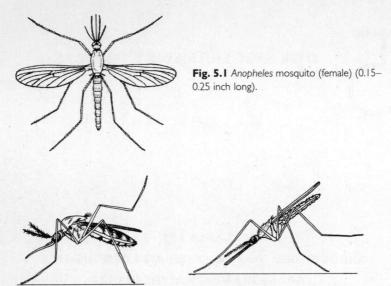

Fig. 5.1 *Anopheles* mosquito (female) (0.15–0.25 inch long).

Fig. 5.2 Resting positions of mosquitos: *Culex* (left); *Anopheles* (right). Anopheles mosquitoes can be recognized by their characteristic posture.

medication as well as by taking careful precautions against mosquito bites.

> **Dr. Hans O. Lobel** *has for many years been in charge of the surveillance of malaria at the Centers for Disease Control and Prevention, Atlanta, and originated the malaria hotline service it offers to travelers; he is the Secretary of the International Society of Travel Medicine.*

Malaria is a parasitic disease spread from person to person by the bite of *Anopheles* mosquitoes (Figs. 5.1 and 5.2). Worldwide, between 300–500 million clinical cases of malaria are estimated to occur each year, and an additional 200 million people carry the parasite; around one million infants and children die annually from malaria in Africa alone.

Travelers may acquire malaria from mosquitoes in the tropics and subtropics (see Map 5.1 and Appendix 2).

Map 5.1 Geographical distribution of malaria and chloroquine-resistant *Plasmodium falciparum* (1993). Note, however, that the exact distribution varies somewhat from time to time. (By courtesy of CDC.)   ▶

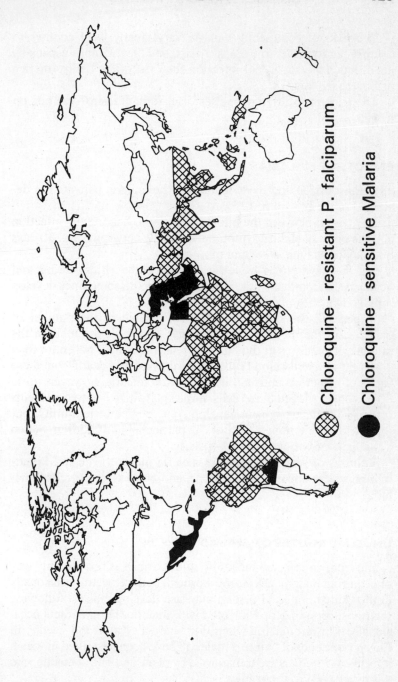

The risks of contracting malaria vary greatly from country to country, and visitors to tropical Africa and New Guinea especially are at much greater risk of infection than visitors to Latin America or Southeast Asia.

There are four different species of malaria parasite—see box on p. 125.

EFFECTS OF MALARIA

The transmission and development of the malaria parasite are described in the box on p. 125.

The period between the bite of a mosquito bearing the infection and the onset of clinical symptoms is usually between 8 and 30 days but may be as long as several months.

The main symptoms are fever, malaise, chills with sweating, and headache; abdominal pains, jaundice, and coma sometimes develop rapidly. Diarrhea may also occur.

In general, the severity of illness is related to the number of parasites in the blood. In *vivax, ovale,* and *malariae* malaria the number of parasites in the blood is relatively small: not more than 1 percent of the red blood cells are parasitized and death from these forms of malaria is unusual. In *falciparum* malaria, however, up to 80 percent of the red blood cells may be parasitized; native residents of malarious areas usually develop some degree of immunity, but those with no immunity—visitors, in particular, and children—often develop severe or even fatal disease.

Features of severe falciparum malaria include liver and kidney failure, severe anemia, convulsions, and coma (from cerebral malaria).

UNUSUAL ROUTES OF SPREAD

A bite from an infected mosquito in the tropics is not the only way of acquiring malaria. Mosquito-borne infections occur occasionally in the United States. A person may also develop malaria following the transfusion of blood infected with malaria. Drug addicts occasionally transmit malaria when they share a syringe and needle. In Europe, episodes of "airport malaria" have been described in which infected mosquitoes are transported by plane and bite someone who has never been to the tropics.

THE MALARIA PARASITE

- Malaria is caused by parasites that consist of single cells (protozoa), called *Plasmodium*. Four different species of *Plasmodium* cause disease in humans: *P. falciparum* (the most serious), *P. vivax*, *P. ovale*, and *P. malariae*. (Other species of *Plasmodium* cause malaria in birds, monkeys, and rodents.)

- When a mosquito carrying malaria bites a person to suck blood, it first injects saliva to prevent the blood from coagulating and blocking its mouth parts. The saliva (which is also responsible for the unpleasant, itchy weal that may develop at the site of the bite) contains infective forms of the parasite (called *sporozoites*).

- After injection, the *sporozoites* pass into the blood, and then into the liver. They infect liver cells, in which they develop further over the next 6–11 days without causing symptoms. (At this stage they are now called liver *schizonts*.)

- When mature the schizonts burst, releasing numerous tiny parasites, called *merozoites*, into the bloodstream. These penetrate red blood cells, and now cause symptoms for the first time. The merozoites develop into ring-shaped *trophozoites*—the form of the parasite that is normally visible under the microscope to doctors trying to detect the disease.

- The trophozoites grow inside the red blood cells, into *schizonts*, which burst and release large numbers of *merozoites*, each able to infect a new red blood cell. Release of each new batch of merozoites coincides with fever; it takes 2–3 days for newly infected blood cells to release further numbers of merozoites, and this explains the intermittent character of the fever which is often seen with malaria.

- Some of the trophozoites also develop into forms called *gametocytes*, which are capable of infecting mosquitoes. The gametocytes are sucked up during a blood meal, and develop in the mosquito's stomach. Between 7 and 20 days later, infective *sporozoites* appear in the mosquito salivary glands, and the mosquito is capable of infecting a person.

DIAGNOSIS

The early symptoms of malaria, of which fever is the most common, are nonspecific. This is why—especially when symptoms do not appear until after the traveler has returned home—the possibility of malaria is not always considered and the diagnosis may be missed.

If malaria is suspected, a blood sample should be taken immediately and examined under the microscope. Detection of parasites under the microscope confirms the diagnosis but it requires experience and skill. Treatment is a matter of urgency, and should not be delayed if such skills are not available. A negative blood sample does not exclude the possibility of malaria.

DRUG RESISTANCE

Chloroquine used to be a very effective drug for treatment and prevention of malaria. However, resistance of falciparum malaria parasites to chloroquine is now common wherever malaria occurs, except in Central America west of the Panama Canal, Haiti, the Dominican Republic, Egypt, and most countries in the Middle East (see Appendix 2). Resistance of vivax malaria to chloroquine has been reported from the island of New Guinea and Indonesia. Resistance of falciparum malaria to pyrimethamine/sulfadoxine (Fansidar) is widespread in Southeast Asia and the Amazon basin of South America, and resistance has also been reported in sub-Saharan Africa. Resistance to mefloquine has been confirmed in Thailand along the borders with Cambodia and Burma (Myanmar); there have been reports from Africa, and it seems likely that resistance will spread further.

TREATMENT

Current U.S. recommendations for the drug treatment of malaria are summarized in Table 5.1.

In the treatment of drug-resistant falciparum malaria, quinine is given for three days, together with tetracycline for seven days. (For infections acquired in Thailand, quinine should be given for seven days and tetracycline for seven days.) Ringing in the ears, nausea, and dizziness may occur from the quinine.

Falciparum malaria can cause severe illness, and special treatment measures are often necessary. An exchange blood transfusion may be life-saving in severely ill patients with levels of parasitemia of more than 10 percent. In severe falciparum infection, intravenous treatment with quinidine gluconate may be necessary.

Treatment with a new drug, halofantrine, is reported to be effective and well tolerated. Halofantrine has recently received FDA approval, but it is not yet available in the United States; it is, however, available abroad. Studies on its safety and effectiveness are still continuing, but it is likely that it will prove to be a suitable drug for travelers to use for emergency self-treatment if symptoms develop. There have been reports of toxic side effects that need further evaluation before the drug can be more widely recommended.

Treatment of infections with falciparum malaria acquired in Cen-

tral America, Haiti, North Africa, and the Near East, and infections
with vivax, ovale, and malariae malaria are treated with three days
of chloroquine. The only exceptions are some vivax infections acquired in New Guinea that may not totally respond to chloroquine.
Such infections require treatment with quinine and tetracycline.

An additional drug, primaquine, is given for treatment of vivax
and ovale malaria because some of these parasites may persist in
the liver and cause a relapse. This drug may cause hemolysis (damage to red blood cells) in people of Mediterranean, African, or Asian
descent, and a blood test for G6PD deficiency needs to be performed
before taking it.

TABLE 5.1 TREATMENT OF MALARIA[1]

Type of malaria	Treatment
Falciparum malaria: Chloroquine-resistant[2]	Quinine 10-mg. base per kg. body weight (usually 650 mg. quinine sulfate in adults) every 8 hours for 3 days, and tetracycline 250 mg. every 6 hours for 7 days (or a single dose of 3 tablets of Fansidar). or Halofantrine 500 mg. every 8 hours for 1 day (total dose 1,500 mg.). May be repeated after 1 week. or Quinidine gluconate given by intravenous infusion if illness is severe.

Chloroquine-sensitive[2]	Chloroquine 1,500-mg. base[3]
	Usual course in adults:
	  Day 1 600-mg. dose
	         300 mg. six hours later
	  Day 2 300 mg.
	  Day 3 300 mg.

Vivax and ovale malaria	Chloroquine as above, then primaquine 15 mg. daily for 14 days to prevent relapses.
Malariae malaria	Chloroquine as above

1. Treatment should preferably be carried out under medical supervision. Anyone with suspected malaria should seek medical help urgently.
2. For information on areas of chloroquine-resistant malaria, see Appendix 2 and Map 5.1.
3. One chloroquine tablet usually contains 500 mg. chloroquine phosphate, equivalent to 300 mg. chloroquine base. All doses in this chapter are expressed as chloroquine base.
Doses given here are for adults.

PREVENTION

Travelers to malarious areas of the world should use personal protective measures and a drug regimen to prevent malaria. However, malaria may still be contracted and anyone who develops symptoms of malaria should seek prompt medical attention.

PERSONAL PROTECTION

An important way of reducing the number of mosquito bites is to apply insect repellent containing DEET (N,N-diethyl-*m*-toluamide) to your skin and clothing, especially in the evening and, when out of doors, at night. Mosquito nets over the bed are an effective way of avoiding bites at night, and nets impregnated with permethrin should be used. A wire mesh across the windows can also be helpful. Measures to avoid mosquito bites are of the utmost importance, and are discussed in greater detail on pp. 180–92.

ANTIMALARIAL DRUGS FOR PROPHYLAXIS

The drugs at present available for prevention of malaria are not true prophylactics because they do not prevent infection. Drugs such as mefloquine, doxycycline, and chloroquine suppress the development of the red-blood-cell forms of the parasite—which is why prophylaxis has to be continued for four weeks after leaving the malarious area.

In almost all countries, both falciparum malaria and the other species coexist and the choice of prophylactic medication is mandated by the presence or absence of chloroquine-resistant *P. falciparum* (See Map 5.1). The following regimens, which are also summarized in Table 5.2, reflect current U.S. recommendations. The drug should be started 1–2 weeks before entry to a malaria-endemic area (except for doxycycline, which can begin 1–2 days before); use of the drug must be continued for 4 weeks afterward.

For travel to areas with chloroquine-sensitive malaria (Central America, Haiti, Dominican Republic, and the Near East):

• *Chloroquine* (Aralen) 300-mg. base once weekly. In most countries chloroquine is available as a syrup for children, and a prescription is often unnecessary; in the United States this is not available, and children's doses can be prepared in gelatine capsules. The side effects of chloroquine include itching, rashes, blurred vision, and dizziness.

For travel to areas with chloroquine-resistant falciparum malaria:

- *Mefloquine* (Lariam) is the drug of choice. It is effective against both chloroquine- and Fansidar-resistant falciparum malaria, except in parts of Thailand and probably Cambodia.

For prophylaxis, the adult regimen is 250 mg. mefloquine weekly. Mefloquine should not be taken by persons who are hypersensitive to it, and should be used with caution in persons with epilepsy or psychiatric disorders (there have been isolated reports of exacerbation of symptoms). Experience with mefloquine in children who weigh less than 33 pounds (15 kg.) and in pregnant women is limited; it should be discussed with the prescribing physician, who may need to seek expert advice. Side effects of mefloquine include dizziness and gastrointestinal disturbance. Mefloquine is considered safe for long-term use by expatriates.

TABLE 5.2 DRUG PREVENTION OF MALARIA[1]

Adults

Areas where falciparum malaria is sensitive to chloroquine[2]
    Chloroquine 300 mg. weekly[3]

Areas where falciparum malaria is often resistant to chloroquine
1. Mefloquine 250 mg. (1 tablet) weekly
or
2. Doxycycline 100 mg. (1 tablet) daily (not in pregnancy, or in children)
or
3. Chloroquine, preferably with proguanil, and with Fansidar in reserve (see p. 130)

Children

As above with doses calculated as follows:

Age less than 1 year	1/4 adult dosage
Age 1–5 years	1/2 adult dosage
Age 6–12 years	3/4 adult dosage

1. Use of prophylactic antimalarial tablets should continue for at least four weeks after departure from a malarious area.
2. For further information on areas of chloroquine-resistant malaria, see Appendix 2 and Map 5.1.
3. One chloroquine tablet usually contains 500 mg. chloroquine phosphate, equivalent to 300 mg. chloroquine base. All doses in this chapter are expressed as chloroquine base.

- *Doxycycline* alone, 100 mg. daily, is an alternative regimen for travel to drug-resistant areas for persons who cannot use mefloquine. Doxycycline is a tetracycline and may cause photosensitivity (an exaggerated sunburn reaction to strong sunlight) or vaginal candidiasis (yeast infection). Gastrointestinal side effects (nausea or vomiting) may be minimized by taking the drug with a meal. Doxycycline should not be taken in pregnancy or by children under eight years of age.

- *Chloroquine*, preferably in combination with proguanil 200 mg. daily, should be taken by persons who can tolerate neither mefloquine nor doxycycline. Travelers using chloroquine (with or without proguanil) are at risk of acquiring malaria and should carry a supply of Fansidar with them to be used for self-treatment (three tablets to be taken as a single dose) at the earliest suspicion of malaria if skilled medical care cannot be obtained quickly. Proguanil (Paludrine) can cause mouth ulcers. It is not available in the United States.

Even if an antimalarial regimen is followed carefully, an attack of malaria may still occur, but it is much less likely to be fatal.

NEW DRUGS

A new drug, PS-15, appears to be highly effective against drug-resistant strains. It is related to proguanil and may be suitable for *prevention*. Research is at an early stage, however.

There have also been some promising results with new drugs for *treatment*. Halofantrine has already been referred to (page 126). An ancient Chinese remedy, quinghaosu, has been under intensive investigation. Several drugs have been derived from it: artemisinin and its derivatives, such as artemether and artesunate. They appear to be dramatically effective in reducing the numbers of parasites present in the blood, with very little apparent toxicity. Because these drugs remain in the bloodstream only for a very short time after being taken, however, they cannot be used to prevent malaria.

PROSPECTS FOR A MALARIA VACCINE

There are many problems, and although prototype vaccines have been developed and tested the prospects for an effective vaccine for humans still remain many years in the future.

SUMMARY OF ADVICE FOR TRAVELERS

- Travelers should reduce the number of insect bites by app
  to exposed skin. It is sensible to be especially vigilant
  Anopheles mosquitoes begin to bite.

- Check current recommendations before departure (see information sources listed in Appendix 8).

- The important point about drug prevention is *to take it*, whatever drug or combination of drugs you prefer. However, prevention is not perfect, and *even the most careful traveler or expatriate may develop malaria.*

- Please remember that falciparum malaria may not start with fever but just a feeling of being unwell. Headache, abdominal pain, and diarrhea may occur. Of course, it can be difficult to differentiate malaria from other infectious diseases, including the common cold. Early treatment of malaria is more crucial than in most other infectious diseases. But if an attack of malaria is treated early, it is seldom fatal.

- If an attack of suspected malaria becomes severe, the patient should urgently ask for a blood test, if possible. Ideally, he or she should try to return to the closest city as soon as possible.

- Treatment in an emergency: see Table 5.1, p. 127.

TRAVELERS AT SPECIAL RISK

MALARIA IN PREGNANCY

Pregnant women should avoid travel to the highest risk malarious areas because no prophylactic regimen is completely safe or effective.

During pregnancy the disease may be more severe and both the mother and the fetus may suffer. Malaria in pregnancy increases the rate of miscarriage and the likelihood of stillbirth.

Chloroquine is the only drug that may be used for prophylaxis in pregnancy because the other drugs are potentially hazardous to the fetus.

FORMER RESIDENTS FROM ENDEMIC AREAS

People who migrate from malarial areas to countries where they are no longer exposed to malaria will quickly lose any immunity to infection that they may have built up. If they then return to their untry of origin for a visit, they will be at high risk of serious illness unless they take adequate preventive measures.

SPLENECTOMY
Malaria and other infections are a greater risk in people who have had their spleens removed (splenectomy).

ARBOVIRUSES: YELLOW FEVER AND DENGUE

Arboviruses are a motley group of infections confined mainly to the tropics. Vaccination can be given against yellow fever; otherwise prevention depends mainly on avoiding insect bites.
Dr. Philip Welsby is Consultant Physician in Communicable Diseases at the City Hospital in Edinburgh, U.K.

Arboviruses (*Arthropod-Borne-Viruses*) are viral infections that mainly affect animals but are occasionally spread to humans. As their name implies, the infections are transmitted to humans by arthropods (insects and their close relatives), especially mosquitoes, ticks, and flies, which introduce the infection into the human bloodstream by their bites. The mosquito, in particular, is well suited to the transport and spread of infection, because it has to obtain blood to enable it to reproduce, and because mosquitoes have a wide distribution throughout the tropics. They also have the remarkable ability to fly backward and upside down while avoiding raindrops!

Table 5.3 (on p. 133) details a few of the 80 or so arboviruses currently known to infect humans.

SOME GENERAL CONSIDERATIONS

RISK OF INFECTION
Particular arbovirus infections are often given specific place names (Rift Valley fever, for example) that may help warn a traveler where the possibility of infection exists. Because certain arbovirus infections are prone to cause inflammation of brain tissue—an encephalitis—this attribute is often also included in the name of the disease (Japanese encephalitis, for example).

In areas at risk any large outbreak of infection will leave the local human population relatively immune from further infection, though they may be unknowingly surrounded by infection in the local wild animal population. Few human cases will then occur in local inhabitants, except in those with no previous exposure to the infection— i.e., young children and visitors to the infected area. *Thus travelers should not be reassured by statements that "there have only been a few cases" in the areas they intend to visit.*

ARBOVIRUS ILLNESSES

The incubation period of arbovirus infections ranges from a few days to about two weeks. Most resulting illnesses tend to have two phases, the first when the virus is invading host cells, and the second a few days later when the body's immune system is fighting the infection. In the second phase of illness, virus and antibody produced by the body's immune system may be deposited in and cause

TABLE 5.3. SOME ARBOVIRUS INFECTIONS AND THEIR GEOGRAPHICAL DISTRIBUTION[1]

Virus name	Areas of distribution[1]
Chikungunya	South Africa, East Africa, Far East
O'nyong nyong	Africa
Kyasanur Forest disease	India
Eastern equine encephalitis	North America
Venezuelan equine encephalitis	North and South America
Western equine encephalitis	Belize, North and South America
Japanese encephalitis	Far East
Yellow fever	Africa, Americas, Caribbean
Crimean hemorrhagic fever	Commonwealth of Independent States (formerly the USSR), Bulgaria, Romania
Tick-borne encephalitis	Forested areas of Eastern and Central Europe (see p. 511)
Rift Valley fever	Africa
Louping ill[2]	UK

1. The geographical distribution of many of these diseases changes somewhat from time to time.
2. Louping ill is a rare occupational disease of shepherds, who acquire their infection from their sheep via tick bites. It is the only arbovirus infection native to the UK.

damage to the blood vessels—this explains why arboviruses often cause bleeding.

GEOGRAPHICAL OCCURRENCE

The incidence and geographical occurrences of most arbovirus infections are impossible to estimate as they vary considerably from time to time: the widespread presence of insects and other arthropods ensures that travelers to the tropics and subtropics will almost certainly be at risk of at least one kind of arbovirus infection. Fortunately not all arbovirus infections cause serious illness.

TREATMENT AND PREVENTION

With a few exceptions the treatment of arbovirus infections is of symptoms and complications, if any. Vaccination is available only for a few arbovirus infections, there are no specific antiviral drugs, and serum containing antibody from patients who have survived an infection is of limited use. As there is no cure, *prevention is essential*, which in practice means measures to avoid or deter insects including the use of mosquito netting at night, insecticides, insect repellents, and protective clothing (including pajamas at night). See also pp. 180–92.

As with every febrile illness acquired in the tropics, the possibility of malaria will also need to be considered.

YELLOW FEVER

Yellow fever is essentially a disease of monkeys living in tropical rain forests: humans are infected by rain forest mosquitoes, causing "jungle yellow fever." If an infected person then enters a densely populated area, infection may be spread from person to person by other types of mosquito, causing "urban yellow fever."

The world distribution of yellow fever—and also the distribution of mosquitoes capable of spreading the disease—is shown in Map 5.2 (p. 136). Interestingly, yellow fever is unknown in Asia despite the presence of mosquitoes capable of transmitting the virus.

THE ILLNESS

Many infections are mild and thus go unrecognized, but severe life-threatening illness is not uncommon. After an incubation period of three to six days, fever, headache, abdominal pain, and vomiting develop. After a brief recovery period, shock, bleeding, and signs related to kidney and liver failure develop. Liver failure is associated with jaundice—hence the name yellow fever.

No specific drug is available to combat yellow fever virus directly, so treatment is aimed at relieving the symptoms and complications. Overall, about 5 percent of patients may die, but in epidemics or in infections in nonvaccinated people the mortality rate may rise to 50 percent. Those who recover do so completely and are immune thereafter.

PREVENTION

Fortunately yellow fever is one of the few arbovirus infections for which vaccination is available (see pp. 503–5). A single injection of a live weakened (and therefore harmless) virus stimulates immune defenses: the vaccine is highly effective and confers protection for at least 10 years. *It is a vaccination not to be omitted for those visiting risk areas.* The vaccination has to be given at specialized centers where adequate storage of the vaccine is guaranteed.

Vaccination of pregnant women or of children less than nine months of age is best avoided unless areas of particularly high risk have to be visited. Other people who should not be vaccinated include those with impaired defenses against infections (people with HIV or malignant tumors, for example) and those receiving medical treatment with certain drugs including corticosteroids.

Reactions to vaccination are rare and relatively trivial—redness or swelling at the site of injection, or headache. The International Certification of Vaccination becomes valid for 10 years from 10 days after vaccination, or immediately on revaccination within 10 years. This certificate is required by many countries for entry of travelers coming from or through the yellow fever zones of Africa and South America, although precise requirements may vary from time to time according to which other countries currently have epidemics.

DENGUE

Dengue probably causes as much illness as all the other arboviruses put together: it is an unusual arbovirus infection because no animals, other than humans and mosquitoes, play a significant part in perpetuating infection.

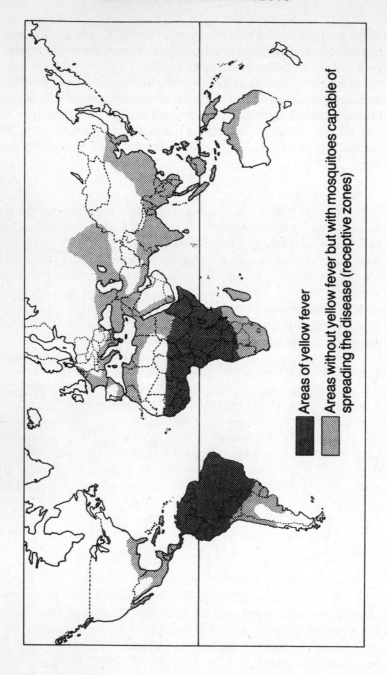

Areas of yellow fever

Areas without yellow fever but with mosquitoes capable of spreading the disease (receptive zones)

Dengue is present in Southeast Asia, the Pacific area, Africa, and the Caribbean. There has been a steady increase in activity in northern South America, particularly Colombia, Venezuela, and Brazil. The more severe, hemorrhagic form of the disease has also started to appear there, and there have been dramatic outbreaks. The geographical distribution is shown in Map 5.3.

THE ILLNESS

Illness is spread from person to person by *Aëdes aegypti* mosquitoes (Fig. 5.3) and, after an incubation period of five to eight days, there is a sudden onset of fever, headache, and severe joint and muscle pains—the latter giving rise to the popular name of "breakbone fever." The initial bout of fever resolves only to recur, and a rash usually appears between the third and fifth days of the illness. The rash starts on the trunk and spreads to the limbs and face, and consists of small spots. Within a few days the fever subsides and recovery follows. Although undoubtedly an unpleasant illness, serious complications are uncommon, and in particular there is no persisting arthritis.

Unfortunately, immunity to infection does not last long, and so second attacks, perhaps with a different strain of virus, are possible. There is no vaccine currently available.

Occasionally a more severe and life-threatening form of dengue may occur in children—dengue hemorrhagic fever—which is thought to be the result of a second infection in patients with some remaining immunity following a first attack. The second attack meets a vigorous immunological response in which severe blood-vessel damage occurs. Dengue is not uncommon in the children of expatriate families, but fortunately dengue hemorrhagic fever occurs only rarely in these families.

PREVENTION

Prevention of dengue, as with most arbovirus infections, and indeed many other tropical infections, involves measures to minimize contact with insects (see pp. 180–92).

◀**Map 5.2** Geographical distribution of yellow fever and of mosquitoes capable of spreading yellow fever.

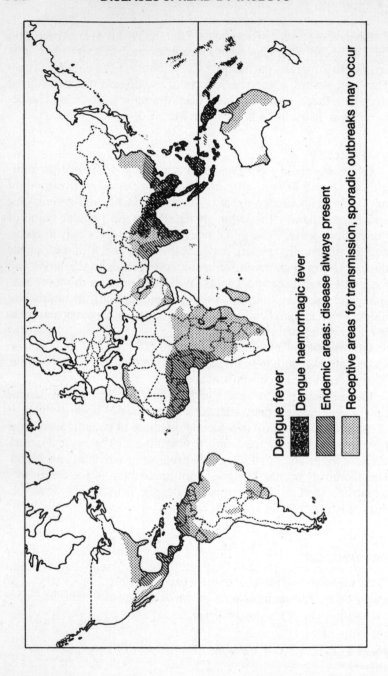

◀**Map 5.3** Geographical distribution of dengue fever. Note, however, that the exact distribution can vary quite significantly from time to time. Sporadic outbreaks occur in the Pacific islands. Reproduced, with slight modification, by kind permission of Dr. C. J. Leake, Department of Medical Parasitology, London School of Hygiene and Tropical Medicine.

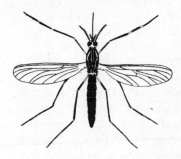

Fig. 5.3 Aëdes aegypti mosquito (female) (0.15–0.25 inch long).

JAPANESE ENCEPHALITIS (JE)

Japanese encephalitis is an infection of the central nervous system that is rare in travelers, but is potentially fatal. An effective vaccine is available, and is recommended for expatriates and certain travelers at high risk.

Dr. Theodore Tsai has been a medical officer with the Centers for Disease Control and Prevention for 15 years. He previously was chief of CDC's Arboviral Disease Branch in Fort Collins, Colorado.

Although Japanese encephalitis is little known outside Asia, this mosquito-borne disease is the region's leading cause of viral encephalitis, causing more than 30,000 cases each year, 5,000 of them fatal (see Map 5.4). Historically, epidemics occurred chiefly in China, Japan, and Korea, but more recently, outbreaks have spread to India and Southeast Asia. Cases occur principally in rural areas and the disease poses little risk to most travelers. Those who are at risk because of extended or frequent travel to endemic areas should consider receiving the vaccine (see pp. 142–43).

HOW IT IS SPREAD

Japanese encephalitis virus is transmitted chiefly in rural areas, among certain *Culex* mosquitoes and domestic pigs and wading birds. The vector mosquitoes that transmit Japanese encephalitis virus breed in irrigated fields and especially in flooded rice paddies. Human infections are incidental to this transmission cycle.

SEASONAL PATTERNS

Disease transmission follows a seasonal pattern that varies in different regions. The disease is transmitted from May to September in temperate areas of China, Japan, and Korea, with slightly longer seasons, from April to October in subtropical zones in the region (southern China, Taiwan, Okinawa, Southeast Asia). In tropical areas (e.g., Indonesia, Philippines) transmission may occur year-round or may follow specific patterns determined by local agricultural practices. Each of the three principal foci on the Indian subcontinent has specific seasonal patterns of transmission: Nepal, Northeast India and Bangladesh, July to December; Central India, September to December; South India and Sri Lanka, October to January; and Goa, May to October.

In endemic areas, nearly all cases occur in children under 10 years; however, all travelers from developed countries are susceptible to the disease because they lack natural immunity.

RISK OF INFECTION

The risk of acquiring Japanese encephalitis during travel is low. Only 24 cases among European and American travelers to Asia have been reported during the last 15 years. Some studies estimate the monthly risk of acquiring the disease during the transmission season to be under 1 per 50,000. However, risk for a given individual is highly variable and depends on factors such as the destination, season, and duration of travel and activities of the individual.

Travel during the transmission season and exposure to rural areas, especially for extended periods, are the principal factors contributing to risk. The majority of travelers to Asia on short trips to cities such as Tokyo, Hong Kong, and Singapore, and on conventional tours to the usual tourist destinations, are at low risk; because of the potential for vaccine side effects, they are *not* considered candidates for vaccination.

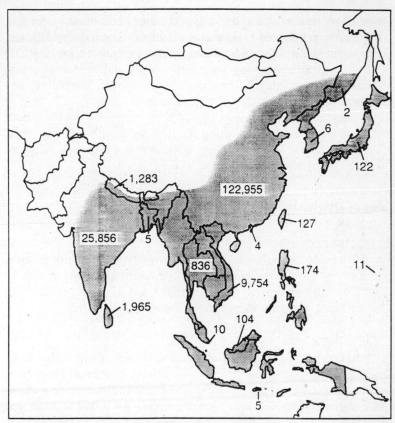

Map 5.4 Reported Japanese encephalitis cases by country, 1986–1990, and regions where viral transmission is proven or suspected.

THE ILLNESS

For reasons that are totally unclear, most infections with Japanese encephalitis virus lead to no symptoms at all, or only to mild, nondescript illnesses. Only one in every several hundred infections results in encephalitis; however, when encephalitis develops, it is usually severe and results in a fatal outcome in 10 to 20 percent of cases.

The illness may be abrupt in onset, with fever, chills, headache, and changes in behavior or coordination. Children often complain initially of nausea, with vomiting and other abdominal symptoms. The illness progresses rapidly and may lead to paralysis, seizures, and coma. One third of surviving patients may be permanently impaired. Although no specific therapy is available, intensive supportive care may improve the chances for survival. The elderly may be more susceptible to developing serious illnesses.

It appears that Japanese encephalitis poses a risk to the unborn fetus when illness occurs during the first six months of pregnancy. Although disease in the pregnant woman is not more severe, spontaneous abortion may occur.

PREVENTION

ANTI-INSECT MEASURES

All travelers should protect themselves from exposure to mosquitoes by using repellents, protective clothing, bednets, and by avoiding outdoor activity in the twilight and evening period when vector mosquitoes are most active (see also pp.180–92).

IMMUNIZATION

Although it is effective, the Japanese encephalitis vaccine is associated with potentially serious side effects in a small proportion of the people who receive it. *Japanese encephalitis vaccine is therefore not recommended as a routine vaccine for travel to Asia, and is advised only for expatriates and certain travelers at high risk.*

The killed Japanese encephalitis vaccine available in the United States (JE-VAX) is purified from brains of infected mice. The vaccine is produced in Japan, where it has been licensed since 1954. Allergic reactions consisting of hives and angioedema (allergic swelling of the face, lips, tongue, and extremities) occur in about 1 in 400 cases.

Reactions may be immediate or may be delayed for as late as two weeks after vaccination. The reactions are transient and can be treated with antihistamines or oral steroids; but, because of their potential seriousness, including the possibility of respiratory distress and hospitalization, the vaccine is recommended only for selected travelers.

Immunization poses a theoretical risk to the developing fetus, and should not be routinely given in pregnancy. Pregnant women who must travel to an area where the risk of JE is high should be immunized when the theoretical risks of immunization are outweighed by the risk of infection to the mother and developing fetus. Safety and efficacy have not been established for infants under one year old, and immunization should preferably be deferred until after this age.

In general, we recommend the vaccine for expatriates (who will be resident in risk areas during the transmission season) and for travelers spending a month or longer during the transmission season in an area where the disease occurs. Others who may be outdoors most of the time (e.g., on a bicycle tour), or who are visiting an area experiencing an active epidemic, should be vaccinated even for brief periods of exposure.

Three vaccine doses are given over a two-week or, preferably, a 30-day period. A booster dose may be needed two years later to maintain immunity. Because of the possibility of delayed allergic reactions, and to allow vaccine immunity to develop, travelers should not begin their journey until two weeks after receiving the last dose of vaccine. Persons with allergies to rodents and to thimerosal (a vaccine preservative) should alert their physicians to these sensitivities.

CONCLUSION

Because the risk of acquiring Japanese encephalitis during travel is generally low, and because the vaccine produces uncomfortable and potentially serious side effects in a small proportion of cases, most authorities feel it is inappropriate to make a blanket recommendation for the vaccine's use in travelers to Asia.

Japanese encephalitis is a serious and potentially fatal disease, and expatriates and selected travelers who are at risk for exposure *should* avail themselves of the vaccine. Because the risk/benefit considerations for this vaccine are so dependent on a given individual's itinerary, circumstances, and perceptions of risk, travelers in doubt about their need for protection should seek specialist advice.

FILARIASIS

Filariasis encompasses a variety of worm infestations confined mainly to the tropics and spread from person to person by insects.

Travelers have little to fear, but precautions must be taken against insect bites.

Dr. David Haddock *was a Senior Lecturer in Tropical Medicine at the Liverpool School of Tropical Medicine. He also worked for long periods in Tanzania, Ghana, Nigeria, and Saudi Arabia, and was a WHO Consultant in Ghana and the Sudan.*

Dr. George Wyatt *is a Senior Lecturer in Tropical Medicine at the Liverpool School of Tropical Medicine.*

Filariasis is caused by long, threadlike worms—up to twenty inches in length—which live in or under the skin and in lymphatic tissues. Several different types of human filarial infections are known: all are transmitted by biting insects, and occur only in warm climates, because the parasite needs high environmental temperatures to complete its development in insects.

Filarial worms may live for up to 20 years in humans, producing larvae that infect insects; but adult worms do not multiply in the body. Severity of disease depends largely on the number of adult worms present in the body, which in turn depends on the number of infective bites received: many people with few worms suffer few or no serious effects. Filariasis affects about 300 million people worldwide but produces significant disease only in some of these and rarely causes death. Drug treatment is effective if given before advanced disease is present.

LYMPHATIC FILARIASIS

Lymphatic filariasis is caused by worms called *Wuchereria bancrofti* and *Brugia malayi* which live in the lymph glands and vessels. Over 200 million people living in Asia, Africa, South America, and Oceania are infected (see Map 5.5). Transmission is by many varieties of mosquito, which become infected with larvae by biting infected people. Often, there are no symptoms; sometimes, however, there are recurrent fevers with painful inflammatory swellings of the lymph glands in the groin or armpit, or the testicles become acutely inflamed. These inflammatory swellings disappear spontaneously within a few days but may recur at intervals for months or years.

A few infected individuals (perhaps 5 percent) develop more serious, permanent disease with incapacitating swelling of legs, arms, or scrotum, called *elephantiasis* because of the resulting resemblance to elephant skin. Elephantiasis occurs only in heavily infected people who have lived for years in areas where the disease is common. Travelers often worry about the danger of developing elephantiasis or permanent genital damage, but these never occur in short-term visitors.

A possible though uncommon result of infection with filarial worms is an asthma-like reaction, with cough, shortness of breath, and alterations in the white cells of the blood. It responds well to treatment with diethylcarbamazine (DEC) tablets.

RIVER BLINDNESS (ONCHOCERCIASIS)

River blindness is caused by the parasitic worm *Onchocerca volvulus*. The adult worm survives for up to 18 years in small nodules under the skin, producing larvae that spread widely in the skin and cause irritating skin reactions. In heavy infections larvae invade the eye, causing damage and sometimes blindness.

The illness is spread by small, biting blackflies (*Simulium*) which breed and live near swiftly flowing rivers in parts of the tropics; their bites are

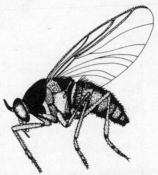

Fig. 5.4 *Simulium* fly (0.06–0.16 inch long).

painful. Approximately 30 million people are affected in parts of tropical Africa, Central and South America, and the Yemen. Travelers visiting infected areas may become lightly infected and develop intensely itchy skin lesions, but they rarely suffer serious eye damage.

Effective treatment with a drug called ivermectin is available but treatment may need to be repeated over several years.

THE AFRICAN EYE WORM (LOIASIS, LOA LOA)

Loiasis is a filarial infection that occurs in the rain-forest areas of West and tropical Central Africa. It is characterized by recurrent, itchy, uncomfortable swellings (Calabar swellings) appearing under the skin. These lumps disappear within a few days. No

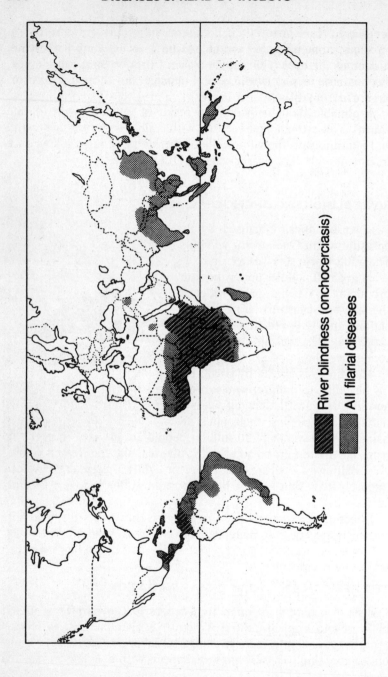

River blindness (onchocerciasis)

All filarial diseases

permanent damage results, but the swellings may recur for up to 15 years. Sometimes the worm can be seen crawling across the surface of the eyes. This causes alarm, irritation, and watering of the eye but no serious damage. Transmission is by the bites of large *Chrysops* flies, which breed in shaded forest pools and bite in daytime.

PREVENTION

All types of filariasis are spread by insects that bite either at night or during the day. Protection against insect bites is important (see pp. 180–92). Screening of houses against insects and sleeping under mosquito nets helps. Wearing long pants and sleeves and using insect repellents on the skin offers some protection. Travelers should not camp near streams where blackflies are breeding. Loiasis can be prevented by taking diethylcarbamazine tablets (DEC, Banocide, Hetrazan) 200 mg. daily for three consecutive days each month while in heavily infected areas, such as parts of Cameroon.

SUMMARY OF ADVICE FOR TRAVELERS

- Travelers occasionally contract filariasis, but, practically always, the infections are only light and not serious. Diagnosis is made by examining blood or small pieces of skin under the microscope, and finding larvae. Most travelers' worries about filariasis are unjustified.

LYME DISEASE

Lyme disease occurs after tick bites that often have not been noticed, and is most commonly recognized by an expanding red rash at the site of the bite.

Dr. George P. Schmid is a physician specializing in infectious diseases at the Centers for Disease Control and Prevention, and took part in some of the earliest studies investigating the cause and global distribution of Lyme disease.

◀**Map 5.5** Geographical distribution of filarial diseases.

Lyme disease (*Lyme borreliosis*) is an infectious disease characterized initially by an expanding red skin rash (called *erythema migrans*, or EM for short), often accompanied by headache, muscle,
and joint aches, and a low-grade fever. The vast majority of cases
occur during the summer and early autumn, and the causative bacterium, *Borrelia burgdorferi*, is transmitted to humans by the bite
of certain ticks; EM occurs at the site of the bite 3–32 days later.
Early cases are successfully treated with oral tetracyclines or amoxycillin, but if the disease progresses to complications involving the
joints, cardiac and nervous systems, antibiotic injections must be
used.

DISTRIBUTION

Lyme disease occurs in much of the United States, throughout Europe, and in selected coastal areas of Australia; cases have also been
reported in China and Japan. Within these countries, the disease
occurs only where the appropriate tick vectors are found, often in
areas of forestation and brush. In the United States, the vectors are
Ixodes dammini (the deer tick), *Ixodes pacificus*, and *Amblyomma
americanum* (the Lone Star tick), and disease is concentrated in
New England and coastal areas farther south to North Carolina;
and also in Minnesota and Wisconsin in the Midwest, Texas, and
the Pacific Coast. Forty-five states have reported cases. In the UK
and the rest of Europe, the vector is *Ixodes ricinus* (the sheep tick)
and cases have been reported from nearly every country. Fewer
cases have been reported from Australia, China, and Japan, suggesting that the disease is unusual in these countries.

   One case of disease has occurred after a mosquito bite and other
insects have been found to be infected, suggesting that additional
arthropods or insects could be vectors.

THE ILLNESS

Clinical illness begins 3–32 days following a tick bite, but only a
minority of patients remember the initial bite. This is because the
Ixodes ticks are quite small and bites are often not noticed. The
first sign of disease is usually a red area at the site of the tick
bite which, over a few days, expands in a circular fashion and
may form a ring as its center returns to a more normal appear-

ance. This expansion occurs as the infecting organisms migrate outward in the skin.

The skin rash is usually accompanied by signs of general infection, as *B. burgdorferi* spreads to other areas of the body. These include a low-grade fever, muscle and joint pain (with spread of *B. burgdorferi* to joints), headache and stiff neck (with spread to the cerebrospinal fluid of the brain), and an irregular heartbeat (with spread to the heart). Additional neurological symptoms, in particular temporary paralysis of the muscles on one side of the face (Bell's palsy) and pain or weakness in specific nerves, may be prominent, although why these symptoms occur is still unknown.

Without treatment, EM and the attendant symptoms will eventually resolve after several weeks in most patients. Many individuals, however, will have persistent or recurrent symptoms. The most common symptoms are recurrent attacks of arthritis lasting about a week, often accompanied by fatigue. Chronic neurological symptoms, such as persistent headache and stiff neck, mental changes, difficulties in thinking or concentrating, or numbness, weakness, or pain in specific nerves of the body may predominate. In a small number of patients, chronic arthritis, usually of the hip and resembling rheumatoid arthritis, may develop months or years following the initial illness.

It is important to note that Lyme disease is highly variable in the symptoms that it causes. Serological studies have shown that many people who have been infected have no prior recollection of illness. Some patients with the later symptoms of Lyme disease seek medical attention because of arthritis or neurological complaints, but likewise do not remember a skin rash. Other people have EM and no other symptoms, while others have associated general symptoms but do not have or notice EM. There are also geographic differences in disease, with neurological symptoms being more prominent in Lyme disease acquired in Europe and arthritis more prominent in disease acquired in the United States.

TREATMENT

The chance of developing Lyme disease after a tick bite is low, and prescription of antibiotics following a tick bite appears to be unwarranted. Instead, anyone who has had a tick bite should be particularly alert to the development of subsequent illness, particularly EM. Patients with EM and/or attendant symptoms should receive antimicrobials, though the optimal regimens are unclear. Tetracycline, 500 mg. four times a day, or doxycycline 100 mg. twice daily for 10 days (or longer) are often recommended; this effectively treats the symptoms and prevents the development of subsequent complications in most patients. If symptoms have not significantly improved by the end of this period, treatment is continued with a second course of tetracycline for 10 days. One study found, however, that lengthening the initial treatment time to 21 days (using doxycycline) prevented long-term complications very effectively, and no patient required retreatment. In this same study, amoxicillin 500 mg. three times a day along with probenecid 500 mg. three times a day, both for 21 days, produced the same excellent result. For patients who are unable to tolerate tetracyclines, amoxicillin appears to be the best alternative. There is a reluctance to use tetracycline for children under eight years, and amoxycillin is most commonly recommended.

For patients with established complications, such as meningitis or chronic arthritis, intravenous penicillin or ceftriaxone are recommended.

SUMMARY OF ADVICE FOR TRAVELERS

- Tick repellents containing DEET (see p. 182) are effective. Individuals in outdoor areas where Lyme disease occurs should also tuck pants legs into socks and examine each other at the end of each day for the presence of ticks.

- If an embedded tick is found, slowly pulling the tick out with tweezers is the best method of removal.

- If the symptoms of Lyme disease, particularly the appearance of a rash at the site of attachment, occur in the succeeding days or weeks, prompt medical attention should be sought.

LEISHMANIASIS

Leishmaniasis can be contracted in Mediterranean countries as well as in the tropics and subtropics, and may have serious disfiguring effects. Avoidance of sandfly bites is the main protective measure.

Dr. Clinton Manson-Bahr *taught and practiced in Africa and the Western Pacific for 23 years. He is a descendant of Sir Patrick Manson, the founder of modern Tropical Medicine, and is the editor of Manson's* Tropical Diseases.

Leishmaniasis is frequently underestimated as a health hazard to travelers, because it rarely causes serious illness. Its importance lies in the fact that when it does occur, doctors and health workers who are unfamiliar with the disease invariably fail to make the correct diagnosis.

Leishmaniasis remains an important public health problem in many parts of the world, and at least 12 million people worldwide are thought to be infected.

WHAT IS LEISHMANIASIS?

Leishmania are tiny single-celled organisms, just smaller than red blood cells. They parasitize *macrophage* cells (part of the immune system) in the skin, spleen, liver, bone marrow, and lymph glands. Their life history involves certain types of sandfly (Fig. 5.5), which bite at night and become infected by sucking the blood of an infected individual. After a two-to-three-week period infective forms of leishmania appear in the biting parts of the insect, and infect a new host during each subsequent blood meal.

Rodents, dogs, foxes, and jackals may also harbor the disease: leishmaniasis is therefore often referred to as a "zoonosis"—an infection that passes between humans and animals. The existence of an "animal reservoir" explains why the disease may be acquired in remote and uninhabited areas, and why it may suddenly occur out of the blue.

CUTANEOUS LEISHMANIASIS

Cutaneous leishmaniasis (also known as Oriental sore, Baghdad boil, or Biskra button) occurs in much of the Middle East, Asiatic regions of the former Soviet Union, North Africa (see Map 5.6, p. 153), and many areas of the tropics and subtropics. The observant traveler may have noticed that in many cities of the Middle East, nearly every inhabitant bears the unsightly scars that are the hallmark of the disease.

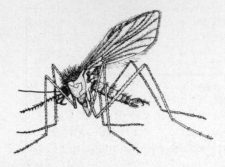

Fig. 5.5 *Phlebotomus* sandfly (0.08–0.2 inch long).

The infection is restricted to the skin at the site of the sandfly bite, and two patterns of disease occur—one in cities, and another in semidesert areas.

The city form, which also occurs in dogs, is found in big cities such as Baghdad and Tehran; it is also found in the Costa del Sol, Spain, the island of Majorca, and the Greek Islands, where it occasionally infects tourists. The reservoir for the rural form is the giant gerbil and other rodents. Travelers and picnickers in the semidesert areas of Israel, Jordan, Libya, Iran, Iraq, and northeastern areas of Saudi Arabia are at risk. At least 20 of the soldiers who took part in Operation Desert Storm developed cutaneous leishmaniasis.

The infection shows itself as one or more chronic skin nodules which appear on the face or arms, and which may ulcerate. The disease is often self-limiting but may persist for up to a year, and can leave a disfiguring scar. Diagnosis is made by examining a smear from the cut edge of an ulcer, and treatment is with an antimony drug.

VISCERAL LEISHMANIASIS (KALA AZAR)

Visceral leishmaniasis or "kala azar" almost disappeared from India as a result of widespread use of insecticides during attempts to eradicate malaria. These efforts have lapsed, however, and it has now returned with a vengeance. The disease is widespread throughout large areas of India, has caused epidemics in East Africa, and is found in many popular tourist destinations around the Mediterranean. There is a major outbreak currently in progress in the Sudan, which has now killed more than 40,000 people.

The parasites responsible for kala azar invade cells in the spleen,

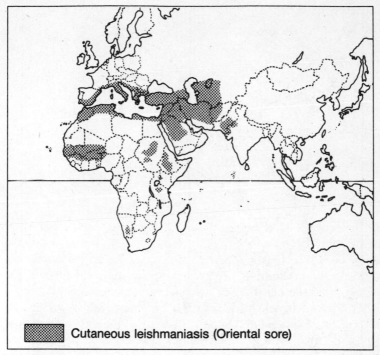

Cutaneous leishmaniasis (Oriental sore)

Map 5.6 Geographical distribution of cutaneous leishmaniasis (Oriental sore and Ethiopian leishmaniasis).

bone marrow, and liver, causing serious illness and, if untreated, death. The disease is rare in travelers, but is an important infection among the inhabitants of eastern India, Africa south of the Sahara, and Brazil (Map 5.7). Tourists to North Africa and parts of southern Spain, France, and mainland Greece (suburbs of Athens and Piraeus) can contract the disease. Although it is rare, travelers should always be aware of the possibility of kala azar, since it mimics many severe diseases, and *deaths have occurred from missing the diagnosis.*

Kala azar in the tourist areas mainly attacks infants and young children. There is prolonged fever, enlargement of the spleen, anemia, and great loss of weight. Consequently, the child will quite likely be suspected of having leukemia or lymphoma and have the spleen removed. A child may become ill in this manner as long as two years after visiting Greece or the Mediterranean; travelers

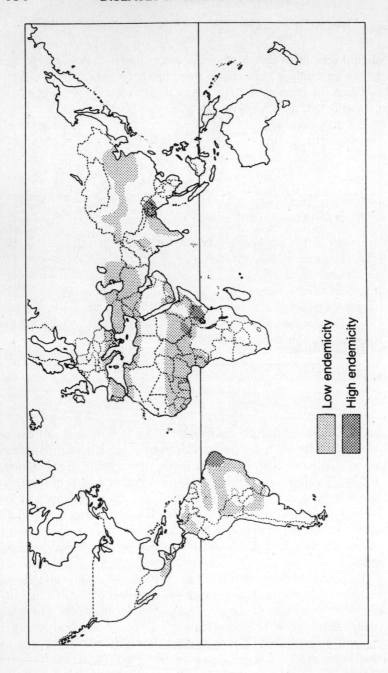

◀**Map 5.7** Geographical distribution of visceral leishmaniasis (kala azar).

should remember this, as should doctors looking after any child in whom leukemia is suspected if there has been any overseas travel.

Once the possibility of kala azar is considered, the diagnosis is easy and treatment is effective. A course of the pentavalent antimony drug sodium stibogluconate (Pentostam) will cure most infections. The diagnosis is established by examining specimens obtained from the bone marrow and a serological test on the blood.

MUCOSAL LEISHMANIASIS AND CUTANEOUS LEISHMANIASIS (AMERICAN)

An American form of cutaneous leishmaniasis is contracted in the lowland forest areas of Mexico and Guatemala (Map 5.8). It is known as "chiclero's ulcer" or gum pickers' ulcer since it is an infection of the forest, especially those parts in which so many Mayan ruins are found. Archaeologists, tourists, and soldiers are at risk. The ulcer is self-healing and is a nuisance only if it occurs on the ear, where it tends to persist for a long time.

Mucosal leishmaniasis (also known as espundia, pian bois, or

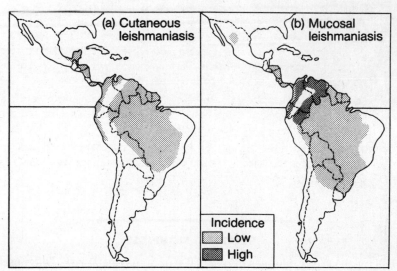

Map 5.8 Geographical distribution of American cutaneous and mucosal leishmaniasis.

forest yaws) occurs in many areas of South America, especially Brazil and the Amazon region. A simple skin ulcer, which may heal, precedes ulceration round the nose and mouth, which can be very destructive.

Travelers should be most suspicious of any skin nodule, whether or not it ulcerates, if it persists for more than a few days—and particularly if (as is often the case) it occurs at the site of known sandfly bites. Severe facial disfigurement may occur.

Mucosal leishmaniasis has hampered many major projects in parts of Brazil—such as road-building and agricultural development. Patients must seek specialized help, since accurate identification of the parasite is important in predicting whether a destructive lesion will develop. Remember the precise areas you visit, and tell your doctor if a suspicious skin nodule develops. Most cases respond well to treatment with sodium stibogluconate.

SUMMARY OF ADVICE FOR TRAVELERS

- Avoid sandfly bites as far as possible. Since sandflies bite at dawn and at dusk, it is especially important to avoid exposure at these times. In the Americas, a useful tip in the forest is to get up late in the morning, and to avoid moving around at dawn when sandflies resting close to the ground can be disturbed and bite viciously. Avoid camping in semidesert country in the Middle East in the vicinity of gerbil colonies—their communal burrows are easy to recognize. Avoid staying overnight in villages where most of the population bear the scars of healed leishmaniasis on their faces. Sleep on the roof where there is a breeze because sandflies are rarely able to jump more than two feet high.

- Sandfly nets are available, but are usually of too small a mesh to permit a comfortable night's sleep in the heat. The best alternative is to use broader mesh netting, impregnated with permethrin.

- Repellents (see p. 182) that last for a number of hours have proved useful in Central America, though repeated applications may have to be made. Repellents can also be impregnated into clothing and netting.

SLEEPING SICKNESS

Travelers to rural areas in tropical Africa may be at risk. Diagnosis and treatment are more difficult than prevention, so travelers should take care to avoid the bite of the tsetse fly.

Dr. George Wyatt *is a Senior Lecturer in Tropical Medicine at the Liverpool School of Tropical Medicine.*

Sleeping sickness, also known as African trypanosomiasis, is an important disease of humans and animals in tropical Africa. It kills cattle readily, and is therefore of great economic concern in large areas of Africa. In humans, the disease is confined to certain rural areas, but within these areas it can be a serious problem, and from time to time major epidemics of sleeping sickness arise. Epidemics often follow social and political turmoil, when control measures break down and people migrate into endemic areas. There has been just such an epidemic in the Busoga area of Uganda since the late 1970s.

Sleeping sickness is not a familiar disease to doctors in developed countries, so infections in travelers may easily remain undiagnosed for some time. Some African countries play down the risks of sleeping sickness so as to avoid frightening away potential tourists.

HOW THE DISEASE IS SPREAD AND ITS EFFECTS

The disease is caused by single-celled organisms called *trypanosomes*. The trypanosomes are spread by the bites of infected tsetse flies.

There are two varieties of sleeping sickness. In East Africa, the Rhodesian form of the disease is primarily an infection of wild animals such as the bushbuck; it is transmitted to people who live or travel near wild animals, by tsetse flies that breed in woodland or bush country.

In West and Central Africa a more slowly developing form of sleeping sickness, the Gambian form, is transmitted directly from person to person by the bites of tsetse flies that breed along the banks of rivers or streams.

The first sign of infection with trypanosomes may be a boil-like swelling which arises at the site of a tsetse bite, five or more days after the bite. Swellings that arise within a few hours of a bite are usually allergic in nature and not a sign of trypanosome infection. Fever (see p. 401) may begin within two or three weeks, and a severe illness may ensue which, unless adequately treated, often leads to infection of the central nervous system, and to the daytime drowsiness so characteristic of the disease.

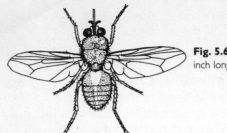

Fig. 5.6 Tsetse fly (female) (0.24–0.6 inch long).

TREATMENT

While the great majority of patients with sleeping sickness can be cured with proper drug treatment, the only effective drugs available are old-fashioned and hazardous to use, so that treatment should be given only by experienced physicians. New drugs are being developed and show some promise for the future.

SLEEPING SICKNESS AND THE TRAVELER

The chief group of travelers at risk from sleeping sickness are those who go on wildlife safaris in East Africa. Each year a handful of tourists among the many thousands who go on such safaris develop

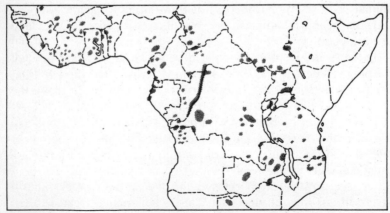

Map 5.9 Distribution of sleeping sickness foci in Africa (from WHO technical report No. 739).

sleeping sickness; the risk is very low in the better-developed tourist areas.

Other travelers who visit remote rural areas in Africa or who work with wild animals may also be at risk.

Map 5.9 shows the known foci of transmission of sleeping sickness.

Travelers who become ill following a safari vacation should make sure that their physician knows which countries they have visited, and if they have been exposed to tsetse bites the possibility of sleeping sickness should be considered.

SUMMARY OF ADVICE FOR TRAVELERS

- Unfortunately there is no vaccine against sleeping sickness, nor is there any likelihood of one being developed in the near future. This is because the trypanosomes are able to change their outer surface coat, thereby escaping the body's immune mechanisms.

- Although drugs are sometimes used as prophylactics against this disease, they cannot be advised for travelers since they do not always work, and when they fail they may mask infection until after the nervous system has been invaded.

- Prevention therefore depends largely upon avoiding the bites of tsetse flies. These flies are active during the daytime and are about the size of a common housefly. They have a pointed "proboscis" projecting forward from their head and at rest sit with their wings folded across their backs. Tsetse flies are attracted to large moving objects and to certain smells and colors such as dark blue. Horizontal stripes provide a measure of camouflage against them.

- Flies soon follow any vehicle traveling through infested areas. When there are tsetse flies about, keep windows closed, and kill any flies entering the vehicle with a "knock-down" *pyrethroid* spray, to which they are highly susceptible.

- Tsetse flies are less attracted to people on foot, and if you ride on horseback they are more likely to bite the horse than to attack you. Insect repellents such as diethyltoluamide (DEET) are of some value against tsetse flies (p. 182) but are not always effective.

CHAGAS' DISEASE

Chagas' disease is a potentially serious infection spread by a South American bug that lives in mud huts. Travelers to rural areas of Brazil are most at risk, but avoidance is reasonably straightforward.

Dr. Clinton Manson-Bahr taught and practiced in Africa and the Western

Pacific for 23 years. He is a descendant of Sir Patrick Manson, the founder of modern Tropical Medicine, and is the editor of Manson's Tropical Diseases.

Chagas' disease is found only in South and Central America (see Map 5.10). The disease is a major problem in Brazil, where it is present in most rural areas: poor peasants living in adobe (mud) huts are at greatest risk. True jungle areas such as the Amazon regions (with a mainly nomadic Amerindian population) tend to be free from the disease. An estimated 16–18 million people suffer from chronic infection, and 50,000 people die from it each year. There are around 20,000 new cases in Brazil each year.

WHAT IS CHAGAS' DISEASE?

Chagas' disease is caused by a small single-celled organism called *Trypanosoma cruzi*, which lives in the blood, and also in macrophage cells (part of the body's immune system) in the heart, intestines, and nervous system. The organism is similar in many ways to the trypanosomes that cause sleeping sickness.

HOW THE DISEASE IS SPREAD

The trypanosome is spread from one person to another by certain types of "cone-nosed" bugs, also known as assassin bugs or kissing bugs (Fig. 5.7 and Table 5.6, pp. 184–85). The bugs become infected by feeding upon the blood of an individual who has the disease. They excrete infective trypanosomes in their feces while biting a subsequent victim, and the trypanosomes enter through the bite wound. Blood transfusion is also a major route of spread.

The bugs live in the walls of mud huts and venture out only at night. They also feed on chickens, which are often kept in pens adjacent to the huts. Opossums and dogs also harbor the infection.

SYMPTOMS

Although infection may be widespread among local inhabitants, only a small proportion ever develop symptoms of disease. Early clues to a possible infection include local swelling around a bite, followed by swelling of the lymph glands or by a fever. At this stage

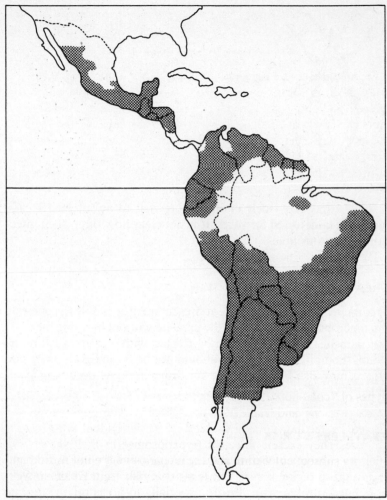

Map 5.10 Geographical distribution of Chagas' disease (South American trypanosomiasis) in South and Central America, 1988. Reproduced by kind permission of the Pan American Health Organization and Dr. F. J. López Antuñano.

it may be possible to detect trypanosomes with a blood test. The early symptoms soon settle.

The long-term complications of infection are serious: damage to the heart may lead to sudden death at a young age, and paralysis of the intestine and esophagus causes severe constipation and difficulty swallowing (megacolon, megaesophagus). A chance infection from

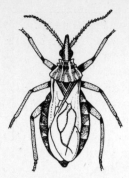

Fig. 5.7 *Rhodnius* "cone-nosed" bug (0.4–1.5 inch long).

a single exposure—such as on a short visit to an infected area—may pass undetected for years. It is not clear how often such infections lead to trouble.

TREATMENT

Treatment is difficult, because at present no drug is able to penetrate the macrophage cells and kill the parasite without harming the host; but parasites in the blood can be treated with a drug called nifurtimox (Lampit), although this should not be given lightly as its side effects may also be serious. Newer drugs are now becoming available.

TRAVELERS AT RISK

Visitors to large cities or to remote jungle ruins are not at risk, and the Amazon region is safe. Those most at risk are travelers to well-populated rural areas in Brazil, especially to areas off the normal tourist track, and include voluntary aid workers or Peace Corps volunteers. Young travelers living rough and sleeping in local adobe huts are also at risk. The bites may be mistaken for bedbug bites, but are uncomfortable and rarely escape attention.

PREVENTION AND PERSONAL PROTECTION

The most important preventive measure is to avoid being bitten by the bugs. This is not difficult because they live in the walls of adobe huts and emerge to feed only at night. The most dangerous parts of the huts are where the occupants usually sleep, and near walls and adjoining the chicken pens. Adobe huts are best avoided altogether, and it is safer to camp some distance away. Always sleep under a mosquito net as this will keep the bugs out, but be careful to tuck the net in completely, all the way round. If it is impossible to avoid spending the night inside, sleep in the center of the room, away from the walls; do not use old rugs, blankets, or sheets from the hut. Blood transfusion from unknown sources should be avoided.

There is little or no prospect for a vaccine, and no preventive drug at present.

CHECKUP (SEE ALSO APPENDIX 7)

The parasite is difficult to detect in the bloodstream once three weeks have elapsed following infection. However, if there is fever or local lymph gland enlargement the parasite can usually be found in the blood or in juice obtained from the lymph gland by needle puncture.

The best check test is a serum test (FAT fluorescent antibody test or ELISA test), which is now specific and accurate. Everyone who has traveled to rural areas of Brazil, or who has had a blood transfusion in Brazil, should have these tests performed on their return home. If they are positive, a course of nifurtimox should be given until the tests return to normal.

PLAGUE

Although plague is still present in several countries, the risk to travelers is very small indeed.

Dr. Thomas J. Quan *has recently retired as a Research Microbiologist with the Bacterial Zoonoses Branch, Centers for Disease Control and Prevention, Fort Collins, Colorado, having worked with plague for more than 30 years.*

Plague, a bacterial infection primarily of rodents, is one of the oldest diseases known. Periodically throughout recorded history, plague has spread to other parts of the world from what appears to be its ancestral home—the Yunnan Province of China. The first written description of the disease is perhaps that given in I Samuel v–vi, which reported an epidemic in about 1320 B.C. Other major outbreaks include the "Plague of Justinian" from A.D. 542–600, the "Black Death" of Europe during the fourteenth century, and the European epidemics of the fifteenth, sixteenth, and seventeenth centuries.

The current worldwide epidemic (pandemic) started in China in the mid-1800s and spread slowly to many other areas via both overland and marine mercantile trade routes. After its introduction in previously uninvolved areas (including the Western USA, South America, and South Africa), the plague organism became established in native wild rodents and persists as a potential public health hazard.

PLAGUE TODAY

In 1977–91, 22 countries in Africa, Asia, Asia Minor, Europe, and North and South America reported 15,540 human plague cases, including 1,474 deaths (Table 5.4).

DISEASE RESERVOIR AND HOW IT IS SPREAD

Human plague cases occur as the result of complex interactions involving four factors:

1. The first is the agent—a bacterium called *Yersinia pestis*.
2. The second is an insect vector (transmitter)—one or more of many types of flea (Fig. 5.8).
3. The third is a rodent or other mammal "host."
4. The fourth is the human host.

The ebb and flow of evident plague activity is closely associated with the natural cycles of its hosts and their fleas and with the weather, climatic, and other ecological factors. Although human cases may occur at any time, most occur in warm (not hot) summer months.

Typically, plague bacteria circulate among rodent hosts that are relatively tolerant of the bacterium's harmful effects. Fleas become infected by feeding on infected rodents or other mammalian hosts. As long as the infection is transmitted only among moderately to highly resistant "maintenance" rodent hosts, plague may remain undetected.

But infected fleas may transfer to and infect other, susceptible rodent species ("amplification" hosts); once the bacterium begins

TABLE 5.4. REPORTED HUMAN PLAGUE 1977–91 (WHO STATISTICS)

Country	Total no. cases (reported)	Deaths	Cases reported 1991
AFRICA			
Angola	27	4	
Botswana	173	12	
Kenya	442	20	
Lesotho	8	8	
Libya	19	6	
Madagascar	1,025	273	YES
Mozambique	109	14	
South Africa	19	1	
Tanzania	4,488	369	YES
Uganda	493	30	
Zaire	1,139	278	
Zimbabwe	5	3	YES
Total	7,947	1,018	
AMERICAS			
Bolivia	296	38	
Brazil	683	9	YES
Ecuador	83	4	
Peru	577	59	
United States	235	34	
Total	1,874	144	
ASIA			
Burma	2,154	119	
China	205	71	YES
Mongolia	19	8	YES
Vietnam	3,334	111	YES
Total	5,712	309	
EUROPE			
Kazakh Republic (formerly USSR)	7	3	YES
Total	7	3	
Grand Total	15,540	1,474	

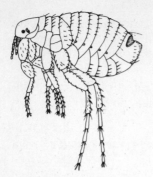

Fig. 5.8 *Pulex irritans* flea (male) (0.1 inch long).

circulating among a sufficiently large population of susceptible rodents and appropriate kinds and numbers of fleas, a widespread
die-off of the hosts may be initiated. Fleas then abandon their dead
or dying hosts and migrate in active search of new hosts, including
humans.

As more susceptible rodents die, progressively fewer are accessible to infected fleas, less contact occurs between infected and
uninfected animals, and eventually the outbreak recedes. Even if
the population of susceptible rodents is large, an outbreak may be
interrupted or stopped by the advent of adverse weather. Long, hot,
dry spells are unfavorable both to the bacteria in the flea and for
the survival of fleas away from their hosts or hosts' nests. During
winter, fleas tend to remain with their hosts (often hibernators) in
underground burrows and nests.

Direct contact with carcasses of animals infected with or dead
from plague may provide another source of infection to scavengers,
carnivores, other animals, or humans. Fortunately, most animals
that die do so in burrows or nests not generally accessible to humans. Most carnivores, except felines, appear to be fairly resistant
to plague but may transport infected carcasses and/or infected fleas
into unaffected areas. A number of human cases in the USA and
South Africa have been attributed to direct contact with infected
domestic cats and dogs as well as wild carnivores. Animals other
than rodents and their predators are not commonly involved in the
transmission of plague to humans. Occasional human cases have
been acquired after direct contact with or ingestion of raw or undercooked camel, sheep, or goat meat in Libya, Afghanistan, and

Saudi Arabia, and an infected antelope was the source of a recent human case in Montana.

SYMPTOMS

In human patients, the onset of *bubonic* plague symptoms is usually sudden, two to seven days after exposure (flea bite or direct contact). The chief symptoms include high fever, headache, muscular aches, shaking chills, and, commonly, pain in the groin or armpit.

The pain is due to the development of a *bubo*, an inflamed lymph node, which may or may not be enlarged until some time after onset of symptoms. Fully developed buboes are excruciatingly painful, and when in the groin may cause marked discomfort on walking. Buboes may also form in lymph nodes elsewhere in the body (in the neck, shoulder, knee, elbow, or deep in the chest or abdomen). In some patients, no buboes are evident: these cases are classified as *primary septicemic* plague.

Untreated bubonic plague progresses rapidly, and bacteria spread via lymphatic and blood circulatory systems to other tissues and organs, including the lungs. When the lungs become involved an infectious pneumonia may develop, allowing person-to-person transmission via coughed-up, bacteria-laden airborne droplets. In the USA transmission by this route has been prevented by the isolation of plague patients, and contacts of patients are given preventive antibiotic treatment; in any case, person-to-person transmission probably requires very close or intimate contact. However, primary plague pneumonia cases have occurred in at least four people exposed to sick domestic pets in the USA.

MORTALITY AND TREATMENT

About 35–40 percent of patients with untreated bubonic plague survive; however, patients with the more severe septicemic and pneumonic forms of plague are unlikely to survive without early, specific antibiotic therapy. Diagnosed early, plague is readily curable. Effective antibiotics include streptomycin (the optimum choice), tetracycline, and chloramphenicol. If these antibiotics are not available, certain sulfonamide drugs, especially sulfadiazine, are also effective.

SUMMARY OF ADVICE FOR TRAVELERS

- Fear of acquiring plague during routine sightseeing, hunting, on safari, or other tourist activities—even in active plague areas—should not prevent such activities or travel, provided that proper precautions are taken to minimize the risk.

- Reports of plague in travelers within or to the United States are uncommon; only 10 out of the 325 cases that occurred in the United States from 1956 to 1990 were reported in persons who were exposed in one state but developed symptoms only after travel to another state. Intrastate travel by patients from the area of exposure to another area occurs more commonly. Only three cases of human plague have been reported in international travelers; one unconfirmed case was in a serviceman who became ill in Texas after exposure to plague in Vietnam. The second case was in a woman, exposed in Africa, who became ill in London while en route to Texas. Her illness was serologically confirmed as plague after her arrival in Texas. The third case occurred in a female biologist exposed in Bolivia while working with rodents and who became ill on return to Washington D.C.

- If you have been in a plague area and develop symptoms similar to those described above, professional medical help should be sought as soon as possible. An account of your travel itinerary and activities (especially of any possible exposure to infected animals or of flea bites) will alert the attending physician and help the correct diagnosis to be made.

- If, and *only* if no such medical help is available within a reasonable time and the drugs are available, oral tetracycline (one 500-mg. tablet four times daily for adults) for 7–10 days can be taken. Professional medical help should be sought urgently, especially if the illness does not improve, or deteriorates.

VACCINATION

Plague vaccines are available commercially, but vaccination for the general public or for casual visitors to plague areas is not practical. Vaccination is urged for persons who work with the organism regularly in the laboratory or those who are regularly exposed to hosts and/or transmitters of the organism in the field.

PREVENTION

The best defense against plague is to avoid fleas and rodents such as rats, rabbits, squirrels, and chipmunks (however attractive some species may be) in plague areas. Appropriate use of insecticides and rodenticides is recommended around permanent or semipermanent dwellings. Regular use of suitable flea powders or dusts on domestic pet animals (dogs or cats) having access to both human and rodent habitats is strongly advised in plague areas. For short-term field excursions in plague areas, use of insect repellents, especially on legs and clothing, may effectively reduce flea infestation.

TYPHUS FEVERS

Typhus may occasionally be a risk to travelers walking or hiking in certain tropical areas, or to those working with refugees.

Dr. George Wyatt is a Senior Lecturer in Tropical Medicine at the Liverpool School of Tropical Medicine.

In the past, epidemic typhus has been one of the most feared diseases. Outbreaks killed many thousands of people during the world wars and under famine conditions both in Europe and in the tropics. At present epidemic typhus is rare except among poor inhabitants of certain tropical highland areas. In recent years most of the world's cases have been reported from the highlands of Ethiopia, Rwanda, and Burundi, with smaller numbers from countries in South America. Epidemic typhus is spread by body lice, but other varieties of typhus spread by other insects are now much more common worldwide.

All varieties of typhus cause fever (see p. 401), severe headache, and a skin rash, but the severity of the illness varies greatly among different types of typhus. These infections respond rapidly to the correct antibiotic provided that it is given early enough in the illness.

VARIETIES OF TYPHUS

All varieties of typhus are caused by *rickettsiae*, which resemble very small bacteria.

EPIDEMIC TYPHUS

The rickettsiae causing epidemic typhus are spread from one person to another by the human body louse (Fig. 5.9); the organisms are passed in the louse feces and cause infection if they are scratched through the skin, or sometimes if the feces are inhaled with dust.

Other kinds of rickettsiae are principally infections of animals and their external parasites. People become infected by close contact with an infected animal or its parasites.

ENDEMIC TYPHUS

This is a disease very similar to epidemic typhus except that it is usually milder. The infection is transmitted in the feces of infected rodent fleas (Fig. 5.8, p. 166). Sporadic human infections occur when people visit rat-infested buildings and are attacked by the rat fleas. Most kinds of typhus are rural infections but endemic typhus often occurs in towns, and occasionally there are sudden outbreaks, such as in Kuwait in 1978.

TICK TYPHUS

Several kinds of typhus are spread to humans by the bites of hard ticks (Fig. 5.12, p. 177). In countries bordering the Mediterranean, dog ticks sometimes transmit tick typhus. In southern Africa, people who walk through the veldt may contract tick typhus from the ticks of cattle or of wild animals.

A severe form of tick typhus known as Rocky Mountain spotted fever occurs in the Americas. Despite the name the disease has been most prevalent in the south Atlantic states of the USA in recent years. Dog and wood ticks are the main vector insects and the disease is most often acquired in the late spring and summer.

SCRUB TYPHUS

This is a disease of Asia and the Pacific islands. The reservoir for this infection is in the rodent population and in the mites that feed on these rodents. Once the mite population is infected, it may remain dangerous for many years because rickettsiae pass directly from one generation of mites to the next. Infected rodents and mites often live in quite small pockets or "mite islands" in "scrub" areas, also known as areas of "secondary" or "transitional" vegetation. People are infected by walking through an area where hungry larval mites are waiting for a blood meal. Rickettsiae cause infection through the bite of infected mite larvae, but infection may take several hours to be transmitted following attachment of the mite.

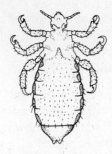

Fig. 5.9 *Pediculus humanus*, the human body (or clothing) louse (0.1 inch long).

TYPHUS AND THE TRAVELER

Epidemic typhus is likely to be a hazard only to people such as refugee workers who come into close contact with poor inhabitants of tropical highlands. A traveler who treks across the veldt in southern Africa may pick up tick typhus, but fortunately this is usually a mild disease except in the older traveler. People who hike in Southeastern Asia are at risk from the more serious scrub typhus, especially if they travel through overgrown vegetation or old plantations. Typhus is very uncommon in the ordinary tourist or business traveler.

SUMMARY OF ADVICE FOR TRAVELERS

- There are at present no commercially available vaccines against any variety of typhus.

- People who walk through tropical bush should inspect their skin carefully at the end of the day and remove any attached ticks (see box, p. 179). Repellents such as dimethyl phthalate, rubbed onto the skin every four hours, give useful protection against ticks and mites. Anyone intending to go walking in bush areas in Southeast Asia should also consider having boots and pants impregnated with a mixture of benzyl benzoate and dibutyl phthalate.

- Dogs are a potential source of a number of infections. It is wise to remove any ticks from pet dogs before they can transfer their infections to you.

MAGGOT INFESTATION (MYIASIS)

Travelers to tropical Africa and South America may occasionally come across this unpleasant condition.

Dr. Clinton Manson-Bahr taught and practiced in Africa and the Western Pacific for 23 years. He is a descendant of Sir Patrick Manson, the founder of modern Tropical Medicine, and is the editor of Manson's Tropical Diseases.

The maggots or larvae of certain tropical flies are able to burrow into human skin, eyes, or the nasal passages, and are an occasional nuisance to visitors to the tropics. The resulting infestation is known as *myiasis*, and two types of larvae are of particular importance.

TUMBU FLY

The tumbu fly is found in many parts of East and Central Africa. It lays its eggs on clothing—especially clothes that bear traces of urine or sweat. Clothes hanging outdoors on the washing line and clothes laid out on the ground to dry are the usual target.

The eggs hatch on contact with human skin. The larvae burrow into the skin and produce a characteristic boil, which contains not pus, but a developing maggot (Fig. 5.10). The boils are usually multiple and are found most often over the back, arms, scrotum, and around the waist.

The breathing apparatus of the maggots can usually be identified at the surface of the boil as a pair of black dots. A maggot can be removed by placing water or oil over its breathing apparatus, and gently squeezing it; the maggot will pop out. This is rather an unpleasant spectacle to witness.

PREVENTION

All clothes dried outdoors should be pressed with a good, hot iron to destroy any eggs that may be present. Clothes should otherwise be hung to dry indoors, in a flyproof environment.

MACAW, OR TROPICAL WARBLE FLY

This tropical warble fly is found throughout South America. Its life history is complex, but the female lays its eggs directly onto mosquitoes' thoraces. When the mosquitoes bite, the eggs hatch, and larvae burrow into the victim's skin.

An inflamed swelling usually results, and this is especially dangerous when it occurs close to the eye; the maggot must then be extracted surgically.

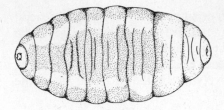

Fig. 5.10 Tumbu fly larva (0.4–0.6 inch long).

Infection is uncommon, but travelers are at greatest risk on the forested eastern slopes of the Andes. General measures to avoid insect bites should always be followed (see pp. 182–92), but no specific precautions are possible. Attempts to wipe out the fly in certain areas have met with a degree of success.

OTHER FORMS OF MYIASIS

Ordinary housefly maggots may appear in the feces when fly-contaminated food has been eaten. This is an alarming sight, but a dose of castor oil is all that is necessary to expel all of the larvae.

Bot flies, which usually lay their eggs in the skin of sheep or cattle, may occasionally attack man; the larvae can be found in the nasal cavity, and can be removed with ephedrine drops or by gargling with a strong salt solution. Infection is a hazard only in rural areas, under the most basic living conditions.

FLEAS, LICE, BUGS, SCABIES, AND OTHER CREATURES

Such creatures often cause annoyance to travelers, but only rarely carry disease. Their attentions can be avoided by a few simple measures.

Rod Robinson *is an entomologist with training in Public Health, and has special interests in lice and scabies.*

Humans provide many insects and other small creatures with both food and shelter from the elements (Table 5.6, p. 184–85). The intimacy of the association varies considerably: some parasites take up permanent residence, while others merely visit temporarily in search of food.

These creatures can be a particular nuisance to the traveler.

Levels of infestation vary from country to country, but in general they are most common where standards of hygiene are low. The human flea is practically extinct in many countries, but our warm, dry homes are ideal for cat fleas. Infestations with lice, bedbugs, and scabies are now comparatively rare in the USA, but are on the increase.

FLEAS

Fleas are small (approximately 0.1 inch long) reddish-brown insects, compressed sideways; they lack wings, but have powerful hind legs for jumping (Fig. 5.8, p. 166). Their larvae are wormlike, and live on organic debris on the floor. Fleas breed wherever their hosts rest, jumping onto their victims to feed. Their larvae form pupae which remain dormant for several months, until vibrations from a passing victim provide a signal to come out and feed.

Some fleas are able to transmit two important diseases—plague ("Black Death") (p. 163) and murine (endemic) typhus (p. 169)—but although fleas are widespread, disease is rare, and is confined to the poorest areas of urban squalor.

Otherwise, flea bites may be an uncomfortable nuisance, but are not dangerous.

JIGGER FLEAS

The jigger (tunga) flea is an unusual flea which lives outdoors in the sand in Central America and West Africa. The female penetrates the skin, usually around the toes, and swells up with eggs, causing inflammation and ulceration. If these are untreated, gangrene can set in. Local people can tell you which places to avoid, but if in doubt wear a good pair of jungle boots.

LICE

There are three types of human louse: the head louse, which lives on the scalp; the clothing louse (body louse), which infests clothing; and the crab louse (see also p. 417), which lives in coarse body hair (i.e., in the pubic region, armpits, in beards, etc.). All three types need to suck blood regularly, and if separated from the body for longer than a few days, they will die. Head and clothing lice are very similar in appearance, are approximately 0.1 inch long, cream to brown in color and lack wings (Fig. 5.9, p. 171). Crab lice are squatter and have prominent claws, giving a crablike appearance.

All three types of louse spread by direct contact between people, and in the case of the clothing louse by two people exchanging clothes. Their eggs are laid at the base of hairs or in seams of clothing, where body temperature enables them to hatch in 7–10 days.

Clothing lice can spread typhus, not by their bite but in their dried feces, which can enter wounds or be accidentally inhaled. Like plague, typhus is restricted to the poorest areas, although it could break out wherever normal hygiene standards collapse.

Louse bites are otherwise merely a nuisance, although long-term infestation can lead to infections of the bites and allergic reactions to the louse saliva.

BEDBUGS

Bedbugs are flat and oval, 0.25–0.4 inches long when fully grown, and reddish-brown in color (Fig. 5.11). They live in bedrooms, in the bedframe, in cracks in walls, and under wallpaper and carpets. They feed only at night, while their victims sleep.

They do not appear to carry any diseases, but their bites can be extremely uncomfortable.

CONE-NOSED BUGS

In South and Central America cone-nosed bugs (Fig. 5.7, p. 162) are common in rural areas where housing standards are poor. They

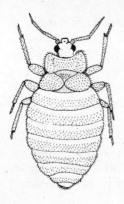

Fig. 5.11 *Cimex* bedbug (male) (0.25–0.4 inch long).

- I am often asked if there is any possibility that insects could carry HIV. This has been the subject of several investigations, but all agree that there is so far no evidence that HIV has been transmitted by any species. However, some laboratory studies have shown that live virus can be recovered from some insects' guts two hours after ingestion; it would therefore be foolish to say that insects will *never* be responsible for spreading AIDS—after all, 20 years ago we had never even heard of AIDS.

- At the moment the answer must be that insects don't spread the disease. There is speculation that, if insects are ever shown to be capable of passing HIV, the culprit will probably be one of the larger blood-suckers (e.g., bedbugs or cone-nosed bugs), after feeding on an HIV carrier and being crushed on a nearby human, with the blood entering a wound or perhaps being scratched in.

are relatively large creatures, 0.75–1.5 inches in length when fully grown, with a thin head and long mouthparts. They can carry Chagas' disease (South American trypanosomiasis, p. 159), and once again it is the feces, not the bite, that is infective.

SCABIES

Scabies is caused by a small mite that tunnels into the outer layers of the skin and causes a characteristic itch. Detecting the mite itself is difficult without a microscope, although with practice one can spot the meandering burrows. The itch itself can be almost unbearable, but the scabies mite does not carry any disease. (See also p. 417.)

TICKS AND MITES

Travelers walking through undergrowth or exploring caves may find ticks or mites attached to their skin (Fig. 5.12). Adult ticks can be alarmingly large when engorged, but they are relatively simple to remove with a pair of tweezers, or nimble fingers. Ticks can carry several diseases (see Table 5.6, pp. 184–85). Rocky Mountain spotted fever occurs in parts of the United States, and so does Lyme disease.

LYME DISEASE
This is a disease of deer and other animals which has recently (1976) been discovered to be capable of infecting man. It is caused

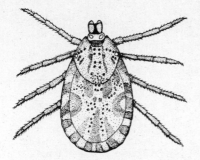

Fig. 5.12 Hard tick (about 0.12 inch long, but up to 0.75 inch when engorged with blood).

by bacteria, and is spread by the bite of several tick species, found in woods, marshes, parks, and grassland across mainland Europe, the UK, and the Eastern USA. If untreated, it can lead to arthritis, heart problems, and neurological disorders. The disease is discussed in greater detail on p. 147.

There is some evidence to suggest that Lyme disease is rarely passed from tick to human until about 18 hours after the tick has begun to feed. It is therefore important to remove ticks as soon as possible, without causing the tick any trauma which might cause it to vomit its intestinal contents (which contain the bacterium) into the wound. For this reason, the old techniques of applying chloroform, oil, or a lighted cigarette are no longer recommended. Instead, grip the tick with tweezers firmly under the head end (where the mouth parts are embedded), push down carefully to disengage the "teeth" from the skin, and gently pull away. Be patient—rock the tick slightly from side to side if it does not come away immediately. Once the tick has been removed, treat the bite area with an antiseptic and keep the tick, if possible, for future reference.

MITES

Mites can be dealt with in a similar manner, but in some species only the tiny mite *larvae* attack people, and they are difficult to spot. They attach themselves to the skin at the waist and ankles, leaving red weals. In Southeast Asia they can spread relapsing fever (a form of typhus).

SOME HINTS ON DIAGNOSIS

Flea bites tend to occur in groups, along clothing constrictions and around the ankles.

TABLE 5.5 TREATMENT OF PERSONAL PARASITES

Parasite	Preferred Treatment	Technique
Head lice	Shampoo or lotion containing pyrethrins (Rid, A-200) or lindane (Kwell, Kwell shampoo); or an aqueous solution of malathion (available in some countries as Derbac)	*Lotions:* apply the lotion liberally to the hair and rub in (avoid contact with eyes). Leave to air dry. Wash hair after at least eight hours with any shampoo. One treatment is usually sufficient. *Shampoos:* use the shampoo as an ordinary shampoo, except that it should be left on the head for at least four minutes. A course of at least three treatments, at three-day intervals, is recommended. *Neither treatment* will remove the eggs (nits) but these will be dead, and of no consequence.
Crab lice	As above	As above, except *all* hairy parts of the body should be treated, including beards, legs, chest, etc.
Clothing lice	Dry heat from dryer, hot wash, or leave alone in plastic bag for two weeks minimum	Place clothes *dry* into tumble dryer for ten minutes at hottest setting. Alternatively, wash clothes in water hotter than 130°F (55°C) (too hot to keep hands in). Clothes can otherwise just be left in a bag for at least two weeks, so lice starve to death. Rotate sets of clothing at one- to two-week intervals, thereafter. *No* treatment of the person is necessary, unless other parasites are found.
Scabies	Lindane-based lotion (Kwell); permethrin 5% cream (Elimite); an aqueous solution of malathion (available in some countries as Derbac)	Apply the lotion thoroughly over all the body from the neck down. Leave to air dry for 5–10 minutes. Wash off after 8–10 hours. Only one treatment is necessary, even when itching persists. Antihistamine tablets may relieve the itch.
Ticks and larger mites	Tweezers or fingers	Hold the tick firmly by the head end. Push down the head to disengage the teeth, then pull away. If the tick does not come away immediately, try rocking it from side to side. This process may have to be repeated several times: patience is the key.

TREATMENT AND PREVENTION: SUMMARY OF ADVICE FOR TRAVELERS

- Treatment of the "personal" parasites—lice and scabies—is the same, and consists of applying an insecticidal lotion to the affected areas (Table 5.5). In many parts of the world lice are resistant to organochlorine insecticides, so a lotion containing malathion, carbaryl, or pyrethroids should be used instead. With scabies, the itch will persist for a week or so, even after all the mites are dead, but can be alleviated somewhat with antihistamine tablets.

- Fleas and bugs can be controlled with insecticide sprays, which are best applied by experienced personnel. Flea bites may be prevented by tucking bedclothes into the mattress, because fleas can jump only six inches vertically at a time, and by discouraging fleas and bugs from climbing up bed legs by standing these in containers of water. If a vacuum cleaner is available it will be very useful in keeping down the flea population, and thorough cleaning will also help.

- If bedbugs are also suspected, move the bed away from the wall and leave a light on in the room for the whole night because bedbugs prefer to feed in the dark.

- Head lice can be discouraged simply by regular use of an ordinary pocket comb; washing hair, by itself, will only produce cleaner lice.

- Clothing lice are easily killed by putting the clothes *dry* into a tumble dryer for ten minutes, or else washing them in water that is hotter than 130°F. (55°C.) (just too hot to keep hands in). Alternatively, the louse needs a period of two to three weeks to develop from egg to adult, so changing clothes once a week will prevent an infestation from becoming established.

- Crab lice and scabies may be detected on close inspection of prospective partners, although this may be difficult to accomplish discreetly!

- Ticks and mites can be discouraged from attaching by the use of repellents, as described in the next chapter. Dimethylphthalate (DMP) is a more effective mite repellent than diethyltoluamide.

Bedbugs bite on the face, arms, and legs, where these protrude from the bedclothes.

Fleas and bugs often pass out undigested blood, leaving telltale bloodstains on the sheets. Pyrethroid flysprays, if available, can be sprayed into cracks and crevices and around bedframes to check for bedbugs; although the bugs are not killed by the spray, it irritates them enough to drive them from their hiding places.

Head lice bite only on the scalp, and crab lice on the body's hairy regions, whereas clothing lice may bite anywhere under the clothes. The best indicator of a louse infection is the discovery of white, empty eggshells, called nits, firmly glued to hairs or in the clothes.

In order to catch *scabies* it is necessary to be in close physical contact with an infected person for a prolonged time, and consequently the primary sites of infection are the hands, arms, legs, and sexual organs. The itch develops about six to eight weeks *after* infection, and is due to an allergic reaction. It is often worse at night, and often involves the sides of the body and between the legs, even though no mites are present there. A rash may also develop around the middle of the body.

Ticks and mites are often noticed by the traveler only after they have attached to the body. Travelers should take precautions against ticks by tucking pant legs into thick socks, using a repellent, and wearing light-colored clothes if possible, which will make a better background to see ticks against. It is a good idea to get into a routine of examining your body for ticks and mites at a regular time, for example, just before getting into bed, when traveling in an area of high risk. Better still, get someone else to check you over and to look at your back.

PERSONAL PROTECTION AGAINST INSECT PESTS

Many serious diseases in the tropics and elsewhere are spread by insects. Personal protection against insects is among the most important of all health precautions for travel.

Dr. Christopher Curtis *is a geneticist and entomologist, and has worked for several years on the application of genetics to tsetse fly and mosquito control. He is now involved in developing "appropriate technology" for mosquito control.*

Several types of insect—as well as related creatures like ticks and mites—obtain all their food by sucking blood from humans or animals, i.e., "biting." In certain other kinds of insects, including mosquitoes, the females require a blood meal in order to produce each batch of eggs. (See Fig. 5.13 for method of distinguishing male and female mosquitoes.)

INSECT BITES

The pain and discomfort that arises as a "by-product" of insect bites is due to an allergic reaction to saliva introduced by the insect

- In medieval Europe, travelers would take along pigs, which they would leave in their beds as soon as they arrived at an inn. By the time the traveler had dined, and was ready for bed, the fleas, bugs, and other insects in the room would— theoretically—have satisfied their appetite by feeding upon the unfortunate pig. Such measures are, I hope, not necessary today.

during bloodsucking. Such bites should be distinguished from the stings of bees, wasps, or ants, which have a different biological function, namely to deter intruders from approaching their nests (see pp. 218–20). This distinction may appear somewhat academic to the unfortunate victim! The severity of skin reaction in different people to bites and stings varies greatly, and people also differ widely in their apparent "allure" to biting insects. (Treatment—see p. 527–28.)

DISEASES SPREAD BY INSECTS

The nuisance of biting insects can be at least as great in the arctic summer as it is in the tropics. It is mainly only in the tropics that insect-borne diseases are still an important health hazard, though more has been heard recently of two tick-borne diseases that are a slight risk in certain parts of North America and Europe (Lyme disease and tick-borne encephalitis). The viruses, bacteria, proto-zoa, or worms responsible for these diseases take advantage of the biting habits of insects and ticks to enable themselves to be trans-ported from the bloodstream of one victim to another.

Some insects and ticks hatch from their eggs already infected with viruses or somewhat larger organisms called *rickettsiae* (see pp. 169–70) which can cause human disease, but this is the excep-

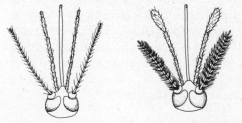

Fig. 5.13 Heads of female (left) and male (right) *Anopheles* mosquitoes. Unlike the fe-males, male mosquitoes do not bite and can be recognized by their bushy antennae.

tion rather than the rule. Most insects become infected when biting an infected individual and pass the disease on to someone else during a subsequent feed, or with some diseases, by defecating onto the skin.

Table 5.6 gives a summary of the commoner biting insects and the diseases they may carry. The list of diseases may appear daunting, but the only ones commonly contracted by visitors to the tropics are malaria (see p. 121) and, in certain places, dengue (see p. 135) and cutaneous leishmaniasis (see p. 151). Of these, malaria presents by far the most serious risk. The other diseases need be considered only by travelers who will be living for a considerable period in a tent, or in tropical villages, urban slums, or refugee camps. In such cases it would be wise to take local advice about the particular risks and possible countermeasures.

Insects spread many diseases for which drug treatment is difficult, dangerous, or nonexistent, and for which we do not yet have vaccines. **Prevention of insect bites is the single most sensible and effective precaution a traveler can take to avoid these diseases.**

PROTECTION FROM INSECT BITES OUTDOORS

Quite apart from the hazard of disease, insect bites themselves can be more than a trivial nuisance in some places—in Howrah, near Calcutta, 500 bites by *Culex* mosquitoes per person per night (about one a minute throughout the night) are usual—and in such situations few visitors would need encouragement to take measures for personal protection.

REPELLENTS
A chemical repellent is the best, and perhaps only suitable personal protection against outdoor biting insects. As far as is known, repellents act by interfering with the sense organs with which insects locate their victims. Most of the commercially available insect repellent preparations contain diethyltoluamide (commonly known as DEET), ethylhexanediol, or dimethylphthalate (DMP). These preparations come as lotions, sticks, gels, creams, or in aerosol cans or pump-action dispensers. In Australia, a mosquito repellent soap has been developed.* This leaves a residue on the skin that can be washed off with water when no longer required.

---

* Simmons Pty. Ltd., Box 107, Chadstone, Victoria 3148, Australia.

DEET and DMP are harmful to some hard plastics and paint, cause a stinging sensation if they get into the eyes, and taste unpleasant: they should be applied with care. Conventional toxicity tests when DEET first came onto the market in the 1950s were reassuring, and DEET has been used without harm by millions of people. More recently, however, occasional reports have appeared of serious reactions in a few individuals. Anyone who suspects an adverse reaction to DEET should stop using it immediately and seek medical advice.

DEET is apparently effective against all free-flying biting insects, although the dose required may depend on the species of insect. When applied to the skin, DEET remains effective for only a few hours. However, when impregnated into cotton (not synthetic) material it remains effective for several weeks if the material is kept in a plastic bag or a can when not in use. The chances of an adverse skin reaction are presumably much reduced if DEET is impregnated into clothing rather than applied direct to the skin.

Clothes can be impregnated by using an aerosol or, more economically, by making a suspension of concentrated DEET in water and pouring it over the garment (1 ml. DEET and 8 ml. water per 4g. cotton or around 25 ml. DEET and 200 ml. water for an average-sized shirt) and then hanging it up to dry. Concentrated DEET can be obtained from some pharmacies and camping goods stores or by mail order.* Clothing can also be impregnated with permethrin (see p. 191).

It is possible to impregnate ordinary clothing covering especially vulnerable areas such as the ankles, wrists, and neck; or an impregnated netting (approximately 0.4 inch mesh) overgarment may be preferred, which can be put on only when needed and minimizes skin contact with the chemical. Such a garment, with a hood, gives off sufficient DEET vapor to protect the face from biting even in areas heavily infested with mosquitoes. Netting jackets may snag and tear if much used in dense undergrowth.

When one is sitting on a chair, most mosquito bites occur on the ankles or feet. Cotton ankle bands, 4 inches wide and each impregnated with 4 ml. DEET, have been found to give 80-85 percent reduction in biting by several species of tropical night-biting mos-

---

* Concentrated DEET is sold as "Repel 100," "Cutter's," and Johnson's "Off!" liquid.

TABLE 5.6. INSECTS, MITES, AND TICKS THAT BITE OR BURROW IN THE SKIN, AND RISK OF DISEASE TRANSMISSION IN DIFFERENT TROPICAL AND SUBTROPICAL AREAS
(Also some parts of Europe and North America in the case of two tick-borne diseases)

Pest	Rough guide to identification of adult	Time and place of biting or burrowing	Disease	Risk of disease transmission (x = slight risk; xx = moderate risk; xxxx = high risk)			
				Africa	Asia	Americas	Western Pacific
Mosquitoes *Anopheles*	head and body in straight line and at an angle to surface (Figs. 5.1, p. 122 and 5.2, p. 122)	night; indoors or out; mainly rural	malaria	xxxx	xx	x	xx
			filariasis	x			x
Culex	body parallel to surface, head bent down, whining flight; dull brown (Fig. 5.2, p. 122)	evening and night; indoors or out; urban or rural	filariasis	x	x	x	x
			encephalitis		x	x	x
Aëdes	body shape as for *Culex*; but tropical species are black and white (Fig. 5.3, p. 139)	day; indoors or out; urban or rural	dengue	x	xx	x	x
			yellow fever	x		x	
			filariasis				xx
Mansonia	as *Culex*; but with patterned wings and legs	night; outdoors; rural	filariasis		x		
Tsetse flies	brown fly with proboscis projecting in front of head (Fig. 5.6, p. 158)	day; outdoors; rural; tropical Africa only	sleeping sickness	x			
Blackflies	0.06–0.16 in., stout and black, with humped body (Fig. 5.4, p. 145)	day; outdoors; rural	onchocerciasis	x		x	
Phlebotomine sandflies	tiny hairy flies (Fig. 5.5, p. 152)	evening; indoors or out; rural or urban	leishmaniasis	x	x	x	
			sandfly fever	x	x	x	
			bartonellosis			x	

Type	Description	Habits	Disease			
Biting midges	tiny flies with spotted wings	evening; outdoors; rural		×		
Gadflies, horse-flies, stable-flies	as large or larger than house-fly; fast-flying	day; outdoors; rural	loiasis	×	×	×
Ticks	eight-legged creatures which attach tightly to skin and swell up with blood to pea size (Fig. 5.12, p. 177)	day or night; cling to long grass or hide on cave floors and attach to passers-by or sleepers	relapsing fever	×	×	×
			typhus	×	×	
			Lyme disease	× (N.E. USA and N. Europe)		
			encephalitis	× (E. and C. Europe)		
			? hepatitis B	×	×	
Bedbugs	0.25–0.4 in.; brown beetle-like; but wingless (Fig. 5.11, p. 175)	night; in beds				
Triatomine bugs	0.4–1.5 in.; cone-like head; long legs (Fig. 5.7, p. 162)	night; in beds	Chagas' disease		×	
Fleas	0.1 in.; brown, flattened sideways; run and jump (Fig. 5.8, p. 166)	night or day; indoors	bubonic plague	×	×	×
Lice	0.1 in.; cream or brown; claws often visible; flattened top to bottom; crawl (Fig. 5.9, p. 171)	night or day; on body hair or clothes for their whole life-cycle	typhus	×	×	×
			relapsing fever	×	×	×
Tumbu fly	robust; yellow-brown; non-biting fly (Fig. 5.10, p. 173)	larvae attach to clothing while it is being dried on the ground and burrow into skin	myiasis	×		
Mites	tiny eight-legged creatures	climb onto skin from undergrowth or from other people and cling to or burrow in skin	typhus		×	×
			scabies	×	×	×

CHOOSING AN INSECT-REPELLENT PRODUCT

- The most effective chemical repellents are those that contain DEET. The choice between sprays, liquid, gel, etc., is largely a matter of personal preference. Whatever you choose, it is worth comparing brands on the basis of how much DEET you are getting for each dollar you spend—calculated from the weight of the product and the concentration of DEET that it contains.

- DEET is generally diluted using a volatile (usually alcohol-based) vehicle that evaporates quickly, leaving concentrated DEET on your skin. Thus, applying a spray that contains 30 percent DEET, for example, presumably achieves the same result as using a 100 percent spray more sparingly.

- 100 percent DEET is generally more economic and more convenient to travel with; it should always be used sparingly, and over clothing in preference to spraying it over large areas of skin.

- Newer formulations of DEET (Ultrathon, 3M) use polymer microencapsulation or other chemical methods to reduce absorption through the skin and retard its evaporation, and are claimed to provide protection for as long as eight hours. Reports of independent tests with these products have so far been limited, however, and you should be prepared to test out manufacturers' claims for yourself. In particular, it does not appear to have been established whether these products would remain effective throughout a night's sleep, or whether they would be rubbed off on the sheets or pillow and thus cease to protect the sleeper.

quitoes. One impregnation remains effective for several weeks if the ankle bands are sealed up when not in use. You can make your own, or you can buy ready-impregnated sets by mail order from MASTA (see Appendix 8).

Citronella oil is distilled from a tropical grass and is used as a soap perfume. It has long been sold as an insect repellent but does not remain effective for as long as DEET. However, some people prefer its lemony smell to the less agreeable smell of DEET.

Mosquitoes tend to be diverted away from a person wearing a repellent (or naturally unattractive to mosquitoes) toward a nearby person not using repellent (or naturally more attractive to mosquitoes). This might suggest that the best protection would be to sleep with someone more attractive to mosquitoes than yourself!

BUZZERS
Electronic buzzers have been advertised widely as mosquito repellents. Manufacturers claim that they simulate the sound of a male

REPELLENTS: PREVENTING TOXIC EFFECTS

Although DEET-containing repellents have been widely used for more than 30 years, there has recently been increased attention to their potential for causing side effects, particularly in children. In high concentrations, DEET can irritate the skin and produce deep ulcerations. More worrisome are rare cases of encephalopathy and seizures, principally in children, that have followed even brief exposures to DEET. To minimize these risks, the following guidelines are advised:

- Apply repellents to clothing, and where ticks are a problem, on shoes and camping gear. Permethrin-containing repellents are best because they kill as well as repel insects and ticks and they are relatively water-fast; treated clothing will remain effective after laundering. Permethrin repellents are not approved for use on skin. (Shampoos and creams containing permethrin are approved to treat head lice and scabies respectively.)

- Use repellents sparingly and apply only to skin not covered by treated clothing. Wear long sleeves, long pants, and a hat when possible.

- Formulations containing more than 30 percent DEET should be avoided or should be used with great care; they should be applied only sparingly to the skin, and only over small areas.

- Toxicity has occurred after inhalation or ingestion of DEET; use aerosols only in an open area. Safeguard containers to prevent accidental ingestion.

- Avoid applying repellent to hands of young children, who may rub them into their eyes or mouth.

- Pregnant women and nursing women should minimize use of repellents. Repellents containing ethylhexanediol may cause fetal abnormality, and are best avoided by pregnant and nursing women.

- Never use repellents on wounds, irritated skin, or mucous membranes.

- Use repellents sparingly; one application will last 4–6 hours and saturation does not increase efficacy. New formulations (e.g., Skeedadle and microencapsulated DEET) may lengthen effectiveness and reduce potential for absorption and systemic toxicity.

- Wash repellent-treated skin after returning indoors.

- If a suspected reaction to insect repellent occurs, wash treated skin and seek medical attention. Bring the repellent to the attending physician.

Dr. Theodore Tsai

mosquito, and that such a sound is repellent to hungry mated females. There is no scientific evidence at all to support this story and in any case the buzzers are set at a far higher pitch than the beat of a male mosquito's wings. Another device that has sold large numbers in the USA was claimed to simulate the sound of the dragonfly—a mosquito predator; this was recently demonstrated to be ineffective in tests conducted for Condé Nast *Traveler*. Some users believe that these devices work, but every time their effectiveness has been put to the test under controlled conditions, no difference has been found between the biting rate with the device on and with it off. More than a dozen accounts of such experiments have been published in scientific journals by entomologists from six different countries. All agree that these devices are completely useless.

CLOTHING

Long sleeves and long pants have for many years been recommended to be worn after dark to minimize the risk of mosquito bites. Canvas mosquito boots can be purchased that make it impossible for mosquitoes to bite the ankles. Denim jeans are thick enough to be impenetrable to the probosces of blackflies, which prefer to attack the lower legs. Blue clothing is said to be very attractive to tsetse flies and should be avoided in the tsetse-infested areas of Africa; the reverse is said to be true of striped patterns—which are believed to provide zebras with natural protection from tsetse flies.

- Detailed information about the contents and active ingredients of all repellent and insecticidal products can be obtained by calling the National Pesticide Telecommunications Network (NPTN) Tel. (800) 858-7378. NPTN operates 24 hours a day, seven days a week, and also provides medical information about adverse reactions.

PROTECTION AGAINST INSECTS BITING INDOORS

In addition to the repellents already described, several other useful countermeasures can be employed when the "target area" is confined to a house or hotel room.

Tight closure of well-fitting windows keeps out most mosquitoes but would be an uncomfortable proposition in a hot climate unless the room is air-conditioned. Ceiling fans help to distract the blood-seeking flight of insects, especially weak fliers such as phlebotomine sandflies.

SCREENS

Windows kept open for ventilation should be screened: fiberglass netting coated with PVC is more durable, more easily fitted, and less expensive than wire netting. The netting should have 15 to 17 threads per inch (6 or 7 threads per centimeter) width to keep out mosquitoes and should be closed before sunset, when *Culex* and *Anopheles* mosquitoes become active.

Similar netting should be used to keep mosquitoes from laying eggs in domestic water containers, in which their larvae could flourish. In cities such as Bombay the screening of roof water tanks, etc., is a strictly enforced legal requirement to prevent the breeding of the urban malaria mosquito *Anopheles stephensi* and the dengue-carrying mosquito *Aëdes aegypti*. The screening of vent pipes and other apertures to cesspits, septic tanks, and pit latrines helps to prevent the mosquito *Culex quinquefasciatus* from breeding in these collections of polluted water, to which it is attracted.

A 0.4-inch-thick floating layer of expanded polystyrene (Styrofoam) beads (as used in the manufacture of packing material) is highly effective in preventing mosquito breeding and lasts for years in such sites.

SPRAYS, COILS, AND VAPORIZING MATS

Screening windows is seldom completely effective in keeping mosquitoes out of rooms, so other lines of defense may also be needed. Aerosol spray cans of insecticide are available in many tropical countries. They usually contain pyrethroids, which are synthetic near-relations of the natural product pyrethrum and are very safe, although they should not be used over uncovered food. They do not harm pets or domestic animals.

Aerosols are good for clearing out mosquitoes that are lurking in a room before one goes to bed, but they have no residual effect on mosquitoes that enter later on during the night. The old-fashioned, but still effective, way of dealing with these insects is to light a slow-burning "mosquito coil," which will smoke gently, giving off pyrethrum or pyrethroids for six to eight hours. These are available cheaply in many tropical countries. However, tests have shown that some fraudulent brands contain no pyrethrum or pyrethroids. Local advice should be sought about good local brands, or some simple tests carried out for oneself.

A modern, smokeless version of the same idea is a small electrically operated heating plate that slowly vaporizes a "mat" or tablet containing pyrethroids. They are more effective than mosquito coils, but a reliable electricity supply and a supply of the tablets may not be available in some parts of the tropics. Heaters for vaporizing mats running off a 12-volt battery or off methylated spirit (without a flame) are available by mail order from Travel Accessories, Box 10, Lutterworth, Leicestershire LE17 4XF, UK.; Tel. 0455-558877, Fax 0455-552240.

Vapona strips slowly give off vapor of the insecticide dichlorvos without any need for heating.

The vapor emitted by coils, vaporizing mats, or vapona strips kills mosquitoes in sealed rooms, but in comfortably ventilated rooms the vapors may do no more than repel or stun insects so that they do not bite. Care may be needed to achieve even this—for example, on a porch or veranda one should always place the source of vapor upwind of those to be protected and perhaps at floor level, to deter mosquitoes heading for the ankles.

MOSQUITO NETS

The use of a mosquito bednet is strongly recommended wherever there is any risk of bites from *Anopheles* mosquitoes that carry malaria and bite at night, or the nuisance of *Culex* mosquitoes. It is well worth buying a good-quality net, because slippage of the weave would allow mosquitoes to enter. Tears should be repaired or blocked with cotton wool and the net should be tucked in carefully under the mattress.

The net should be checked after getting into bed, using a flashlight to make sure that no gaps are left. Take care not to sleep with any part of the body resting against the net—mosquitoes feed through nets, and never miss an opportunity. Rectangular nets are safer in this respect than the "tent" type.

Increased security can be achieved by impregnating nets with

The right holes...

Modern nets are made of lightweight synthetic fabric, usually polyester. Choose the right mesh size: too small, and the net becomes uncomfortably hot to use.

Standard mosquito netting uses a mesh size of 0.06 inches (1.5 mm.) (hole plus adjacent thread), equivalent to 18 holes per inch (7 holes per centimeter). A coarser mesh is possible if the net is treated with permethrin—0.16 inches (4 mm.).

permethrin* (a pyrethroid) which is effective for several months in killing or repelling mosquitoes which contact it. A dose of 0.2 gram per square meter is sufficient, which can be achieved by dipping the net in a 1-percent emulsion made by diluting an emulsifiable concentrate of permethrin with water. The net is wrung out and laid to dry on a plastic sheet. If the liquid concentrate cannot be obtained, an alternative is to use permethrin spray (sold as Permanone). Because many of the mosquitoes making contact with a permethrin-treated net are killed, one person using such a net has been shown to provide some degree of protection to a companion in the same room, but not using the net. This contrasts with the situation where only one person uses a repellent (see above) or an untreated net. There is a communal benefit when almost all the inhabitants of a village are using permethrin-impregnated nets—the risk of a malaria infective bite to those in the village only temporarily or permanently not using nets was found to be reduced by 90–95 percent in experiments in Tanzania.

Many hotels in the tropics provide mosquito nets. If in doubt it

*Permethrin is available as a 0.5 percent aerosol from Fairfield American Corporation, 201 Route 17 North, Rutherford, NJ 07070; or from Coulston International Corporation, Easton, PA 18044-0030; or from some Wal-Mart stores. The aerosol is recommended for treatment of clothing against ticks and mites which crawl on the skin. In case of difficulty, permethrin liquid emulsifiable concentrate can also be obtained by mail order from MASTA (Appendix 8). Nets already impregnated with permethrin are not sold in the USA; they can be obtained by mail order from Oasis Mosquito Nets, 1 High Street, Stoke Ferry, King's Lynn, Norfolk PE33 9SF, UK (Tel. 0366-500466; Fax 0366-501122) and cost approximately £30. After six months' use the company recommends that the net is sent back to them for re-treatment, which costs approximately £5; also from International Supplies, Alpha Place, Garth Road, Morden, Surrey SM4 4LX, UK (Tel. [081] 337-0161).

may be worth taking your own, and if suitable anchorage points are not available you should ask the management to provide some.

OTHER MEASURES

Ornamental ponds should be stocked with small fish to eat any mosquito larvae that may start to develop there. Other water containers around houses are likely to be rubbish and should be removed, buried, flattened, or punctured so that they cannot hold water.

It almost goes without saying that residents should always cooperate with any community-wide insect-control measures run by local authorities.

CONTROL OF DOMESTIC NONBITING PESTS

Although they do not bite, houseflies, roaches, ants, and termites are often worrying pests in the tropics, and some may be a serious health hazard. Flies, for example, are able to carry more than 100 different types of harmful disease-producing organisms, and may transfer them directly from excreta to food and children's faces. In the kitchen, exposed food, unwashed plates, crumbs, and garbage are an open invitation to flies, roaches, and ants. Very attractive foods such as sugar and jellies should be kept in the refrigerator and others, such as breakfast cereals, cookies, or bread, should be kept in screw-topped containers.

FLIES, ANTS, AND ROACHES

Houseflies breed in rotting garbage, and if garbage is not regularly collected by the local authorities it should be buried under a thick layer of soil. Screening of the vent pipes of pit latrines and cesspools is a most effective measure against *Chrysomya* blowflies, because light attracts them into the pipes and they are unable to escape. Mothballs on bathroom drain grilles discourage roaches from emerging from the drain. Ants' nests can often be located by following the trail of ants back to its source, and can then sometimes be destroyed with boiling water or, if the nest is in a small object such as a book, by placing it in an oven.

Old-fashioned sticky flypaper can help to keep a fly infestation in check, but in the event of a persistent fly problem, periodic use of insecticide aerosol spray cans may be necessary. These pyrethroid insecticides may also be effective in irritating roaches and driving them out of the crevices in which they hide. Otherwise, the best insecticidal approach for a roach infestation is to scatter a carbamate insecticide such as "Baygon" in powder form near crevices, drain-inspection covers, and in the bottoms of cupboards and closets.

TERMITES

In the many tropical areas where there is a serious termite problem, houses should be protected by pouring a persistent insecticide such as dieldrin into a trench around the foundations and impregnating timber with this insecticide. Before starting long-term occupation of a house, it is wise to inquire whether such precautions have been taken. For the short-term resident, termite infestation will be revealed by sinuous earth-covered tunnels adhering to the walls.

Termites can completely destroy books and other objects from within, and before this happens, the trails should be followed to where they reach ground level and liquid "Baygon" or a similar insecticide should be poured down any crevices. As an additional precaution, bookcases can be stood on bricks placed in basins of water covered in an oil film to reduce evaporation and prevent them becoming breeding places for *Aëdes aegypti* mosquitoes.

6

ANIMAL BITES; RABIES; VENOMOUS BITES AND STINGS

ANIMAL BITES; RABIES; VENOMOUS BITES AND STINGS

Snakes and scorpions may spring most readily to mind as a fearsome zoological hazard to travelers, but in practice dog bite is a much more common problem: in many countries it carries a formidable risk of rabies, and in all cases requires prompt and careful treatment. Bathers and swimmers in tropical and temperate seas should be aware of the various types of venomous marine animals, and individuals allergic to bee and wasp stings must also take special precautions.

Professor David A. Warrell *has treated animal bites and stings in five continents. He is Professor of Tropical Medicine and Infectious Diseases and Director of the Center for Tropical Medicine, University of Oxford, Honorary Clinical Director of the Alistair Reid Venom Research Unit at the Liverpool School of Tropical Medicine, and a Consultant to the WHO. The illustrations in this chapter were drawn by Professor Warrell.*

Encounters with animals can produce the following medical problems, all of which are uncommon but potentially fatal: mechanical injury, envenoming, infection, infestation, and allergic reactions. Only the first three of these will be discussed in detail in this chapter.

INJURIES: ATTACKS BY LARGE ANIMALS

Many species of animals are equipped with claws, teeth, tusks, horns, or spines capable of inflicting serious mechanical injuries which may prove fatal. With the one exception of bites by domestic dogs, these accidents are very rare and are easily avoided by treating all large animals with respect and avoiding unnecessarily close contact with them.

Most wild animals, unless they are ill or starving, avoid confrontation with humans. Visitors to game parks in the tropics or to safari parks in the temperate zones should take local advice about where and when it is safe to walk (see also p. 392). Strolls between dusk and dawn without a light invite attacks by large carnivores. It is usually safe to approach large carnivores in a hard-topped vehicle, but under some circumstances this may not be a safe place from which to view elephants or rhinoceroses.

Animals in zoos or safari parks should not be assumed to be tamer and therefore safer. Two keepers have been killed by tigers and two by elephants in British zoos or safari parks during the last few years; in the last 15 years, tigers have killed 659 people in Sunderbans Reserve Forest, in West Bengal; and between 1967 and 1986, 12 people were killed by grizzly bears in Banff, Glacier, and Yellowstone National Parks, with 126 attacks by these bears in North American National Parks during the first 80 years of this century.

Other mammals known to have killed or severely mauled humans include lions, leopards, wild cats, wolves, hyenas, hippopotamuses, camels, buffaloes, and wild pigs. Recently, a man was killed by an ostrich in Zimbabwe.

Sharks claim about fifty lives each year out of 100 reported attacks, mostly between latitudes 30°N. and 30°S. Much smaller fish may pose a greater threat to human life in some parts of the world. Garfish, for example (which have long spearlike snouts), have been known to leap out of the water and impale fishermen in parts of the Indo-Pacific Ocean. Moray and conger eels, groupers, barracudas, and stingrays can also produce severe mechanical injuries with their teeth or spines.

Fish capable of delivering electric shocks are found in freshwater rivers of South America ("electric eel"—*Electrophorus electricus*) and Africa (electric catfish—*Malopterurus electricus*) and in the sea (e.g., torpedo rays). The electric eel can discharge up to 650 volts at 1 ampere 400 times per second and is capable of killing an adult human. The electric catfish can discharge 90 volts at 0.1 amp and is not dangerous, but the torpedo ray produces a dangerous shock in salt water of 80 volts at high amperage. Victims should be given cardiorespiratory resuscitation as in other cases of electric shock.

It is foolhardy to wade, bathe, or swim in rivers or lakes in the tropics unless they are known to be safe—not only from bilharzia (p. 94) but from crocodiles as well. Crocodiles continue to take a small toll of human life. Riverine populations in the Sudan, Central Africa, and Southeast Asia are at risk. The annual mortality from the Nile crocodile in Africa may exceed 1,000 and small numbers of accidents caused by the saltwater or estuarine crocodile are reported from Indonesia, Sarawak, and northern Australia.

The giant pythons (reticulated python of Indonesia, African rock python, and anaconda of South America) are certainly capable of killing a human and there are a few reliable reports of fatal attacks.

Travelers, however, are at far greater risk of receiving injury from a dog bite before leaving their home country than from a wild animal on their travels.

In the USA there are now more than a million dog bites each year requiring some sort of hospital attention; the number is increasing. In Liverpool and Sunderland, in the north of England, about 500 people per 100,000 population go to the hospital each year because of dog bites. Reports of 11 deaths from dog bites were collected in a two-year period in the USA, and there have been several in the UK during the last few years. Domestic cattle (especially bulls), rams, pigs, cats, and even ferrets have also killed people.

TYPES OF INJURY

Teeth and claws produce lacerating and destructive injuries to soft tissues. Tusks, horns, and antlers can tear and produce serious penetrating injuries resulting in blindness, pneumothorax, and hemothorax (leakage of air and blood into the lining of the lungs), perforation of the intestines, and bleeding from the liver and spleen. Even dog bites are capable of producing compound fractures (where the broken bone ends protrude through the skin).

All bites, gorings, and maulings carry a heavy risk of infection with bacteria, viruses, and other microorganisms present in the animal's mouth or contaminating its claws, horns, etc. Large mammals may trample and kneel on the human victim, producing severe crush injuries.

FIRST AID

A guide to the treatment of mammal bites, licks, and scratches is given in the box on p. 199. Mild superficial injuries should be cleaned thoroughly. Anyone who has suffered a serious attack should be taken to a hospital for proper assessment. The use of antibiotics, antitetanus, and antirabies treatments may need to be considered.

RABIES

Rabies, or "hydrophobia," is a virus infection of mammals that can be transmitted to humans in a variety of ways, but usually as the result of a bite by a domestic dog.

Rabies probably causes at least 50,000 human deaths each year, although only a small fraction of these are reported to official bodies such as the WHO. At least 10 human cases are known to have occurred in travelers returning to the USA between 1980 and 1992, but hundreds of travelers have had to undergo post-exposure treatment.

In areas where rabies exists, the infection is usually established and circulates only in a few particular animal species. These may include domestic animals, particularly dogs, and/or wild animal species, for example, skunks, raccoons, foxes, and insectivorous bats in North America (in the USA, rabid bats have been reported from every state except Alaska and Hawaii, and have caused rabies in at least 18 humans); foxes in the Arctic; mongooses and vampire bats in the Caribbean; vampire bats in Central and South America; foxes, wolves, raccoon dogs, and insectivorous bats in Europe; and wolves, jackals, and small carnivores such as mongooses and civets throughout most of Africa and Asia.

Humans may contract rabies from any rabid animal, domestic or wild, but because of the particularly close association between humans and dogs the most common cause of human rabies worldwide is the bite of a rabid domestic dog (which may itself have contracted the virus from another dog, cat, or from a rabid wild animal). In the USA, canine rabies has been largely eliminated through measures such as immunization, but there is still a risk to people who come in contact with rabies-affected wild animal populations— naturalists, animal trappers, and people on expeditions, for example. Thus a bite from a skunk in the Midwestern USA or from a jackal in Africa could involve a very significant risk of rabies. A little girl died recently from rabies, following contact with an unidentified wild animal in New York state.

GEOGRAPHICAL DISTRIBUTION

Rabies occurs in most parts of the world, in Greenland, Canada, and North America, throughout the Commonwealth of Independent States (formerly the USSR), China, and New Territories of Hong Kong, as well as in the main tropical regions.

The following areas are free of rabies at present: Britain and Ireland, mainland Norway, Sweden, and Iceland, peninsular Malaysia, New Guinea, Taiwan, Japan, Oceania, Antarctica, Australia, and New Zealand. Human and animal rabies is most common in parts of South America, the Indian subcontinent, Thailand, Vietnam, and the Philippines.

HOW INFECTION OCCURS

Rabies infection can occur when the normal protective barrier provided by healthy, unbroken skin is breached by a bite or scratch, and the wound is contaminated with the animal's saliva containing rabies virus. Rabies virus can penetrate unbroken mucous membranes such as those covering the eye and lining the mouth or nose. On a few occasions, rabies has developed after the virus has been inhaled—in the air of bat-infested caves in Texas—and as the result of a laboratory accident. On at least four occasions, recipients of corneal transplants from patients dying of unsuspected rabies have later developed rabies themselves.

After the virus has entered the body, it may be killed by antiseptics used to clean the wound or by the person's own immune defense mechanisms. Unless this happens within a few days of the bite, the virus is likely to spread to the nerve endings in muscles and along the nerves which lead to the brain and spinal cord; it then multiplies and causes a severe infection of the central nervous system (called an encephalomyelitis), which is almost invariably fatal.

Rarely, it seems that the virus may become permanently or temporarily inactive after it has reached the nervous system; in the latter case the infection may flare up again, and progress months or even years after the initial bite, following some kind of stress. This may explain the occasional reports of very long incubation periods.

The incubation period—the time interval between the bite and

TREATMENT OF MAMMAL BITES, LICKS, AND SCRATCHES

First aid
- Scrub with soap or detergent and running water for at least five minutes.
- Remove foreign material (e.g. dirt, broken teeth).
- Rinse with plain water.
- Irrigate with a virucidal agent, such as povidone iodine (Betadine), 0.01 percent aqueous iodine, or 40–70 percent alcohol (gin and whisky contain 40 percent). Note: hydrogen peroxide, mercurochrome, and quaternary ammonium compounds—the brightly colored antiseptic dyes still popular in some countries— are not suitable for this purpose.

At the hospital or dispensary
A medical attendant should:
- Check that first-aid measures (above) have been carried out.
- Explore and irrigate deep wounds (if necessary, under local or general anesthesia). Dead tissue should be cut away, but wound excision is rarely necessary.
- Avoid suturing (stitches) and occlusive dressings.
- Consider tetanus risk and treat accordingly:
- Give a booster dose of tetanus formol toxoid (0.5 ml. by intramuscular injection) for those fully immunized in the past and boosted within the last 10 years; give human tetanus immune globulin (250 mg. by intramuscular injection) for severe or grossly contaminated wounds that have been left untreated for more than four hours in a previously unimmunized person.
- Consider risk of infection with other bacteria, viruses, and fungi particularly associated with mammal bites. Preventive antibiotic treatment is advisable for severely contaminated wounds, e.g. a broad-spectrum antibiotic such as amoxycillin (500 mg. three times a day for five days) (see pp. 200–1).
- If the exposure occurred in a rabies-endemic area, consider post-exposure rabies vaccination.

the first symptoms of rabies—is usually two to three months but can vary from a few days to many years. The earliest symptom of rabies infection of the central nervous system is itching, irritation, tingling, or pain at the site of the healed bite wound. The disease advances rapidly, producing headache, fever, spreading paralysis, and episodes of confusion, aggression, hallucination, and hydrophobia (literally fear of water). Attempts to drink water induce powerful contractions of the neck muscles and the muscles involved in swallowing and breathing in. These spasms are associated with indescribable terror. The patient dies in a few days.

Some species of animals such as mongooses, skunks, and vampire bats can recover from rabies encephalomyelitis, but in humans the infection is almost invariably fatal. During the last 15 years, two patients with probable rabies and only one with proven rabies have recovered after prolonged intensive care.

The prospect of an agonizing death from this untreatable disease should encourage everyone to do everything possible to prevent rabies.

PRE-EXPOSURE VACCINATION

Pre-exposure vaccination against rabies should be considered in the case of travelers who run a high risk. These include cave explorers, animal collectors, zoologists, botanists, hunters, and also those whose work involves walking and cycling in urban or rural areas, as well as travelers spending a prolonged period in endemic areas. One of the safe new tissue-culture vaccines, such as the Connaught/Institut Merieux human diploid cell strain vaccine (HDCV) and purified vero cell rabies vaccine (PVRV) or Behring-werke purified chicken embryo cell vaccine (PCEC) should be used (see Table 6.1, p. 202). Expense can be reduced by giving one-tenth of the normally recommended dose by intradermal rather than intramuscular or subcutaneous injection, but this regime is not satisfactory if chloroquine or mefloquine is being taken (e.g., for malaria prophylaxis) at the time of immunization.

Travelers within a rabies-endemic area should avoid close contact with domestic or wild mammals. They should be particularly wary of wild animals that appear tame, for this change in behavior is a common early sign of rabies in animals.

ACTION FOLLOWING A BITE

Irrespective of the risk of rabies, all mammal bites, scratches, and licks on mucous membranes or broken skin should be cleaned immediately and vigorously (see box, p. 199). Mammal bites (including human bites!) are usually contaminated by a variety of bacteria, some of which can cause serious infections.

In the case of deep penetrating or contaminated wounds, it is wise to take a prophylactic antibiotic (such as amoxycillin 500 mg. three times a day for 5 days, tetracycline 500 mg. four times a day for 5 days, trimethoprim/sulfamethoxazole [Septra, Bactrim] 1 tablet twice a day for 5 days, or cefuroxime axetil [Ceftin] 250 mg. twice a day for 5 days)—all *adult* doses. The risk of tetanus should always be considered: all travelers should be fully protected with a course of tetanus toxoid before starting their journey. An animal bite warrants a booster dose of tetanus toxoid (tetanus formol toxoid 0.5 ml.).

POST-EXPOSURE VACCINATION

The aim of post-exposure vaccination is to neutralize the rabies virus introduced by the bite before it can enter the nervous system. Treatment should be started as soon as possible, but although the chances of preventing rabies decrease with delay, vaccination is still worthwhile even weeks or months after the bite. The decision about vaccination should be made by a physician, who will need the following information:

1. When, where, and in which locality the bite occurred; the circumstances—was it unprovoked?
2. The severity and site of the bite;
3. The species, appearance, behavior, and fate of the biting animal; whether it had been vaccinated against rabies during the last year.

This information should allow some assessment of the risk of exposure, but if there is any doubt it is safest to give a full course of vaccine with or without passive immunization (see p. 202). The first dose of vaccine should be tripled and divided between several sites on the body if there has been more than 48 hours' delay in starting vaccination, if passive immunization has been given more than 24 hours before vaccine, if the patient is elderly, malnourished, or believed to be immunodeficient or immunosuppressed, and if passive immunization is not available.

The newer tissue-culture antirabies vaccines such as HDCV carry no serious risk of reactions, unlike the older vaccines, which consisted of animal nervous tissue.

Passive immunization (see p. 202) should never be omitted in cases of severe bites or high risk of exposure unless the patient has had pre-exposure vaccination. "Ready-made" rabies-neutralizing antibody in the form of human rabies immune globulin (HRIG) or equine antirabies serum (EARS) is necessary to provide immediate activity against rabies virus during the interval of about seven days between vaccination and the first appearance of antibody produced by the body itself in response to the vaccine. HRIG is free from side effects, but equine antirabies serum is complicated by allergic reactions such as serum sickness in up to 10 percent of those treated.

Travelers who are exposed to the risk of rabies (mammal bites, licks, scratches, etc.) should seek immediate help at the time of the incident, and not wait for days (or even months) until they return home before considering post-exposure treatment.

Only orthodox/Western medical practitioners should be consulted about rabies, *not* herbalists, homeopaths, traditional practitioners, monks, priests, or other practitioners of "fringe medicine." In some countries even Western-style practitioners may not give

TABLE 6.1. RABIES IMMUNIZATION SCHEDULES

Pre-exposure vaccination
Merieux (Connaught) human diploid cell strain vaccine (HDCV)
1 ml. by intramuscular (*im*) injection* on days 0, 7, and 28
+ boosters of 1 ml. by *im* injection every two years if there is continued high exposure *or* have antibody test.

Post-exposure vaccination (Do not forget wound cleaning! See box, p. 199).
A *For those who have been given pre-exposure vaccination:*
No passive immunization (human immune-globulin/equine antirabies serum) is needed.
HDCV PVRV or PCEC 1 ml. by intramuscular (*im*) injection on days 0 and 3.
B *For those not given pre-exposure vaccination:*
HDCV, PVRV, or PCEC 1 ml. by *im* injection on days 0, 3, 7, 14, and 30.[†]
AND
Passive immunization with human rabies
immune-globulin 20 units/kg body weight
or   half infiltrated round
Equine antirabies serum   the bite wound, half
40 units/kg body weight   by *im* injection

---

*An economical regimen using 0.1 ml. by intradermal (*id*) injection rather than 1 ml. by *im* injection is effective, but is recommended only if the patient is being vaccinated in the United States.
[†]Two other regimens are effective and can be recommended:
   (1) 8-site intradermal regimen: 0.1 ml. HDCV given at 8 sites (deltoids, suprascapular, abdominal, and thighs) on day 0, 4 sites on day 7, and single sites on days 28 and 90. This is very economical and induces antibody rapidly.
   (2) 2-1-1 regimen: 2 × 1 ml. *im* injections on day 0, single 1 ml. injections on days 7 and 21. This is quite economical and requires only three vaccination sessions.

RABIES PREVENTION FOLLOWING EXPOSURE IN A RISK AREA

MINOR EXPOSURE

including licks of the skin, scratches or abrasions, minor bites:

▶ *Unprovoked attack by cat or dog:*

- Vaccine
- Stop treatment if animal remains healthy for ten days.
- Stop treatment if laboratory test on animal's brain proves negative.
- Administer serum on positive diagnosis and complete the course of vaccine.

▶ *Attack by wild animal or by domestic cat or dog unavailable for observation:*

- Serum and vaccine

MAJOR EXPOSURE

including licks on mucosa or major bites (multiple or on face, head, fingers, or neck):

▶ *Unprovoked attack by cat or dog or attack by wild animal, or domestic cat or dog unavailable for observation:*

- Serum and vaccine
- Stop treatment if domestic cat or dog remains healthy under observation for five days.
- Stop treatment if animal's brain fluorescent antibody test proves negative.

adequate treatment. *No one exposed to rabies should allow themselves to be fobbed off with tablets or a single injection.*

In the USA, expert advice and materials for post-exposure treatment are available from local or state health departments, or from the Division of Viral Diseases at the Centers for Disease Control and Prevention, Tel. (404) 329-3095 (24-hour service).

VENOMOUS ANIMALS

Many animals possess venoms that can be injected into the unfortunate traveler by a variety of mechanisms. The normal purpose of envenoming is to discourage enemies or to immobilize prey.

Some people become sensitized to venoms if they are stung or bitten repeatedly. In this case, the allergic reaction to the venom may prove far more dangerous than its toxic effects, and in some parts of the world, such as Europe and North America, there are more deaths from allergic (anaphylactic) reactions to bee and wasp stings than from lethal snake, scorpion, and spider venoms.

Tropical regions have the richest venomous fauna, and travelers to these areas often regard snake bite and scorpion sting as the two greatest medical hazards of their journey. However, it is nearly always the indigenous population, rather than the traveler, that falls victim to venomous animals.

Snakebite is a major cause of death among South American Indians who hunt barefooted in the jungle, and among rice farmers in Southeast Asia who work barefooted and barehanded in the paddy fields. Travelers are usually less exposed and better protected, and there has been no report of American or European travelers dying from a venomous bite or sting in recent years. However, a German tourist came close to death after being bitten by a cobra in central Bangkok, several other Europeans have been severely envenomed in the jungles of South America and Southeast Asia, and a number of scientists working in the jungles of Central America have also been severely envenomed.

Anyone planning to travel off the beaten track in a tropical country should find out about the venomous fauna well before leaving home. An expedition to a particularly remote and snake-infested area may want to take its own supply of antivenom. Usually, this can be supplied only by a national center of antivenom production; contact will have to be made with the center well in advance. Many antivenoms available in Europe and in tropical countries are of dubious potency. Information supplied with commercial antivenoms (the "package insert") may be misleading or even dangerous! It is also important to find out something about the quality of local medical services or referral centers in the larger cities.

Information and advice about venomous fauna and availability of antivenoms can be obtained from the centers listed at the end of this chapter.

VENOMOUS SNAKES

Venomous snakes have one or more pairs of enlarged teeth, the fangs, in the upper jaw. Venom is conducted from the venom gland just behind the eye, through a duct to the base of the fang, and then through a channel to its tip.

DANGEROUS SPECIES
Important venomous snakes belong to four families:

The Hydrophiidae, sea snakes (Fig. 6.1A).

The Elapidae, which include cobras (Figs. 6.1B and 6.2), kraits (Fig. 6.3), mambas (Fig. 6.4), coral snakes, terrestrial Australasian snakes, and the South African ringhals and African and Asian spitting cobras, which can eject venom from the tips of their fangs as a defensive strategy.

The Viperidae, which are the largest and best-known family of venomous snakes and include the subfamilies *Viperinae,* the Old World vipers (Figs. 6.1C and 6.5) and adders; and *Crotalinae,* the New World rattlesnakes, moccasins, and lance-headed vipers (Fig. 6.6), and Asian pit vipers.

The Colubridae, of which some members have small fangs at the back of their mouth (Fig. 6.1D). Effective bites in humans are very uncommon but a few species, such as the African boomslang and bird, twig, or vine snake have caused some fatalities.

The Atractaspididae, burrowing asps or stiletto snakes, are found in Africa and the Middle East. They strike sideways, with one long fang protruding from their mouth (Fig. 6.1E).

Venomous snakes do not occur at high altitudes (more than 16,000 feet or about 5,000 meters), in the Antarctic, or in a number of islands such as Ireland, Iceland, Crete, New Zealand, Madagascar (where there is a mildly venomous rear-fanged colubrid snake—*Madagascarophis*), and most Caribbean and Pacific islands (see Map 6.1). Sea snakes inhabit the warmer oceans within latitudes 40° north and south, except for the Atlantic (see Map 6.2).

The incidence and medical significance of snakebite has been underestimated because it is a problem of the rural tropics, often little known to academic centers in the capital cities even of countries where it is particularly common. As mentioned above, the incidence of snakebite is highest among native populations who are forced to live and work, relatively unprotected, within the snake's chosen environment. Epidemics of snakebite can result from flooding and invasion of a snake-infested region by a large human work force.

EFFECTS OF SNAKE VENOM

Snake venoms are complicated substances which contain a large number of harmful components. The main clinical effects of snake venoms are summarized below:

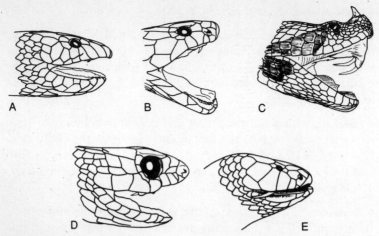

Fig. 6.1 Fangs of the five families of venomous snakes. A: sea snake (*Hydrophis cyanocinctus*, family Hydrophiidae), very small front fang; B: Thai spitting cobra ("*Naja atra*," family Elapidae), erect front fangs; C: Gaboon viper (*Bitis gabonica*, family Viperidae), long, hinged front fangs; D: boomslang (*Dispholidus typus*, family Colubridae), rear fangs; E: burrowing asp or stiletto snake (*Atractaspis aterrima*, family Atractaspididae).

- *Local swelling, bruising, blistering, and necrosis (gangrene) of the bitten limb* with enlargement of local lymph glands (e.g., in the armpit or groin) are seen particularly with *Viperidae* and some cobras. Fluid and blood leaks into the tissues of the bitten limb. Swelling starts soon after the bite and may spread to involve the whole limb and adjoining area of the trunk.

- *Bleeding and blood-clotting disorders* occur mainly in patients bitten by *Viperidae, Colubridae,* and Australian venomous snakes. The commonest sites of bleeding are the gums, nose, and stomach.

- *Shock (fall in blood pressure)* may occur in patients bitten by *Viperidae.*

- *Paralysis ("neurotoxicity")* is first manifest by inability to open the eyes (ptosis), but later spreads to other muscles, particularly those responsible for swallowing and breathing. The *Elapidae, Hydrophiidae,* and a few of the *Viperidae* have neurotoxic venoms. Venoms of *Hydrophiidae,* Australian snakes, and of several species of the *Viperidae* may cause extensive direct muscle damage, with painful stiff muscles and paralysis.

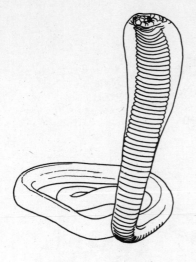

Fig. 6.2 Egyptian cobra (*Naja haje*) in typical threatening/defensive posture.

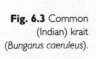

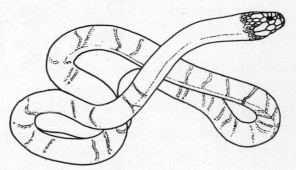

Fig. 6.3 Common (Indian) krait (*Bungarus caeruleus*).

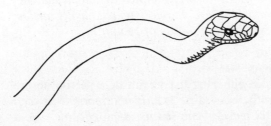

Fig. 6.4 Black mamba (*Dendroaspis polylepis*).

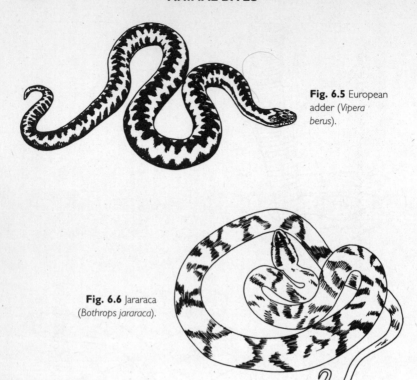

Fig. 6.5 European adder (*Vipera berus*).

Fig. 6.6 Jararaca (*Bothrops jararaca*).

- *Kidney failure* resulting from clotting of blood in the small blood vessels, prolonged shock, or a direct action of the venom is a major feature of bites by Russell's viper, and some of the *Crotalinae* in the Americas.

Despite this formidable repertoire of toxic effects, many people bitten by venomous snakes suffer *negligible* or *no* envenoming. It may be that the snake's strike is not well adapted to human anatomy and that *a large number of bites are therefore mechanically ineffective and fail to inject significant amounts of venom.*

MANAGEMENT OF SNAKEBITE
First aid for snakebite, either by the victim or a person on the spot, is summarized in the box on p. 212. *It is important to keep calm, immobilize the bitten limb as far as is practicable, avoid*

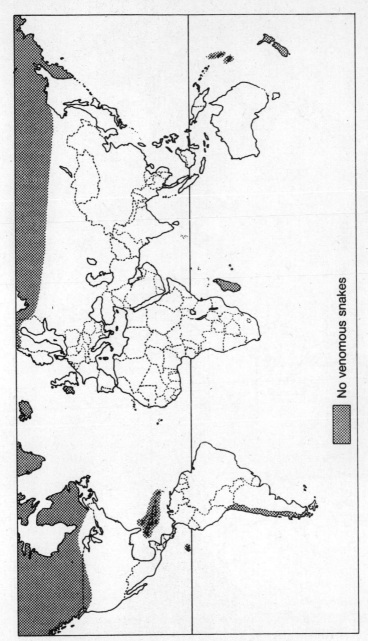

No venomous snakes

Map 6.1 Areas where there are no venomous snakes.

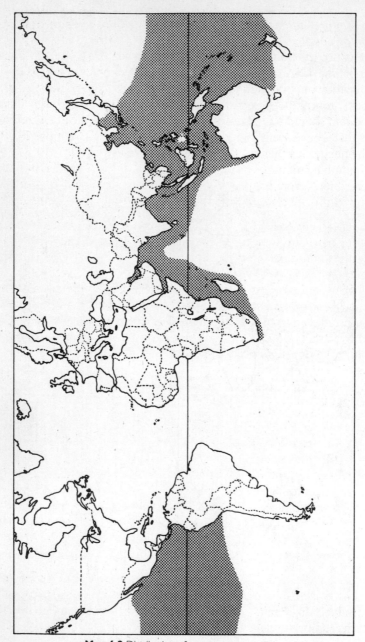

Map 6.2 Distribution of venomous sea snakes.

harmful first-aid measures and get to the hospital or dispensary as soon as possible.

Most of the traditional first-aid remedies for snakebite still popular in the USA and elsewhere, such as suction, local incisions, application of potassium permanganate crystals, cold packs, electric shocks, tourniquets, herbs, and snake stones, do more harm than good and should not be used. All commercially produced snakebite kits that I have seen, including vacuum extractors, are more likely to be dangerous than useful.

Immobilization of the bitten limb is important, because muscle contraction (exercise) promotes the systemic spread of venom via veins and lymphatics.

Tourniquets and bandaging are not generally recommended. The only circumstance in which compression bandaging or a tourniquet might be considered is following a bite by a dangerously neurotoxic elapid (such as some cobras, mambas, kraits, coral snakes, or Australasian elapids) or sea snake. In such cases ace, biscard, or cotton stretch bandaging and splinting of the whole bitten limb is more comfortable and possibly more effective than applying a pressure pad over the wound or a conventional tight (arterial) tourniquet around the upper arm or thigh. However, the use of compression may increase the local effects of necrotic venoms such as those of cobras and Viperidae. No tourniquet should be left in place for more than two hours.

Reassurance is a most important part of treatment. Most snakebite victims are terrified, but only a minority of bites, even by dangerously venomous species, produce serious envenoming.

The speed of the lethal effects of snake venoms has been greatly exaggerated. To kill a man, lethal doses of venom usually take hours in the case of neurotoxic species such as cobras, mambas, and sea snakes, or days in the case of vipers and rattlesnakes, not seconds or minutes as is commonly believed. This interval between bite and death is usually sufficiently long to allow effective treatment.

Pain If pain is a problem, a safe pain-killing drug for snakebite victims is acetaminophen (Tylenol)—the dose is one or two 500-mg. tablets for adults. Aspirin should never be used in snakebite victims as it may cause stomach bleeding.

Medical treatment At the hospital or dispensary, medically trained

SNAKEBITE: FIRST AID

1. Reassure the patient.

2. Immobilize the bitten limb with a splint or sling.

3. Move the patient to the hospital or a dispensary as quickly as possible.

4. Avoid harmful measures such as incisions, suction, potassium permanganate crystals, electric shocks, and tourniquets (except as below).

5. Use acetaminophen *not* aspirin to treat pain.

6. If you have your own supply of antivenom, take it with you to the hospital or dispensary.

7. If the snake has been killed, take it along with you to the hospital or dispensary, but do not handle it with your bare hands, even if it appears dead.

8. Only if the patient has definitely been bitten by a dangerously neurotoxic species (e.g., cobra, mamba, krait, coral snake, Australian elapid, sea snake) firmly ace-bandage and splint the bitten limb or apply a tight tourniquet around the upper arm or thigh.

staff should examine the patient and dead snake if brought, and decide about further treatment. The only specific remedy for snakebite is antivenom (also known as antivenin, antivenene, or antisnakebite serum), which is made in animals, usually horses, by immunizing them with increasing doses of snake venom. Although most modern antivenoms are refined and purified, injection of "foreign" protein (i.e., from another species of animal) always carries the risk of potentially serious reactions. To be optimally effective, antivenom must be given by a slow intravenous injection or infusion.

Not all people bitten by snakes require antivenom. Since the decision about antivenom treatment, the administration of antivenom by the intravenous route, and the treatment of antivenom reactions all require clinical skill, lay people should not undertake the medical treatment of snakebite except under most unusual conditions (for example, a serious bite in a member of an expedition in a very remote area).

As a life-saving measure, antivenom may be given by intramuscular injection (the dose divided between the upper outer quadrants of both buttocks), followed by massage to promote absorption of the antivenom into the bloodstream. *However, this is certainly not recommended as a general rule!*

Patients who need antivenom are those in whom there is evidence that venom has been absorbed and is circulating throughout the body to produce severe general effects ("systemic envenoming"). The important signs are loss of consciousness, low blood pressure, failure of the blood to clot, bleeding from the nose or gums or vomiting blood, generalized pain and stiffness in the muscles, and paralysis.

The earliest sign of neurotoxic poisoning is an inability of the upper eyelids to retract when the bitten person tries to look up ("ptosis"). Slight bleeding from the site of the bite and mild local swelling and bruising are not normally regarded as justification for antivenom treatment, but massive local swelling involving more than half the bitten limb (for example above the knee and above the elbow in bites of the foot and hand respectively) indicate that significant amounts of venom have been injected and that antivenom is probably required, especially if the snake is known to have a venom that causes necrosis (gangrene).

Administration of antivenom by a medically qualified person For intravenous injection, freeze-dried antivenom is dissolved in sterile water for injection (usually 10 ml. per ampoule) and liquid antivenom is given neat. The injection should be given slowly, at a rate not more than 2 ml. per minute. A method that is easier to control, but requires more equipment, is to dilute antivenom with "normal"/isotonic saline or 5 percent dextrose solution, making up the volume to 200 ml. This is given through an intravenous giving set and is infused over about 30 minutes, starting slowly (30 drops per minute), then speeding up after about 10 minutes if there is no reaction. The dose of antivenom varies with the manufacturer and the severity of envenoming. It is usually not less than five ampoules. **THE SAME DOSE SHOULD BE GIVEN TO CHILDREN AS TO ADULTS!**

Antivenom should never be given, even by medically qualified staff, unless epinephrine (0.5 ml. of a 1 mg./ml. or 1 in 1,000 solution by subcutaneous injection) is available to treat antivenom reactions.

The commonest symptoms of an antivenom reaction are itching, the appearance of a raised reddened rash (urticaria), and a throbbing headache. More serious symptoms include coughing, vomiting, wheezing, and fall in blood pressure leading to unconsciousness. At the first sign of a reaction, epinephrine should be given by subcutaneous injection.

Epinephrine is dangerous if given by other routes. An antihistamine drug should also be given, preferably chlorpheniramine maleate (Chlor-Trimeton) 10 mg. by intravenous injection. Allergic patients (those suffering from asthma, hay fever, and eczema) are more likely to develop severe antivenom reactions than other people. Unfortunately there is no reliable way of predicting, by the use of a skin test, whether or not someone will develop a reaction.

Although I would strongly discourage lay people from giving antivenom themselves, it may be worth some expeditions taking a small supply (5–10 ampoules) of antivenom* to be given by a local physician or dispensary if the need arises. Unfortunately, the supply of antivenom to rural hospitals and health centers in the tropics is often very unreliable.

Infection There is a small but definite risk of tetanus and secondary bacterial infection following snakebite. A booster dose of tetanus toxoid and a course of penicillin should therefore be given.

PREVENTION OF SNAKEBITE

Fortunately, travelers can virtually exclude the risk of being bitten by a snake if they heed the following advice.

Snakes and snake-charmers should be avoided as far as possible. If you happen to see a snake, do not disturb, corner, or attack it, and never attempt to handle a snake even if it is said to be a harmless species or appears to be dead. Even a severed head can bite!

---

* *Principal antivenom manufacturers* Wyeth-Ayerst Laboratories, Box 8299, Philadelphia, PA 19101-1245, USA (North America and Mexico); Instituto Clodomiro Picado, Universidad de Costa Rica, Ciudad Universitaria, Rodrigo Facio, San José, Costa Rica (Central America); Instituto Butantan, Caixa Postal 65, 05504 São Paulo, Brazil (South America); Pasteur Merieux serum et vaccin, 1541 Av. Marcel Merieux, 69280 Marcy l'Etoile, Lyon, France (Europe, Middle East, Africa); Behringwerke AG, Postfach 1140, D-3550 Marburg/Lahn 1, Germany (Europe, Middle East, Africa); Institute of Immunology, Rockerfellerova 2, Zagreb, Croatia; South African Institute for Medical Research, P.O. Box 1038, Johannesburg 2000, Republic of South Africa (Africa); Haffkine Biopharmaceutical Corporation Ltd., Acharya, Donde Marg, Parel, Bombay 400012, India (Indian Subcontinent); Thai Red Cross Society, Queen Saovabha Memorial Institute, Rama IV Road, Bangkok, Thailand (Southeast Asia); Commonwealth Serum Laboratories, 45 Poplar Road, Parkville, Victoria 3052, Australia (Australasia).

If you should happen to find yourself confronted with a snake at close quarters, try to keep absolutely still until it has slithered away: snakes strike only at moving objects.

Never walk in undergrowth or deep sand without boots, socks, and long pants; and at night always carry a light. Unlit paths are particularly dangerous after rainstorms or floods. Never collect firewood or move logs and boulders with your bare hands, and never push your hands or sticks into burrows, holes, or crevices. Avoid climbing trees and rocks that are covered with thick foliage and never swim in overgrown rivers or lakes (there are a good many other reasons for not swimming in lakes and rivers in the tropics!).

If you are forced to sleep in the open or under canvas, try to raise your bed at least one foot off the ground or else use a sewn-in groundsheet or mosquito net that can be zipped up or well tucked in. Snakes never attack man without provocation but will strike if grabbed, trodden on, or even if someone rolls onto them in their sleep. Snakes are sometimes attracted to human dwellings in pursuit of their prey (domestic chicks, rats, mice, toads, and lizards). Sea snakes bite only when they are picked out of fishing nets or trodden on by waders.

It has not proved possible, nor would it be desirable, to exterminate venomous snakes. The Burma (Myanmar) rice farmer may regard the Russell's viper as his enemy, but in fact the snake protects his livelihood, the rice crop, by controlling the rodent population.

VENOMOUS FISH

Fish sting by impaling their supposed aggressor on venomous spines which may form part of the dorsal and pectoral fins and gill covers or may be separate appendages situated in front of the dorsal fins or on the tail. Tropical coral reefs, especially of the Indo-Pacific region, harbor the greatest number and diversity of venomous fish. Fish stings can also occur in temperate waters such as along the coasts of the UK and Europe (e.g., Adriatic and Cornish coasts).

DANGEROUS SPECIES

Members of at least five families of fish have caused human deaths: sharks and dogfish, stingrays and mantas, catfish, weeverfish, scorpionfish, and stargazers.

Stingrays (Rajiformes) cause many stings in North America. Waders and bathers may tread on these fish as they lie in the mud or sand. The tail, armed with a formidable spine up to a foot long in some species, is lashed against the intrusive limb, causing severe mechanical trauma and releasing venom into the wound.

Weeverfish (Trachinidae) occur in temperate waters of the North Sea, Mediterranean, and north coast of Africa.

Scorpionfish (Scorpaenidae) include the very dangerous stonefish (which lies motionless and well camouflaged on the bottom, resembling a roughly textured lump of rock) and the attractive zebra or lionfish (Fig. 6.7). They occur throughout the Indian and Pacific oceans.

EFFECTS OF FISH VENOM

Fish stings can produce excruciating pain radiating from the wound, some local swelling, vomiting, diarrhea, sweating, fall in blood pressure, and irregularities of the heartbeat.

Treatment To relieve the intense pain the stung limb, finger, or toe should be immersed in water that is hot enough to be uncomfortable but not scalding (just under 120°F., or 65°C.). Alternatively, a local anesthetic such as procaine (Novocain) or lidocaine can be injected. The most effective way to deal with a stung finger or toe is to apply a "ring block" of local anesthetic—a simple procedure that any physician should be able to perform. The stinging spine and mem-

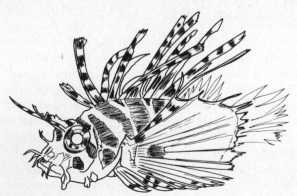

Fig. 6.7 Lionfish (*Brachirus* species, family Scorpaenidae) from Papua New Guinea.

If hot water is not available to treat a fish sting, make a hot compress by heating a wet towel on the engine block of a car or boat motor that has recently been used, and then apply its clean side to the wound. Alternatively a heat-lamp effect can be achieved by using a boat spotlight: hold the affected area close to the spotlight. Be careful, however, not to allow the skin to touch either the spotlight or the engine block directly, because this can produce a burn.

Dr. Stanley Schwartz, Fort Myers, Florida

branes should be removed to prevent secondary infection of the wound. If the patient loses consciousness, stops breathing, and no arterial pulse can be felt, mouth-to-mouth respiration and external cardiac massage should be used.

Antivenoms for *Scorpaenidae* and *Trachinidae* are manufactured in Australia and in the former Yugoslavia. Waders and bathers can avoid stepping on stinging fish by using a shuffling gait in sand or mud, and prodding in front of them with a stick. Footwear is protective, although not against stingray spines. Skin divers should be aware of the dangers of stinging fish, especially in the neighborhood of coral reefs.

FOOD POISONING AND MARINE ANIMALS

See pp. 60–69 (Poisons and contaminants in food).

VENOMOUS JELLYFISH AND RELATED ANIMALS

Jellyfish, sea wasps, Portuguese men-of-war, polyps, hydroids, sea anemones, sea nettles, and corals all belong to a group of animals called the *Coelenterates*. The tentacles of these often brightly colored and beautiful animals are armed with myriads of stinging capsules (called nematocysts) which discharge when touched by a swimmer. In many cases the worst that can occur is an itchy skin rash, but some jellyfish can cause a severe sting. The most dangerous species is the box jellyfish (*Chironex fleckeri*) of the Indo-Pacific region. Severe stings produce violent shivering, vomiting, and diarrhea with fall in blood pressure, paralysis of breathing muscles, and fits.

TREATMENT

Fragments of tentacles must be removed from the skin as soon as possible without causing a further discharge of stinging capsules. Commercial vinegar or dilute acetic acid effectively inactivates the capsules.

In the case of box jellyfish stings, a tight tourniquet should be applied in the hope of delaying absorption of the venom until the patient has reached the hospital. Resuscitation (mouth-to-mouth respiration and cardiac massage) has proved effective in several cases as a first-aid measure, as the most severe effects of the toxins may be extremely transient. An antivenom for box jellyfish is manufactured in Australia.

PREVENTION

Coelenterate stings could be prevented if swimmers avoided the water during seasons when large numbers of jellyfish are washed inshore.

OTHER VENOMOUS MARINE ANIMALS

The venomous spines and grapples of echinoderms (starfish and sea urchins) can produce dangerous poisoning, and their spines can be a painful nuisance. All spines and grapples should be removed methodically from the wound after softening the skin with 2 percent salicylic acid ointment.

A few molluscs (snails, slugs, sea cones, and octopuses) are also venomous. Cone shells and the Australian blue-ringed octopus (Fig. 6.8) can produce fatal envenoming. No specific treatment is available but a tight tourniquet might delay absorption of venom until the patient reaches a hospital.

BEES, WASPS, AND HORNETS

Stings by bees, wasps, and their relatives are very common events throughout the world. Transient pain, local swelling, and redness are usually the only effects. People are occasionally attacked by swarms of bees. A rock climber in Nigeria fell to his death when attacked by bees, and in Thailand one child died of kidney failure and another of swelling and blockage of the windpipe after being

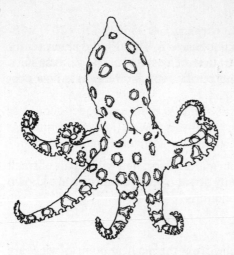

Fig. 6.8 Venomous spotted octopus (*Octopus lunulatus*) from Papua New Guinea (similar to the Australian blue-ringed octopus *O. maculosus*).

stung hundreds of times. In Zimbabwe, however, a man survived being stung 2,243 times by an angry swarm.

ALLERGY

About 1 in 200 people develops an allergy to bee or wasp venom such that a single sting may produce a severe and even rapidly fatal effect. In the USA, many more deaths occur from severe allergic reactions (anaphylactic reactions) to insect stings than from snakebites. Anyone who is allergic to bee or wasp venom may notice progressively severe responses to successive stings. Suggestive symptoms include tingling of the scalp, flushing, dizziness, fall in blood pressure, wheezing, and swelling of the lips, tongue, and throat. The diagnosis of venom hypersensitivity can be confirmed by special skin tests.

TREATMENT

Embedded stings should be scraped out with a fingernail or knife blade, not grasped between the finger and thumb or tweezers (which may inject more venom into the skin). Aspirin is an effective painkiller.

Insect-sting anaphylaxis should be treated with epinephrine 1 mg./ml. solution in a dose of 0.5–1 ml. given by subcutaneous injection. People who know they are allergic to stings should carry an identifying tag such as provided by Medic-Alert Foundation International (P.O. Box 1009, Turlock, CA 95381, Tel. [209] 668-3333) in case they are found unconscious. They should always carry equipment for self-administration of epinephrine (e.g., Ana-Kit). Effective desensitization using purified specific venoms is now possible.

VENOMOUS SPIDERS

Almost all spiders have venom glands associated with a pair of small fangs near the mouth, but only about a hundred species are known to be capable of severe envenoming.

DANGEROUS SPECIES

The most important species from the medical point of view are the following:

Latrodectus tredecemguttatus, which occurs in Mediterranean countries and was known historically as tarantula.

Latrodectus mactans, the black widow spider of North America.

Latrodectus hasselti, the Australian red-back spider.

Loxosceles reclusa, the brown recluse spider of North America.

Phoneutria (Fig. 6.9), the banana spider of South America.

Atrax robustus, the Sydney funnel-web spider of Australia.

Spider venoms cause two groups of symptoms—neurotoxic, with painful muscle spasms and stimulation of the autonomic nervous system (*Latrodectus, Phoneutria* and *Atrax*), or local necrosis (gangrene) and hemolysis (*Loxosceles*).

TREATMENT

Local infiltration of lidocaine (1–2 percent) is effective for painful bites (e.g., *Phoneutria*).

Neurotoxic symptoms may develop very rapidly in some cases, so a tight tourniquet or crepe bandage should be applied to delay spread of venom until the patient reaches a hospital.

Spider antivenoms are manufactured in a number of countries. Calcium gluconate (10 ml. of 10 percent solution given by slow intravenous injection) is said to relieve painful muscle spasms dramatically in cases of *Latrodectus* bite.

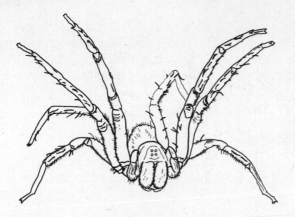

Fig. 6.9 "Banana spider" (*Phoneutria keiserlingi*) from Brazil, in defensive posture.

VENOMOUS TICKS

In Northwestern North America, Eastern USA, and eastern Australia, children and sometimes adults have become progressively paralyzed following attachment of hard or soft ticks. The tick may not have been spotted because it is hidden in a hairy area or even inside the ear. The victim may vomit and eventually die from paralysis of the breathing muscles unless the tick is found and removed. The tick should be detached without being squeezed: paint it either with ether, chloroform, paraffin, gasoline, or turpentine or prise it out between partially separated tips of a pair of small curved forceps. In Australia, an antivenom is available against the venom of the common dog tick.

VENOMOUS SCORPIONS

Dangerously venomous scorpions are found in South Africa, North Africa, Asia, North, Central, and South America (Fig. 6.10), and the Caribbean. Scorpion stings are common in North Africa, Mexico, South America, the Caribbean, and India. In Mexico, scorpions kill ten times more people than do snakes. Mortality is particularly high in young children. Scorpion venoms produce symptoms such as sweating, vomiting, and diarrhea (due to the stimulation of the autonomic nervous system). Damage to the heart muscle may cause a fall in blood pressure, irregular heartbeat, and development of heart failure.

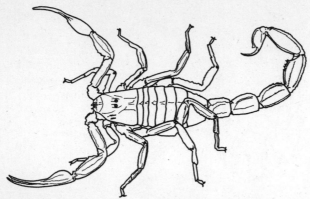

Fig. 6.10 Scorpion (*Tityus serrulatus*) from Brazil.

TREATMENT

Local pain is very severe in all scorpion stings, even those that are not particularly dangerous. This is best treated with local anesthetic given by a ring block in the case of stings on fingers or toes (pp. 216–17). Emetine is effective but may cause necrosis. If this does not control the pain, a powerful analgesic such as meperidine (Demerol) (50–100 mg. by intramuscular injection for an adult) or even morphine may be needed. Antivenoms are made in the USA, South America, the Middle East, North Africa, and South Africa.

MILLIPEDES AND CENTIPEDES

Millipedes can secrete an irritant liquid which may produce blistering of the skin or more severe effects if it gets into the eyes. Centipedes can produce painful venomous bites but are rarely, if ever, dangerous.

ANTS, BEETLES, AND CATERPILLARS

Ants, beetles, some hairy caterpillars, and a variety of other insects and their larvae can produce irritation of the skin and conjunctiva on contact, with pain, inflammation, and blistering. Serious effects caused by fibrinolytic venoms are common in some parts of Venezuela and Brazil. Hemolymph of blister beetles (family Meloidae) contains the vesicant substance cantharidin which is emitted in defense or if the insects are crushed. Beetles may be trapped inadvertently in body crevices and skin creases such as under the arm or in front of the elbow. Painful blisters are produced. The most famous species is *Lytta vesicatoria*, misleadingly known as "Spanish fly." Treatment of the blister with magnesium sulfate or methyl alcohol has been suggested.

LEECHES

Leeches can be a severe nuisance to travelers, particularly in damp rain-forest regions of Southeast Asia.

Land leeches wait in low vegetation near game tracks or paths until a large warm-blooded animal approaches. With incredible speed and efficiency they sense their victim and attach themselves. In humans they usually suck blood from the lower legs or ankles, easily penetrating long pants, socks, and lace-up boots. An anticoagulant is secreted so that even after the leech has been removed or has fallen off, replete with blood, there is persistent bleeding.

Aquatic leeches attack swimmers and crawl into the mouth, nostrils, eyes, and other small openings into the body.

TREATMENT

Leeches are best removed by application of salt, alcohol, vinegar, or a lighted match or cigarette. If they are pulled off forcibly their mouthparts sometimes remain in the wound, which may then become infected.

PREVENTION

Infestation with leeches can be prevented to some extent by smothering boots, socks, and pant legs with dibutylphthalate or N,N diethyl-*m*-toluamide (DEET, see p. 182). Coarse tobacco rolled into the top of the socks and kept soaked is also effective. Aquatic leeches are best avoided by refraining from swimming or bathing in forest streams and pools.

USEFUL ADDRESSES

USA

Poisondex
Rocky Mountain Poisons Center
645 Bannock Street,
Denver, CO 80204
Tel. (303) 629-1123

Arizona Poison Control & Antivenin
    Index
University of Arizona,
Tucson, AZ 85721
Tel. (602) 626-6016

UK

Poisons Unit
Avonley Road
New Cross
London
UK
Tel. (071) 955-5095
Fax (071) 639-2101

Liverpool School of
Tropical Medicine
Pembroke Place,
Liverpool L3 5QA,
UK
Tel. (051) 708-9393
Fax (051) 708-8733

Centre for Tropical Medicine,
University of Oxford
John Radcliffe Hospital,
Headington,
Oxford OX3 9DU,
UK
Tel. 0865-220968,
221332, 60871
Fax 0865-220984, 750506

7 AIR AND SEA TRAVEL

AIR TRAVEL

Most health problems in air travelers are minor, and can usually be anticipated. All travelers should know about the possible effects of reduced cabin pressure.

Wing Commander Richard Harding is author of the book Survival in Space. His research interests include advanced oxygen systems and the medical problems of manned spaceflight.

Air travel is remarkably safe: it is a tribute to the technological and practical skills of aircraft designers, airlines, and air-traffic controllers that of well over 1 billion people who traveled on scheduled passenger flights during 1992, only 929 were involved in just 9 fatal accidents. The previous decade's annual average fatalities and accidents were 1,063 and 39 respectively during a period in which world airline departures increased by over 30 percent and the number of passengers by over 50 percent; and 1984 was the safest year for air travel since the earliest days of flight.

PREPARATION FOR THE JOURNEY

IMMUNIZATIONS AND MEDICINES

Even the seasoned air traveler should double-check requirements and recommendations for immunization and malaria prevention—not just for the ultimate destination, but also for any stopover points en route (see Appendixes 1 and 2). Don't forget to carry any medical supplies you may need for the trip in hand luggage at all times, and it may also be sensible to take along a prescription or certificate, signed by your physician, confirming the details of your medical treatment. Passengers taking regular medication (such as those with diabetes mellitus or epilepsy) should remain on "home time" during a long journey, and readjust timings only after arrival.

FEAR OF FLYING

Flying is an exciting and exhilarating experience but some people may also be anxious and, occasionally, frightened by it. This is particularly likely in inexperienced passengers, although fears usually abate very quickly once they are airborne.

For the habitually fearful passenger, mild sedation may be advisable for a few days before and during the flight. Such treatment can be discussed and prescribed on a pre-trip visit to your physician, and minimizes the personal misery that can surround an impending air journey. Remember that sedatives enhance the effects of alcohol, so avoid alcohol when taking these drugs.

Once at the airport, the hustle and bustle increase tension for many people, particularly the elderly, and if at all possible a "dummy run" to the airport some weeks before flying is one way to reduce this. So too is arrival in good time on the day of travel, and prompt transfer to the departure lounge, where the surroundings are usually much calmer.

PACEMAKERS

The security devices through which passengers must pass in most international airports work by detecting changes in an electromagnetic field made by metal objects passing through it. The intensity of the field is set, in the USA and other Western countries, at a level that will not induce changes in the electrical components of cardiac pacemakers, but machines used in developing countries may not be so innocent. People fitted with pacemakers should mention the fact to security officials: this will enable a personal body check instead, and remove any possibility of interaction.

FITNESS TO FLY

The presence of a pacemaker and indeed of *any* other serious medical condition should be notified to the airline at the time of booking. This useful precaution is as much for the benefit of the passenger as for the airline and, if in doubt about whether or not to notify a condition, ask your family physician to contact the airline's medical department for advice.

Patients may well be advised not to fly when suffering from a disease or condition that will be affected by the environmental changes produced by ascent to altitude. Ascent carries with it certain physiological problems, the most important of which is a *fall in atmospheric pressure* from 760 mm. mercury (mm. Hg) at sea level to about 600 mm. Hg at 6,000 feet (a realistic cabin "altitude" for a civil aircraft, maintained by the pressurization system regardless of the actual height of the aircraft).

The fall in *total* pressure may cause problems for passengers because it allows gases in body cavities to expand. But the associated fall in pressure of each constituent gas in the air, and in particular the reduced oxygen pressure, is also highly important.

At sea level, the *partial* pressure of oxygen contained in the lungs is about 103 mm. Hg and this pressure allows healthy individuals to function normally. At 10,000 feet, however, the partial pressure of oxygen falls to only 60 mm. Hg. In fact, because of the peculiar way in which oxygen is bound to blood, healthy people are virtually unaffected by this reduction, but the health of people who have any difficulty obtaining sufficient oxygen at sea level will be further compromised by the fall in pressure, and they may develop symptoms of *hypoxia* (lack of oxygen).

Aircraft designers build in a safety margin which ensures that cabin altitude is held well below 10,000 feet and, as mentioned above, typically at 6,000 feet, where the partial pressure of oxygen in the lungs is a "safer" 74 mm. Hg. If the cabin were not pressurized in this way, passengers would be obliged to breathe oxygen from face masks whenever the aircraft altitude exceeded 10,000 feet. In addition, they would be unable to enjoy any freedom of movement within the cabin. Cabin-pressurization systems also allow the cabin temperature to be controlled.

MEDICAL CONDITIONS UNSUITED TO FLYING

Table 7.1 on pp. 230–31 lists many of the preexisting medical conditions that may be affected by hypoxia and/or pressure changes associated with even the modest climb to 6,000 feet. It also lists certain other conditions that should be discussed with a physician before a flight is contemplated *and* about which the airline's medical department would wish to know.

Such prior notification enables the airline to support needy passengers during embarkation/disembarkation procedures, and to provide wheelchairs and escorts if appropriate. Extra seats and special arrangements may be required for those wearing large plaster casts or with orthopedic problems, or for whom a stretcher is needed. The cabin staff will also wish to know of any passengers who might need oxygen during the flight. The airlines normally make no additional charge for such supporting services, but passengers are expected to pay for any extra seats occupied.

PHYSIOLOGICAL EFFECTS OF FLIGHT

Fortunately, the vast majority of passengers do not have a serious preexisting illness and are fit to withstand the rigors of air travel. They are not, however, immune from certain other risks.

HYPOXIA

Hypoxia may affect those who are heavy smokers, because carbon monoxide in cigarette smoke reduces the oxygen-carrying capacity of the blood; it may also affect drinkers (because alcohol enhances and mimics the effects of hypoxia) as well as those who are fatigued or have minor illnesses such as acute head colds. The last group should avoid or delay flying if at all possible, while heavy smokers and drinkers should avoid these vices, at least while airborne! The effects, such as acute irritation of the respiratory tract, and the effects of "secondary smoking" on nonsmoking passengers, are minimized by both segregation of smokers and by efficient cabin air conditioning. By mid-1987, however, national regulating bodies in many countries had gone further, prohibiting smoking on most internal flights: a move that has met with widespread approval.

The symptoms and signs of mild hypoxia are subtle and insidious, and resemble the early stages of alcoholic intoxication: personality change, euphoria, impaired judgement, mental and muscular inco-ordination, and memory impairment may all be features, along with blueness of the lips, earlobes, and nail beds. The treatment is administration of oxygen, and this should be given by the cabin staff whenever hypoxia is suspected.

HYPERVENTILATION

A more common, but happily less sinister, problem is hyperventilation, which may best be described as inappropriate overbreathing. The symptoms and signs of this condition are similar to those of hypoxia and, indeed, hypoxia can cause hyperventilation. But the commonest cause is emotional stress, and the picture is usually one of an obviously anxious passenger who becomes increasingly agitated, breathes rapidly, and then complains of light-headedness, feelings of unreality and anxiety (which reinforce the condition), pins and needles, and visual disturbances.

All of these features are the result of an excessive loss of carbon dioxide by overbreathing and, since carbon dioxide controls the acidity of the body, this loss leads to increasing alkalinity of the tissues.

The treatment is to rebreathe the expired air (traditionally from a paper bag!), which will minimize the loss of carbon dioxide. Reassurance, explanation, and firm instructions to breathe more slowly should also be given. Habitual hyperventilators may require mild sedation during the flight.

GAS EXPANSION

Gas expansion on ascent may manifest itself in healthy individuals by a tighter than normal waistband, particularly if much alcoholic or carbonated drink is consumed or if gas-producing foods such as beans, cabbage, turnips, and curries are eaten. Moderation in drinking and gastronomic habits is therefore advisable, and comfortable, loosely fitting clothes are recommended. (Women who are susceptible to cystitis should in any case not wear tightly fitting pants for long flights.)

TABLE 7.1. PREEXISTING MEDICAL CONDITIONS UNSUITED TO OR REQUIRING SPECIAL CONSIDERATION FOR AIR TRAVEL

Condition	Reason	Comments
Conditions made worse by hypoxia (lack of oxygen)		
Respiratory disorders e.g., chronic bronchitis } causing emphysema } breathlessness bronchiectasis } at rest	lower partial pressure of oxygen at altitude compromises already impaired oxygenation	may fly if able to walk about 150 feet and climb 10–12 stairs without symptoms
Severe anemias of any sort		
Cardiovascular disorders e.g., severe heart failure severe angina heart attack		should not fly within 2 weeks
Neurological disorders e.g. stroke		risk improves with time but wait at least 21 days
hardening of the arteries in the elderly, causing confusion at night		should be accompanied
epilepsy		drug dose may need to be increased
Conditions made worse by pressure changes		
Recent ear surgery inner (e.g., stapedectomy)	risk of severe damage	wait at least 2 weeks, ideally two months
middle		wait until eardrum healed
Recent abdominal surgery	gas expansion may cause disruption of the wound	wait at least 10 days
Recent gastrointestinal bleeding	re-bleeding may occur	wait at least 21 days
Recent chest surgery	trapped gas may expand and reduce lung function	wait at least 21 days
Collapsed lung (pneumothorax)	trapped gas may expand and compress lung tissue	wait until lung re-expanded
Recent cranial procedures	trapped gas may expand and compress brain tissue	wait at least 7 days
Fractured skull (with air entry)		wait at least 7 days
Plaster casts	trapped air in plaster may expand and compress limb	consider splitting plaster for long journeys

Other conditions requiring special consideration

People with colostomies/ileostomies	increased gas venting may occur
Psychiatric disorders	novelty of airport and flight environments may exacerbate conditions
	carry extra bags and dressings
	trained escort needed
Diabetes mellitus	problems with control may occur, possibly complicated by motion sickness
	remain on home time during flight; consider anti-nauseant treatment; see pp. 245–52.
Facial surgery	at risk of asphyxia if jaws are wired and vomiting occurs
	should be accompanied by a person trained to release wires quickly
Pregnancy	aircraft are not ideal delivery suites
	no flying after 34–35 weeks of pregnancy on international routes and after 36 weeks on domestic routes
Newborn infants	at risk from hypoxia if lungs not fully expanded
	should not fly until over 48 hours old
Terminally ill	death in-flight is distressing to other passengers and is legally most complex
	may be allowed to fly on humanitarian grounds or for urgent treatment but not if likely to die on board
Infectious diseases and disease characterized by offensive features such as vomiting, diarrhea, copious sputum, or severe skin disfigurement	Cabin staff have neither the training nor the time to act as nursing attendants; they also have to handle food

AIRPORT RADIATION RISK

A delegate at a travel-medicine conference reported the recent case of a young Eskimo mother who had never flown before, traveling with an infant swaddled to a cradleboard. Airport security staff insisted on passing the unfamiliar bundle through their X-ray machine.

R.D.

DEHYDRATION

Continuous plying with drinks is partly a legitimate attempt by the cabin staff to counteract dehydration caused by the dry circulating cabin air. Water and juices are the preferred means of fluid replacement because of the problems with alcohol and carbonated drinks. The dryness of cabin air may also affect wearers of contact lenses and such passengers should be aware of accelerated drying of both soft and rigid lenses (see p. 388). Dehydration increases the risk of thrombosis.

EARS AND SINUSES

During ascent, gas expansion will also take place in the middle-ear cavities and the sinuses, and some gas must escape to the outside; the middle-ear cavities vent gas via the eustachian tubes, which open into the back of the throat, and the sinuses vent via tiny holes, called *ostia,* into the back of the nose. Such venting during ascent is entirely normal, and will be noticed when the ears "pop": it should be neither unpleasant nor painful and does not require the help of chewing or other maneuvers.

Unfortunately, the same cannot be said of the pressure changes that take place in these cavities as the aircraft descends. The volume of a gas decreases as the pressure increases, so that there is a "contraction" of gas inside the middle-ear cavities and sinuses on descent. If the eustachian tubes and ostia are reasonably clear, air passes freely into the cavities, and the pressure inside rises to equal the pressure outside. If, however, the tubes and ostia are closed or are only partially clear—because, for example, they are inflamed and swollen as the result of a cold—air cannot enter the cavities and a *pressure differential* develops.

In the case of the middle-ear cavity, this differential is across the eardrum, which is pushed inward: slight deafness and feelings of fullness are followed by discomfort and increasingly severe pain. Similarly, if the ostia are blocked, severe pain develops in the sinuses above the eyes or in the cheeks. Such *barotrauma* (trauma due to pressure) may happen to anybody, but is clearly more likely in those with a severe head cold.

Prevention of this kind of problem is one of the principal reasons for the slow rates of descent adopted by passenger aircraft. Sinus involvement is uncommon, but middle-ear barotrauma is a relatively frequent event.

Fortunately, the ability to "clear the ears" by forcible opening of the eustachian tubes relieves the pressure differential, and correct use of maneuvers for achieving this will prevent much airborne misery. Helpful maneuvers include pinching the nose and, with the mouth shut, blowing out hard or swallowing; pinching the nose and drinking; moving the lower jaw from side to side; yawning, or simply opening the mouth wide. Such techniques should be repeated during descent at regular intervals when pressure on the eardrum is felt, and it is therefore advisable not to be asleep during this time.

Nasal decongestant sprays or drops may help keep both the eustachian tubes and ostia clear, but there is no voluntary means of opening the latter. Babies and small children are less affected by barotrauma because of the anatomy of the ostia and eustachian tubes, but crying or sucking will also help!

AIR SICKNESS

Many people worry about motion sickness, but only a small number of passengers suffer symptoms.

Prevention with medication is a realistic approach, and motion sickness is discussed further on pp. 245–52.

IMMOBILITY

Prolonged sitting encourages swelling of the feet and legs (*postural edema*) which in turn is responsible for the familiar sight of people struggling to replace footwear at the end of a flight. Postural edema and stasis or stagnation of blood flow in the legs predispose to development of deep vein thrombosis (DVT)—painful clotting of blood in the deep veins of the calves—especially in those with a past history of such problems. This may, on rare occasions, lead

THE ECONOMY-CLASS SYNDROME

Crossing the globe by air is less arduous—and less of an adventure—than traveling the same distance by any other means, though it somehow never feels that way at the time. New research by doctors from the German airline Lufthansa has shown that factors like reduced cabin pressure and low humidity are in fact less important on long flights than was previously thought: many symptoms long-haul passengers experience can be linked to airline seating conditions—what some people call the "economy-class syndrome."

The Lufthansa team used a mock-up of a Boeing 747 interior; they studied 12 volunteers in economy-class seating on four simulated 12-hour flights (two daytime and two nighttime), during which physiological tests were performed. The experiments were then repeated at 35,000 feet, in a real 747 on a 10-hour flight, using the same volunteers; a total of 35,000 samples were taken and analyzed.

Key observations included significant movement of fluid out of the bloodstream and into the tissues of the lower body—evident as the ankle swelling with which many air travelers are all too familiar. Volunteers' weight increased considerably during the flights—some individuals gained as much as 4–5 pounds—an increase attributed almost entirely to the tissue fluid. There was remarkably little difference between the measurements in the air, and those recorded from the "passengers" who stayed on the ground, but there were significant differences between passengers who stayed in their seats and those who walked about the cabin or took exercise.

These findings suggest that the dehydration or fluid loss usually associated with flying, responsible for so many other symptoms, is in fact caused or made worse by sequestration of fluid in the tissues by gravity, during prolonged immobility in a seated position under cramped conditions.

The economy-class syndrome contributes to other problems, too, including deep-vein thrombosis (p. 233); it is not related to class of travel—there are documented links with business-class seating too! The ideal solution would be to provide air travelers with much more space and freedom of movement, with (horizontal) sleeping facilities on long-haul flights. Hardly any airlines do this, so here are some tips for comfort:

- Avoid crowded flights; travel the highest class you can afford; choose an aisle or bulkhead seat, or find empty seats and put your feet up; bring your own pillow or cushion; perform isometric exercises in your seat, and stand up, stretch, and walk about the cabin every hour; request prompt removal of your meal tray when you have finished eating.

- Drink plenty: ideally at least 1 pt. (water, fruit juice) every three hours. Small "airline-sized" cans of soda are not enough. Alcohol, tea, and coffee have a diuretic (fluid-losing) effect; if you drink them you'll need to drink extra water. Airline food is low on water content and low in fiber: consider bringing your own picnic, and include some fresh fruit.

R.D.

to pulmonary embolism (caused by movement of the clot from the leg to the lungs), which is a very serious and potentially fatal condition (see also p. 444).

EMERGENCIES IN THE AIR

ACCIDENTS (see also pp. 262–73)

When in your seat, it is always as well to keep the lap strap loosely fastened: this not only prevents injury should the aircraft suddenly encounter turbulence, but also prevents any likelihood of being sucked out of the aircraft should it decompress rapidly!

Airborne emergencies are very rare, but do occur occasionally. So pay attention to safety briefings given by cabin staff before take-off, and take careful note of the description of the emergency oxygen system (some masks deliver oxygen only after they have been firmly pulled onto the face), the location of emergency exits, and to any other advice offered. You should also be aware of the danger of fires on board caused by illegal smoking in the lavatories.

An article in the *Journal of the American Medical Association* prompted a spate of letters from physicians involved by chance in flight emergencies: many complained about poor first-aid kits on board—they are now being improved. So what was the most fruitful source of in flight medication? Other passengers, it seems: tranquilizers, sleeping tablets, nitroglycerine, bronchodilators, antiemetics, insulin, diuretics, painkillers—even tracheal tubes—have been supplied by fellow passengers. On one flight, a single appeal for medication yielded more than 20 bottles of Valium, and a suitcase full of brand-new stethoscopes from a traveling salesman.

R.D.

In the unfortunate event of an in-flight emergency, passengers can do little more than follow instructions carefully, stay calm, and help one another. Should a crash landing be announced, pay particular attention to crash posture since survival will depend upon being fully conscious and mobile immediately after landing; most crash landings are survivable, but deaths have commonly occurred because of toxic fumes generated by post-crash fires. Again, in the aftermath of several "survivable" tragedies of this nature, the regulating bodies have acted to insist upon the use of fire-blocking and

The Indian government is waging war on rats, despite the fact that they are regarded as holy by some Hindus. The problem is that rats have been chewing through electrical circuitry and control cables on aircraft, in places no human can reach. According to newspaper reports, several Indian aircraft have been affected; there is also a constant battle to keep them away from airline food preparation facilities.

R.D.

less toxic materials for cabin furnishings, and upon the assessment of other aids to survival and escape (e.g., fire extinguishers, exit route lighting, smokehoods, etc.). Speedy and panic-free evacuation is of the greatest importance, however. Once at the foot of the escape slide, move quickly out of the way of following passengers in order to avoid the risk of a collision injury.

ILLNESS DURING A FLIGHT

The statistics available are difficult to interpret, but the "attack rate" for illness in passengers during a flight is of the *order* of one in 13,000—increasing to one in 350 for passengers who have a previously notified disability. This means around one medical emergency in every four or five flights.

The most common problems are associated with the central nervous system, including stress and anxiety, the gastrointestinal system, the cardiovascular system, and the respiratory system. Of these, the cardiovascular disorders are the most serious and include angina, heart attacks, and heart failure.

The chances of a physician being on board any flight have been variously estimated at 40 percent on domestic routes to 90 percent on international flights. The all-important decision, after any necessary or possible first aid has been administered, is whether or not to divert the aircraft if help can possibly be obtained sooner than at the intended destination: an expensive and inconvenient course to take. The decision is ultimately that of the aircraft captain, but he will naturally take advice from any available professional source.

DECOMPRESSION SICKNESS FOLLOWING SCUBA DIVING

An unusual form of in-flight medical emergency, normally only a risk to scuba divers, is decompression sickness (often known as the "bends"), which is caused by the release of nitrogen bubbles in body tissues as pressure is reduced. Decompression sickness does not occur in healthy individuals at altitudes below 18,000 feet and is very rare below 25,000 feet. Passengers within a pressurized aircraft are not, therefore, at risk *unless* they have been scuba diving shortly before undertaking a journey by air.

Diving allows compression of more nitrogen than normal into the body tissues, some but not all of which will evolve on return to the surface; the rest may evolve during ascent in an aircraft. Symptoms and signs include joint pains, itching, and rashes (see also p. 339).

Subaqua enthusiasts should avoid any dive requiring a decompression "stop" in the 24 hours preceding their flight and should not dive at all during the two to three hours preceding their flight. Most divers will or should be aware of these precautions and what constitutes a dive requiring "stops," but if in any doubt, a foolproof rule is to avoid diving to a depth greater than 30 feet (9 meters) in the 24 hours before the flight.

The risk of decompression sickness affecting passengers after a failure of cabin pressurization is also remote, since the aircraft will rapidly be flown to a safe altitude.

JET LAG

Finally, modern air travel can cause disruption or desynchronization of many physiological and psychological rhythms. These circadian rhythms are governed or entrained in part by environmental cues— clock hour, temperature, day and night. Rapid passage across several time zones outstrips the ability of environmental factors to readjust these rhythms: desynchronization occurs and "jet lag" develops.

Jet lag is discussed in further detail in the next section. Simple methods to minimize its effects include sleeping on the aircraft, with or without the effect of short-acting sleeping medication (but remember the interaction with alcohol) (see also p. 526), avoiding heavy meals and excessive alcohol, avoiding important commitments for at least 24 hours after arrival, and generally being aware of the inevitable reduction in performance for a few days. Sensible behavior along these lines will help make your trip a successful one.

FOR EXTRA SAFETY ON AN AIRLINE FLIGHT:

- Buy tickets for children under two and place them in child-restraint seats. Do not carry an infant on your lap throughout a flight to avoid the cost of a ticket. (For details of child-restraint seats, obtain the FAA's "Child/infant safety seats recommended for use in aircraft"—call the FAA at [202] 267-3479 to order.)

- Choose an aisle seat for faster evacuation in an emergency; there is no evidence that one section of the aircraft is safer than any other.

- Memorize the number of rows between your seat and the nearest emergency exit door, as well as an alternate exit.

- Read the emergency card in the seat pocket, and learn how to open the emergency exit doors.

- In an emergency evacuation, leave all possessions and move quickly toward the exit, keeping your head as low as possible if the cabin fills with smoke or toxic fumes. Don't get down on your hands and knees—you might be trampled.

- Keep your seat belt buckled during the flight: even in fine weather, the plane could hit clear-air turbulence and you could be thrown about the cabin.

Gary Stoller, Associate News Editor
Condé Nast *Traveler* magazine

JET LAG

An understanding of the underlying mechanisms is the most helpful basis for developing your own strategy to minimize the effects of jet lag. Many different remedies for jet lag have been proposed, but their effectiveness varies and may differ from one individual to another.

Air Commodore Anthony Nicholson *is Consultant Adviser in Aviation Medicine at the Royal Air Force Institute of Aviation Medicine, Farnborough, UK, and has for many years been involved in the problems of sleep disturbance in aircrew.*

Peta Pascoe *is a Principal Scientific Officer at the Royal Air Force Institute of Aviation Medicine.*

Present-day aircraft operating round northern and southern latitudes cross time zones at almost the same rate as the earth rotates, and it is these rapid transmeridian transitions that lead to the syndrome commonly referred to as jet lag. On arrival at their destination, travelers find themselves out of synchrony with the social and time cues of the new environment and, until they adapt, may experience symptoms like malaise, gastrointestinal disturbance, loss of appetite, tiredness during the day, and poor sleep. The severity and exact nature of the problems vary with the direction of travel and the number of time zones crossed, and some individuals react more unfavorably to intercontinental travel than others. Nevertheless, with increasing numbers of passengers undertaking such journeys, there is considerable interest in strategies to reduce jet lag or to facilitate acclimatization.

Among the most frequent complaints are those relating to sleep and to alertness during the day, as these are most likely to impair the individual's capacity to function efficiently after a time zone change. We will now consider in more detail the effects of transmeridian flights, in particular on circadian rhythmicity and on sleep and wakefulness, and will discuss some of the treatments that have been proposed to relieve the symptoms of jet lag.

UNDERLYING MECHANISMS

CIRCADIAN RHYTHMS

The reason why there may be difficulty with sleep and, possibly, impaired alertness for several days after a transmeridian flight is that the body's functions vary with time in a regular manner. The natural period of our rhythms is greater than 24 hours, but is normally entrained to the 24-hour solar day by external environmental synchronizers or *zeitgebers*. The principal zeitgebers are light and darkness, though others such as meals and social activities also have an influence. Many variables, including body temperature, hormone levels, and alertness, demonstrate circadian periodicity, and it is the sudden disengagement of these rhythms from those of the environment after transmeridian flights that is the major factor leading to jet lag. In addition, symptoms may be worsened initially by sleep loss during the flight itself and, during the next few days, by internal desynchronization as the biological rhythms adjust to the new time zone at different rates.

SLEEP AND WAKEFULNESS

After transmeridian flights, people often complain of feeling tired, and sleepiness is experienced at inconvenient times of the day.

Sleep may be disturbed: the individual may have difficulty in falling asleep when it is the local time for rest, and there may be spontaneous awakenings during the night, or early awakening in the morning. Such difficulties can be attributed to the shift of the day or night that occurs after a time zone change. Journeys between North America and Europe, for example, can be completed within a few hours. After eastward flights, which tend mostly to be overnight, it would be eight o'clock in the morning on arrival in London, for example, but only three o'clock in the morning in New York. After a westward flight, on the other hand, when it is eight o'clock in the evening in London, it would be only three o'clock in the afternoon on arrival in New York. It is not surprising, therefore, that alertness may be impaired during the morning and early afternoon after traveling eastward, and in the late afternoon and evening after a flight in a westwardly direction.

As far as sleep is concerned, it is relatively easy to fall asleep after a westward flight: the traveler is going to bed later than usual as the overnight rest period has been delayed. Also, the day of the journey itself has been lengthened, and this contributes to faster sleep onset on the first night. However, wakefulness during sleep may be increased toward the end of the night, with the local time of rising corresponding to much later in the home time zone. There are also subtle changes in the normal stages of sleep, such as rapid eye movement (REM) sleep and slow-wave sleep. Slow-wave sleep may be related to the length of prior wakefulness and, after westward flights, there may be an increase in slow-wave sleep during the first night due to the delay to the rest period. REM sleep, on the other hand, is influenced by the timing of sleep and increases after travel in a westerly direction, but the normal temporal pattern is reestablished after two or three days.

Sleep disturbance may be more persistent after an eastward flight. For many days it can take longer to fall asleep as travelers attempt to sleep earlier in their sleep-wakefulness cycle. However, many eastward flights are overnight and, without sleep during the journey or during the day of arrival, the loss of sleep may overcome any difficulty in falling asleep on the first night in the new location. There may also be an increase in wakefulness and the number of awakenings for several days, and sleep efficiency declines. Slow-wave sleep may be reduced, and REM sleep is decreased due to the displacement of sleep to earlier in the natural rhythm of sleep and wakefulness.

In general, the immediate effect of a transmeridian flight is determined by sleep loss during the journey and the delay to the first rest period, the subsequent disturbance being determined largely by the direction of travel. Westward flights, which are mainly daytime, may be followed by wakefulness during the latter part of the night, but probably for no more than a day or two. Eastward flights, however, may lead to more persistent impairment of sleep, and certainly travelers should at least try to plan their sleep during the journey and immediately afterward to ensure some degree of tiredness before the first night. The relatively slow adaptation after eastward flights is believed to be related to the natural period of the circadian rhythm, which is longer than 24 hours. This may well encourage individuals to lengthen their day, as after a westward flight, but may lead to difficulty when they need to shorten their day, as after an eastward flight.

REDUCING JET LAG

Various approaches have been proposed to reduce the impact of time zone changes on the traveler. It has been suggested that some strategies alter the rate of resynchronization through an action on the mechanisms that control the underlying circadian rhythms themselves. However, until firm evidence is available, it is probably more reasonable to assume that most countermeasures simply relieve some of the symptoms of jet lag, thereby facilitating adaptation to the new environment. Some of the approaches involve manipulation of diet or rest and activity, while others employ measures to reinforce the influence of the environmental zeitgebers. Though some strategies may be more soundly based than others, no single approach has yet been shown to be completely and consistently effective and, in the same way that the severity of jet lag differs from one individual to another, so the success of the treatments varies. It is, essentially, up to the traveler to choose the method that he or she finds best.

The most relevant issue for the intercontinental traveler is adapting to the new time zone, when the drive for sleep and wakefulness only adjusts slowly to the local pattern of rest and activity. Attention to basic aspects of "sleep hygiene" is the first step toward coping with sleep disturbance after transmeridian flights. Both caffeine and alcohol should be avoided during the hours before bedtime as these are known to disrupt sleep, and some individuals benefit from relaxation techniques or exercise during the evening. Exposure to the zeitgebers of the new environment, particularly daylight, is also important.

Light exposure Research has shown that bright light may encourage circadian rhythms to shift, and it has been suggested that travelers may even prepare themselves for a time zone change by carefully regulating their exposure to daylight before and during the trip (see box).

Meals and diet There may certainly be some benefit in adopting local times for meals on arrival, and some individuals find it helpful to adjust their eating pattern (and also their rest patterns) during the flight itself in anticipation of the new time zone. Other dietary measures are related to the constituents of the meals, and include those proposed by Ehret and Scanlon in their book, *Overcoming Jet Lag*, in 1983. According to their "jet lag diet," protein and carbohydrate intake is scheduled in an attempt to enhance the synthesis of the brain's "wake" and "sleep" neurotransmitters at appropriate times. It is suggested that protein-rich meals that are high in tyrosine, at breakfast and lunchtime, increase catecholamine levels during the day, while an evening meal high in carbohydrates provides tryptophan for serotonin synthesis at night. Recommendations in favor of tyrosine and tryptophan supplements, to be taken in the morning and evening, respectively, have been developed on a similar basis. The diet is difficult to follow, and is considered by many to be ineffective.

Aromatherapy products are also available for the treatment of jet lag, and are offered to passengers by at least one major international airline. Combinations of essential oils have been formulated for use at different times of the day and, when added in small amounts to a bath, are reported to improve subjective ratings of sleep quality and well-being after a time zone change.

Sleeping medication The use of sleeping medication is an important question for the intercontinental traveler.One of the most disturbing effects of jet lag may be the inability to maintain sleep, and in this context medication may be useful for the first night or two after a westward flight and for a few nights after flying eastward. What is needed is a drug which is likely to sustain sleep without residual effects or "hangover," and which is free of accumulation on daily use. Some travelers also find that sleeping medication is helpful during long flights, particularly when there are reclining seats or a

MELATONIN AND LIGHT

Melatonin, a naturally occurring hormone, may one day be used routinely in alleviating jet lag. In animals, it is a "seasonal synchronizer," responsible for controlling rhythms like seasonal breeding cycles and winter coat growth; it is produced during darkness, and is thought to act by signaling day length. It is produced by the pineal gland, situated in the brain; in humans, this has always been thought of as some kind of evolutionary remnant, rather like the appendix; but in hamsters and ferrets, seasonal events, such as preparation for sexual activity, are controlled by melatonin output, which in turn varies according to the amount of daylight. In a primitive creature called the lamprey, the pineal is actually a "third eye."

Early research on melatonin was performed in laboratory animals, and seemed promising, but as one seasoned traveler commented at the time, "Not many rats fly the Atlantic, and hardly any attend conventions on arrival." There have been further reports of human experiments. One was on 17 volunteers who flew from San Francisco to London; prior treatment with melatonin—which in theory would help them adapt to a shorter day—did in fact relieve symptoms and improve performance in some of the travelers. Another was on 20 volunteers who flew between Auckland and London. Melatonin is still used mainly in research and has not been licensed in any country as a treatment for jet lag.

There is a fascinating link between melatonin and research based on the effects of exposing volunteers to different patterns of darkness and light. It has been found that different patterns of exposure under laboratory conditions can make rapid and dramatic adjustments to the natural body clock.

Air travelers do not travel in sleep laboratories, and these findings do not translate easily into practical advice. However, melatonin levels rise as darkness descends, and reach a peak around midnight, falling again through the rest of the night: it seems that exposure to light in the evening and early part of the night—9:00 p.m.–3:00 a.m.—(on what would be "old time") tends to delay melatonin secretion, and delays the body clock (for westward travel); conversely, early morning exposure—5:00 a.m.–11:00 a.m.—would tend to bring secretion to an end and advance the body clock (for eastward travel). Following this pattern of exposure for the first few days on arrival in a new time zone, and wearing dark glasses at other times, may aid adaptation. (The ideal eyewear is said to be a pair of welder's goggles, although researchers who have tried to test this theory have found that this can lead to unwelcome attention from airport security personnel!)

R.D.

sleeperette. However, it must be realized that most flights are unlikely to provide an uninterrupted rest period of more than a few
hours, and the dose of any medication used must reflect the duration
of the journey. The lowest dose of the normal therapeutic range is
probably appropriate. If medication is to be used, it should be tried

THE OZOTHERM

Among treatments touted for jet lag is the Ozotherm machine at the Paris Ritz. Not exactly Woody Allen's Orgasmatron, it feels more like being in a washing machine. You recline in a capsule, enveloped in steam, oxygen, a choice of lemon, lavender, or eucalyptus aromatherapy oils, followed by a tepid rinse. Sybaritic, but makes no difference to the jet lag.

Eve Glasberg, *Travel & Leisure* magazine, New York

beforehand, and travelers should seek the advice of their own physician on the most appropriate choice (see pp. 526–27).

Although sleeping medication may be useful to preserve sleep on arrival in the new time zone, there is no evidence that it has a direct effect on circadian rhythms themselves.

Melatonin There has been much interest in melatonin (see box, p. 243), a hormone that is secreted during the late evening and suppressed by light. Studies have shown that melatonin, given at an appropriate time before sleep, reduces sleep disturbance and improves subjective ratings of jet lag, and recent research indicates that some of the body's circadian rhythms may resynchronize more quickly. However, the physiological basis of these effects needs further investigation, and the potential side effects of regular ingestion of melatonin need to be fully explored before it can be recommended for use by travelers.

SUMMARY OF ADVICE FOR TRAVELERS

- Plan the timing of your flight so as to minimize fatigue and loss of sleep; for example, choose daytime flights.
- Avoid caffeine and alcohol during your flight, so as to avoid further sleep disturbance.
- Consider taking a short-acting sleeping medication, on flights that are long enough to permit several hours of uninterrupted sleep.
- Such medication may also be useful in reducing sleep loss on the first two or three nights on arrival at a new destination.
- Plan your trip to avoid important business meetings for the first 24 hours after arrival in a new time zone.

MOTION SICKNESS

Motion sickness is a common problem related to travel itself, and
it is helpful for travelers to understand its underlying mechanisms.

*Dr. Alan Benson is a Senior Medical Officer (Research) and is the Consultant in
Behavioral Sciences at the Royal Air Force Institute of Aviation Medicine, Farnborough.
He has a long-standing interest in vestibular and allied problems in aviation, and
more recently, also in space medicine.*

Motion sickness is characterized by nausea, vomiting, pallor, and
cold sweating, and occurs when humans, in common with other
primates and lower species, are exposed to unfamiliar motion stimuli, real or apparent. There are many types, including sea sickness,
air sickness, car sickness, swing sickness, flight-simulator sickness,
space sickness, even camel sickness and elephant sickness. Despite
the diversity of possible causal environments, however, the provocative stimuli have essential characteristics in common, and so have
our responses to them.

"Motion sickness" is really a misnomer, as symptoms can be
evoked as much by the absence of an expected motion as by the
presence of an unexpected motion, as occurs in some flight simu-
lators or when viewing a movie of a dynamic scene displayed on a
large screen (Cinerama or Imax sickness). Furthermore, motion
sickness is a quite normal response of a healthy individual exposed
for a sufficient length of time to unfamiliar motion of sufficient
severity. Indeed, if the motion stimulus is severe, it is the absence
rather than the presence of symptoms that would be abnormal. Only
individuals with a nonfunctional vestibular system (the balance
mechanism of the ear) are truly immune. It would be more appropriate to label the condition as the "motion maladaptation syndrome."

SIGNS AND SYMPTOMS

The development of motion sickness follows an orderly sequence,
having a time scale determined by the intensity of the stimulus and
the susceptibility of the individual. The initial symptom is usually
discomfort around the upper abdomen ("stomach awareness"),
which is the harbinger of nausea of increasing severity and general
malaise. At the same time, the face or the area around the mouth

becomes pale and the individual begins to sweat. With the rapid worsening of symptoms—the so-called avalanche phenomenon—there may be increased salivation, feelings of bodily warmth, a lightness of the head, and, not infrequently, depression and apathy. Vomiting is then not long delayed, although some people can remain severely nauseous for long periods and do not obtain the transitory relief that many report once vomiting has occurred.

Apart from pallor, sweating, nausea, and vomiting, other signs and symptoms are frequently though more variably reported. Increased salivation, belching, and flatulence are commonly associated with the development of nausea. Hyperventilation (p. 229) sometimes occurs, and alternation of sighing and yawning occasionally precedes the "avalanche phenomenon." Headache is another variable initial symptom, usually affecting the front of the head, and complaints of tightness around the forehead or of a "buzzing" sensation are not uncommon. Drowsiness is an important yet often ignored symptom, even if not necessarily an integral part of the motion sickness syndrome. Feelings of lethargy and somnolence may persist for many hours after the provocative stimulus has been withdrawn and nausea has abated. In certain circumstances a desire to sleep may be the only symptom evoked by exposure to motion, especially when the intensity of the stimulus is such that adaptation occurs without significant malaise.

With continued exposure to provocative motion, as for example when aboard ship in a storm, most individuals experience a progressive reduction in the severity of symptoms as they "adapt" or "habituate" to the motion environment. After two to three days most have obtained their "sea legs" and are relatively symptom-free, although a minority of the population (estimated at about 5 percent) are "nonadapters" and continue to have problems as long as the rough weather persists.

Adaptation to an atypical motion environment carries a penalty on return to stable dry land. Aboard ship, the central nervous system has come to expect—has adapted to—a pattern of motion stimuli that is different from those on land. On coming ashore the motion stimuli differ from those to which the individual is adapted, and this change in sensory input can engender a recurrence of symptoms—the *"mal de débarquement"* phenomenon. Readaptation to the familiar, stable motion environment of dry land is fortunately more rapid than that to the atypical one of ship motion and sickness is rarely severe, although transient illusory sensations of motion may remain present for a day or more.

INCIDENCE

The incidence of sickness in a particular environment is influenced by several factors. They are the physical characteristics of the stimulus (frequency, intensity, duration, and direction), the natural susceptibility of the individual, the nature of the task performed, and environmental factors such as odor.

The incidence of air sickness ranges from a fraction of 1 percent in large civil passenger aircraft (that usually fly above the worst turbulence) to 100 percent during "hurricane penetration flights" in those who have had no previous experience of such severe turbulence; 90 percent of those who have flown in such conditions before may experience the problem again.

Likewise, the incidence of sea sickness varies widely. An extensive questionnaire study of sickness in ferryboat passengers, under a variety of different sea states, found overall that 7 percent of passengers had been vomiting and 21 percent experienced less severe symptoms, although the incidence on any one journey ranged from 0 to 40 percent depending on the sea state. In contrast, in rough seas all the occupants of a life raft or an enclosed survival craft may be seasick.

There is considerable variability between people in their response to provocative motion. However, susceptibility appears to be a relatively stable and enduring individual characteristic. Furthermore, there is evidence that those who are sensitive to one type of motion are likely to succumb when exposed to another. Motion sickness is rare below the age of 2 years, but susceptibility increases rapidly to reach a peak between the ages of 3 and 12 years. Over the next decade there is a progressive increase in tolerance that continues, though more slowly, with increasing age. This reduction in susceptibility with age has been recorded for both sea sickness and air sickness, though the elderly are not immune. About a fifth of those suffering from sea sickness on a British Channel Island ferry were aged 60 years or more.

Females are more susceptible to motion sickness than males of the same age, and a higher incidence of vomiting and malaise is reported by female than by male passengers on ferries. The difference in susceptibility between men and women is in the ratio of about 1 to 1.7. The reason for this, which applies both to children and to adults, is not clear. It may be that females are more ready to admit to having symptoms. Hormonal factors may also play a part as susceptibility is highest during menstruation and is increased in pregnancy.

PREVENTION

Behavioral aspects Avoidance of exposure to provocative motion is the only certain way of preventing motion sickness, the possible, but not practicable, exception being the bilateral destruction of the vestibular apparatus of the inner ear. In the modern world, however, few are prepared to forgo travel by automobile, airplane or boat, or to tolerate the restriction of their mobility imposed by the "go sit under a tree" approach to prevention. Nevertheless, there are a number of things an individual can do that may allay development of symptoms, or in favorable circumstances, prevent them. The passenger aboard ship may be able to move to a position where the motion is least, usually near the middle of the ship on a low deck. The intensity of motion can also be influenced by the way a vehicle is controlled. The driver of a car can take bends gently and avoid frequent and powerful braking and acceleration. Likewise, the captain of a boat may be in a position, by regulating its speed and heading, to provide a more comfortable passage; and the pilot of a aircraft can attempt to avoid flying through turbulent air and making high-rate turns that may discommode his passengers.

There is evidence that head and body movements potentiate susceptibility to motion sickness. Restriction of head movement by pressing the head firmly against the seat or other available support is therefore likely to be beneficial. Likewise, lying down minimizes head movement and also places the vestibular apparatus in a more favorable orientation to the motion stimulus so that sensory conflict is reduced. It is well known, for example, that people with sea sickness have less malaise when made to lie down with their eyes closed.

Procedures to reduce visual/vestibular sensory conflict can also be helpful. When below deck in a boat or in the enclosed cabin of an aircraft, it is better to close the eyes than to keep them open. On the other hand, when able to see out, one should fixate on the horizon or some other stable external orientational reference. Passengers in a car should, like the driver, look at the road ahead. Reading in a car is well known to precipitate motion sickness, so tasks involving visual search and scanning within the vehicle should be avoided.

The person in control of a car, boat, or airplane is less likely to suffer from motion sickness than other passengers, presumably because of a greater ability to anticipate the motion and to make appropriate postural adjustments so that sensory conflict is reduced. A further benefit of being in control may derive from the mental distraction that it provides. There is experimental and anecdotal evidence that symptoms are reduced by mental activity that directs the subject's attention away from features of the provocative motion and introspection about lack of well-being.

In addition to the behavioral measures outlined above, a further important factor in reducing susceptibility is adaptation or habituation to the provocative motion. The phenomenon is familiar to many mariners in whom symptoms of sea sickness commonly abate during the first few days at sea. Likewise, astronauts who develop motion sickness–like symptoms (space sickness) on initial exposure to weightlessness are usually nonsymptomatic by the third or fourth day in space. Adaptation is "nature's own cure" and in many respects is the ideal prophylaxis, although the specificity of adaptation can be responsible for the return of symptoms on transfer from one motion environment to another, such as the *mal de débarquement* mentioned earlier in this chapter.

Therapeutic programs that build up an individual's level of protective adaptation by graded exposure to progressively more intense provocative stimuli have proved to be very successful in controlling air sickness in student pilots and other flying personnel. The procedure is time-consuming (typically 3–4 weeks of twice daily, ground-based exercises and 10–15 hours in the air) and costly. There is a possibility, however, that a self-administered, ground-based desensitization program could be of benefit to the weekend sailor or the light aircraft or glider pilot, whose frequency of exposure to provocative motion is often insufficient to promote an adequate degree of adaptation.

Acupressure Claims have been made that pressure applied to a point above the wrist, known to acupuncturists as the P6 or Nei-Kuan point, is an effective prophylactic against motion sickness. Unfortunately, these claims have not been substantiated in controlled trials in which pressure to the P6 point was applied by elasticated bands, sold as "Sea Bands" or "Acubands." Nevertheless, the placebo effect of any form of treatment, prescribed with conviction, can be beneficial to some individuals.

Static electricity The same argument can be applied to the conductive strips fitted to the rear of cars to discharge to earth static charge accumulated on the vehicle. Even if static electricity were to be of significance in causing car sickness, the charge on a hollow metal box is always on its exterior surface, and its interior is always at zero potential.

Preventive drugs Over the years, many medicinal remedies have been proposed for the prevention of motion sickness, but relatively few are effective and none affords complete protection to all individuals in severe environments. Nevertheless, there are a few drugs that are of proven value in increasing tolerance to provocative motion, and allay the development of the motion sickness syndrome. It should be noted, however, that a number of drugs that are used to treat nausea and vomiting from other causes are either not effective or are of doubtful value in motion sickness prophylaxis; these include metoclopramide, prochlorperazine, ondansetron (a $5HT_3$-receptor antagonist), and root ginger. Table 7.2 lists currently used drugs, with brand name, dosage, time of onset, and duration of action.

The choice of drug to be used depends in part upon the expected duration of exposure and the susceptibility of the individual. In practice, if one drug is not effective or not well tolerated then another should be tried. Where the objective is to provide short-term protection, oral dimenhydrinate or buclizine are the drugs of choice.

Protection over a longer duration is provided by drugs like meclizine, promethazine, and cyclizine. As may be seen from Table 7.2, most of these drugs are not effective until about two hours after ingestion. The duration of action ranges from about eight hours for cyclizine to about 24 hours for meclizine. All of these drugs have antihistaminic and antimuscarinic properties, and none is without side effects. Sedation is common with promethazine and dimenhydrinate, but somewhat less so with cyclizine, although the latter drug can give rise to hallucinations in excessive or repeated dosage. Dryness of the mouth and blurred vision may also occur, particularly with promethazine, meclizine, and buclizine.

An acceptable alternative to repeated oral administration of drugs over an extended period, such as during a long sea voyage in rough weather, is transdermal delivery of scopolamine by means of a skin patch (Transderm-Scōp). This delivers a loading dose of 200 micrograms of scopolamine and controlled release at 20 micrograms per hour for up to 72 hours after the patch is applied behind the ear. Therapeutic blood levels are not reached until some six hours after application of the patch, so it is necessary to anticipate the problem or to take 50 mg. of buclizine or dimenhydrinate orally at the time the patch is applied if exposure to provocative motion is more imminent.

Although the characteristic side effects of oral scopolamine are less when the drug is administered transdermally they are not necessarily absent. In addition to dry mouth and drowsiness there may be impairment of vision (difficulty focusing), particularly in far-sighted individuals, and this effect tends to increase with the length of time the patch is in place. Side effects may persist for several hours after removal of the patch because of the presence of the drug

TABLE 7.2. ANTI-MOTION SICKNESS DRUGS

Drug	Route	Adult dose	Time of onset	Duration of action
Scopolamine (Transderm-Scōp)	patch	one	6–8 hr.	72 hr.
Meclizine hydrochloride (Bonine)	oral	25–50 mg.	2 hr.	24 hr.
Promethazine hydrochloride (Phenergan)	oral injection	25–50 mg. 25 mg.	2 hr. 15 min.	15 hr. 15 hr.
Cyclizine hydrochloride (Marezine)	oral	50 mg.	2 hr.	8 hr.
Buclizine hydrochloride (Bucladin-S)	oral	50 mg.	1 hr.	6 hr.
Dimenhydrinate (Dramamine)	oral	50–100 mg.	2 hr.	6 hr.

in the skin under the patch. Scopolamine is unsuitable for prophylaxis in children or the elderly. Hallucinations, extreme agitation, and psychotic reactions have been reported in children who have received the drug by means of a dermal patch.

Once vomiting induced by motion sets in, treatment by orally administered drugs is unlikely to be effective because of delayed gastric emptying or elimination of the drug by vomiting. If the individual has no duties to perform, as for example a passenger aboard ship, an intramuscular injection of 25 mg. promethazine hydrochloride is the best treatment. The drug may also be given as a rectal suppository. However, if the degree of sedation produced by promethazine is unacceptable, effective blood levels of scopolamine can be achieved, albeit slowly, by the transdermal route. One or even two transdermal scopolamine patches can be applied if exposure to the provocative motion is likely to be prolonged.

Because of the central activity of all effective anti-motion-sickness drugs, irrespective of the route of administration, it is inadvisable to drink alcohol, drive a car, or operate dangerous machinery when under the influence of the drug. Under no circumstances should the sole pilot of an aircraft take any of the drugs detailed above.

HEALTH AT SEA

Cruise liners are generally very healthy places, but travelers may need to take precautions against motion sickness, and certain pre-existing medical conditions are best not taken to sea.

Dr. Peter O. Oliver was the Medical Director of the Cunard Shipping Company, responsible for the medical services on board all Cunard passenger vessels. He has acted as principal medical officer on the QE2 from time to time, and has traveled widely.

Despite the passing of the great passenger liners, cruising has become an increasingly popular form of vacation and is no longer the exclusive privilege of the rich and famous: almost 4 million Americans take cruise vacations every year. Of course, long sea voyages are less common nowadays, and most pleasure cruises are of just one or two weeks' duration, although longer world cruises lasting ten to twelve weeks are still popular.

A cruise on a modern liner can offer many health advantages compared with a land-based vacation abroad—for example, the assurance of hygienic food and water on board and the immediate availability of medical facilities.

Avoidance of currency problems and political upheaval is conducive to relaxation. Modern liners are fully air-conditioned, fitted with stabilizers to reduce the ship's movement in rough weather, and have elevators to all decks; separate toilet and shower or bath are usually also available. These advantages apply, at least, to cruises run by reputable shipping companies on modern liners.

Some cheap package cruises may not offer all the facilities listed above, and conditions and standards of hygiene aboard "flags of convenience" vessels may be questionable. Obviously, careful inquiry is essential in choosing a cruise to suit your individual requirements. As a general rule, you get what you pay for: paying a little more may well be worthwhile to secure peace of mind and a comfortable and safe vacation.

Remember that many cruise vacations operate on a fly-cruise basis, which may involve a long and fatiguing journey by air before reaching one's port of embarkation. For elderly people or those with debilitating medical conditions, a cruise starting nearer to home may well be preferable—special facilities for such passengers such as wheelchairs and assistance at embarkation can usually be provided on request.

Sea travel is one of the safest modes of transport: for example, no serious disaster has occurred to a British passenger vessel since the loss of the *Titanic* in 1912, a record marred only by the loss of the *Herald of Free Enterprise* off Zeebrugge, Belgium, on March 6, 1987, with the loss of 188 passengers. All passenger vessels have stringent safety regulations regarding the number of lifeboats, safety rafts, and life preservers, and routine lifeboat drills are carried out on every voyage.

The most serious fire disaster ever to hit Scandinavian shipping claimed 186 lives on the car-passenger ferry *Scandinavian Star* in April 1991. This, coupled with the sinking of the ill-fated Greek cruise liner *Oceanos* in August 1991, has again highlighted the need for high standards of safety on board, and a well-trained crew. It is reassuring to learn that new, stringent international safety regulations are to be introduced, endorsed by the International Maritime Organization (IMO).

Delays may occasionally occur as a result of rough weather or navigational problems, but at least you are still being well looked after while on board.

Travel on short ferry crossings usually presents few problems, apart from occasional sea sickness. Bear in mind, however, that no medical facilities exist on board such vessels, so take with you anything you require.

PREPARATION FOR THE VOYAGE

Selecting suitable accommodations for your needs can be most important. An outboard cabin is generally preferable to an inboard one especially if you suffer from claustrophobia, and provided your finances allow. The center of the ship, called amidships in seamen's parlance, is more stable and less subject to vibration and movement in bad weather.

IMMUNIZATION AND ANTIMALARIAL MEDICATION

The medical services of most passenger cruise lines can normally provide up-to-date information, and can administer any necessary inoculations on board should you have failed to take the necessary precautions before joining the ship (see pp. 498–514). It is more sensible, however, to arrange for immunization to be completed well in advance—and I would suggest that you aim to complete any immunization schedule at least two weeks prior to departure. Although vaccine reactions are uncommon, they occasionally do occur and may spoil the first few days of vacation, which is always a disappointment. Similar considerations apply to malaria prevention—it is wise to seek advice, and to commence any necessary medication prior to embarkation. With the spread of drug-resistant strains of malaria, it is increasingly important to avoid mosquito bites; make sure you have sufficient insect repellent to protect you during shore visits.

FITNESS TO TRAVEL

Many shipping companies require a certificate of fitness for travel from your own physician if you are over 75 years of age. If you are under treatment from your physician it is essential that you have sufficient medication with you for your cruise. You would be surprised at the number of passengers who, on joining a ship, have forgotten or lost their regular medication, sometimes with serious consequences. Baggage can sometimes go astray—particularly where fly-cruises are involved; retrieving delayed baggage can be difficult when you are at sea. Those with a medical condition that may cause complications should bring a full medical report from their physician. This is invaluable to the ship's doctor should any treatment be necessary. If in doubt about your health, have a checkup with your physician prior to embarkation.

Most major passenger lines have comprehensive medical services ashore from whom advice can be obtained and special facilities arranged for invalids and the infirm, such as special diets, wheelchair assistance, and medical care on board.

The *QE2,* for example, provides a full supportive cardiac unit.

SEA SICKNESS

With the widespread introduction of ship's stabilizers, which largely control the movement of the ship in rough weather, motion sickness is nowadays much less common. However, smaller vessels, like ferryboats, may not be so equipped and you may therefore be affected.

Prevention is better than cure. Try to avoid that farewell party and the undue fatigue of overnight travel. Smoking may aggravate the condition. When necessary, and where possible, lie down and avoid moving your head from side to side.

A wide variety of tablets are beneficial in preventing motion sickness. All these should be taken some hours in advance of the onset of symptoms wherever possible. They are discussed in detail on pp. 250–52.

Once vomiting has occurred I find oral medication next to useless and, in these circumstances, would recommend promethazine hydrochloride (Phenergan) by injection, or, if preferred, by rectal suppository. This drug is highly effective and its failure rate is minimal.

With correct and well-chosen medication sea sickness should not nowadays be a problem.

PREEXISTING MEDICAL CONDITIONS

Generally, cruising presents no special problems to travelers with preexisting medical conditions, provided suitable precautions are taken beforehand and that your physician has approved the vacation you have in mind. Sophisticated radio satellite communications systems now make it possible for passengers to talk directly with their own personal physician if necessary, and make it possible to seek expert medical advice without difficulty.

GASTROINTESTINAL ILLNESS
Patients suffering from active stomach ulceration should not undertake a sea voyage of more than 24 hours' duration as the risk of stomach perforation or hemorrhage is too great, especially in circumstances where expert facilities and blood transfusion are not available. Well-controlled cases, with appropriate medication and diet, are no problem. Patients with a subacute or "grumbling" appendix should never contemplate a sea voyage.

Changes in normal eating habits and the consumption of unfamiliar food and drink, often associated with an alteration in social pattern, may cause considerable upset to colostomy patients, unless well controlled. Remember that cabin accommodation is sometimes shared, so it may be necessary to make special arrangements to ensure privacy.

There is a high risk of diarrhea from eating ashore in certain countries—such as Mexico, for example. It is important to pay constant attention to the food-hygiene precautions outlined elsewhere in this book.

CARDIOVASCULAR DISORDERS
With the ever-increasing number of older passengers taking the opportunity of a cruise, the incidence of heart and circulatory disease is high. Most large passenger vessels provide facilities in the form of electrocardiography, cardiac monitoring, and resuscitation to deal with cardiac emergencies should they occur. Passengers whose preexisting heart condition is well controlled by medication and who have adopted a sensible lifestyle should have no problem.

RESPIRATORY DISEASES
Upper-respiratory infections (coughs and colds) are all too common in the enclosed confines of an air-conditioned ship, where the opportunity for the spread of infection is high. Nevertheless, the risk to individuals who suffer from preexisting lung disease, such as bronchitis or emphysema, is minimal as appropriate antibiotics and medical support at an early stage of the infection is highly

effective. Chest X-ray facilities will usually be available on board should complications develop.

Sufferers from severe emphysema, obstructive-airways disease, and related breathing difficulties are well advised to bring with them their own portable oxygen concentrator. These are readily available and avoid the need to rely on oxygen supplies on board, which may be inadequate to meet individual requirements. Always check that the power supply is compatible. Oxygen cylinders are actively discouraged by most cruise operators in view of the risk of explosion and fire—check regulations well in advance.

Asthmatics prone to severe bronchospasm may run into serious difficulty at sea. Poor air-conditioning in some vessels, combined with a sense of claustrophobia in tourist-class cabins, may aggravate an attack. Oxygen therapy and expert medical treatment may not be available in all cases. Well-equipped ships' hospitals providing steroid therapy can deal effectively with such emergencies, but beware of flag-of-convenience vessels that operate low-cost cruises, which generally have minimal medical facilities. Severe, uncontrolled asthmatics should not travel by sea.

MENTAL ILLNESS

Although a sea cruise can provide an enjoyable and relaxing break from the daily ratrace, ships are poor places to suffer from a psychiatric disorder. Contrary to popular belief, depressed people do very badly at sea: the anticipated improvement from escaping the anxieties of life ashore does not occur. Individuals suffering from severe depression should never travel by sea, where the risk of suicide from jumping overboard is too great.

Seriously disturbed patients may need hospital treatment ashore, with admission to a local hospital; complicated by language and cultural difficulties, this can prove a distressing and traumatic experience, and there may also be problems with repatriation when recovery occurs. Restraint and sedation on board may sometimes prove necessary for the individual's protection, and where the safety of the ship and passengers is affected. This disruption is best avoided. Ships are no place for the mentally disturbed.

EPILEPSY

Attacks present no special danger provided skilled medical help is available on board if needed. Occasionally, the disruption of the normal daily routine and the fatigue of travel may exacerbate the frequency of attacks.

ALCOHOL PROBLEMS
The convivial life at sea, freely available cheap alcohol, and no worries about getting home after an evening's drinking can pose problems to people who have difficulty in controlling their alcohol intake or have a past history of drink problems. The complications of mental disorder and even delirium tremens are not uncommon. If you have had any problems with drink, long sea voyages are best avoided.

DIABETES
Well-stabilized cases usually present no problem. Always ensure you carry with you adequate supplies of your usual insulin regime— suitable products may not be available in the same form overseas. Persons suffering from fragile insulin dependent diabetes mellitus ("brittle diabetes") should travel with care, and ensure that they are well able to cope with unstable glycemic control. Always bear in mind that expert medical assistance may not be available to help reorganize therapeutic regimes.

RENAL DIALYSIS
An increasing number of people with chronic renal failure, especially those on peritoneal dialysis, are now able to undertake cruises. They can normally be accommodated on an individual basis provided they are self-reliant and bring supplies of all they need. The shipping company should always be contacted prior to reservation.

PREGNANCY
Normal pregnancy presents no particular difficulty at sea. Most companies do not accept passengers in an advanced stage of pregnancy, and usually such passengers should not embark if they will be more than 36 weeks pregnant on the day of disembarkation. Women with histories of repeated miscarriages, especially in the first few months of pregnancy, are best advised not to travel. Bear in mind that blood transfusion on board can be a complicated and risky procedure.

All passenger cruise ships arriving at U.S. ports are subject to inspection, and all cruise ships receive a rating on hygiene standards. To obtain a copy of the most recent sanitation report for an individual cruise ship, write to: Chief, Vessel Sanitation Program, Center for Environmental Health and Injury Control, 1015 North America Way, Room 107, Miami, FL 33132, or call (305) 536-4307.

SEXUALLY TRANSMITTED DISEASES

Sexually transmitted diseases are a high risk in overseas ports and have proved the downfall of many a passenger. The prevalence of HIV infection is particularly high among prostitutes at seaports, and HIV is discussed in greater detail on pp. 419–30. Condoms are normally available on board ship.

KEEPING FIT

Keeping fit on a long sea voyage is an ever-present problem, owing to the lack of exercise and the temptation to overindulge in food and alcohol. Fortunately most cruise liners provide gymnasium facilities and swimming pools, and many run organized fitness programs.

DEBILITATING ILLNESS OR INFIRMITY

Sea travel need not present undue concern to those convalescing from a debilitating illness, or to the aged or infirm. Special facilities can normally be arranged, including wheelchairs for the disabled, and assistance at embarkation or at ports of call, although this is not always possible at every port; it is important to confirm this in advance. Disabled passengers should normally be accompanied by an escort. The shipping company should be given plenty of notice to enable arrangements to be made.

Select your cruise carefully with this in mind as disembarkation by wheelchair, or where physical assistance is required at so-called launch ports where the ship cannot come alongside the dock, may cause disappointment or unnecessary discomfort or risk. Only exceptionally, where complications are likely, may travel be refused.

INSURANCE

Most well-run shipboard medical services will endeavor to treat you on board ship and avoid disembarkation to the hospital ashore—

where there may be problems such as language difficulties, non-availability of drugs, the expense of treatment, and possibly questionable standards of care. Be prepared, however, and never travel overseas unless you have taken out adequate health insurance protection, not only for all medical expenses, but for your repatriation should this prove necessary.

With the cost of medical and hospital treatment in some countries escalating alarmingly, it is essential to take out ample insurance cover.

On board ship, medical charges are made on a private practice basis. These vary from company to company and can normally be reclaimed through individual private health insurance.

SUMMARY OF ADVICE FOR TRAVELERS

- Medical hazards at sea are relatively uncommon and do not differ significantly from those ashore. Should you have the misfortune to fall ill, what better place to be than a modern luxury liner! Most major shipping companies provide comprehensive medical services which are concerned not only with treating illness and injury on board but also with maintaining high standards of hygiene and safety throughout the ship. Good luck and *bon voyage*!

8

ENVIRONMENTAL AND RECREATIONAL HAZARDS

EXPLORERS AND SPELUNKERS, BEWARE . . .

- Histoplasmosis is caused by inhalation of spores of the fungus *Histoplasma capsulatum*. Symptoms are a flu-like illness with fever, headache, and a dry cough; the illness usually lasts 3–7 days, and almost always gets better without treatment.

- Spores are found in bird and bat droppings, and in the soil. Cases have occurred in travelers to Central America and within the USA, and are particularly associated with inhalation of dust from bat-infested caves during dry weather, which should be avoided.

ACCIDENTS

Accidents abroad are an underestimated hazard. More travelers die from accidents than any other cause, and most accidents are avoidable.

Dr. Richard Fairhurst is the Chief Medical Officer of The Travelers' Medical Service, the Chairman of the British Association for Immediate Care, and was formerly the Chairman of the British Aeromedical Practitioners Association and Chief Medical Officer of Europ Assistance. He has supervised the medical assistance rendered to more than 70,000 ill or injured travelers abroad, and has logged more than 5,000 flying hours repatriating some of them.

Many travelers abroad will regard exotic infections as the biggest danger to their health, but in fact these represent only a small proportion of medical problems involving travelers. In a survey of 1,369 consecutive cases, 30.9 percent were due to trauma, 53 percent of these being related to road accidents. Only 1.7 percent involved the usually recognized tropical or exotic infections. Such figures are hardly surprising when one considers that accidents are the main cause of death between the ages of 2 and 45, and that more than 45,000 people die each year on U.S. roads alone.

Infectious diseases are important, of course. They are preventable, and a proper program of vaccination as well as the general precautions described elsewhere in this book are vital. However, travelers should also employ similar strategies to protect themselves against injury, the foremost of these being simply to avoid circumstances in which there is a risk of injury.

RISK AND THE TRAVELER

Travelers fall into different categories of risk: many have paid out a great deal of money in the expectation of enjoyment for themselves and their families, and are under pressure to have a good time regardless of inconvenient safety rules and common sense. Others, alone perhaps, and traveling on business, are under pressure to complete the business deal at any cost, to press on regardless with itineraries, and to use dangerous shortcuts to achieve results.

Because of these pressures, and the absence of the usual constraints of home, family, and work, many people behave in a quite reckless, uncharacteristic manner while abroad—exposing themselves to risks they would never dream of taking at home. Of course, a certain amount of risk-taking is all part of the excitement and enjoyment of being on vacation—but if you are to avoid accident and injury, you must examine the hazards to which you are exposing yourself and decide whether these are really justified.

EVERYDAY RISKS

First of all, travelers should realize that they face at least the same risk of everyday accidents abroad as they do at home. Travel does not suddenly remove these dangers; on the contrary, the enjoyment and carefree, escapist attitudes that travel engenders can increase the hazards.

As a general rule, *you should continue to apply your usual safety standards even if the legal requirements in the country you are visiting are lax.* For example, in your home state you may be legally required to wear seat belts, and most car drivers are happy to comply with such rules in the knowledge that this markedly reduces the risk of serious injury; to stop wearing seat belts when you are traveling, just because there may be no legal requirement to wear them, is inviting trouble. The same applies to wearing helmets on motorcycles and mopeds, and observing traffic regulations and speed limits, and using child seats.

The same approach extends to safety in the home, at work, and during leisure activities: in the USA, each year more than 50,000 people die from unintentional injuries unrelated to motor vehicles—falls, drowning, fires, burns, and accidental poisoning (mainly in children) are the commonest causes of death.

These dangers do not just simply disappear because you happen to be on vacation, and they are more hazardous when local safety standards are not as good as they are at home. Antiquated electrical wiring, gas-fueled water heaters that are poorly ventilated, unsafe domestic appliances, medicines and household products like bleach that do not have childproof caps, are just some of the hazards you may come across, and it is up to you to apply your own strict safety code. This is especially important for people who work abroad, where there is often a strong temptation to cut corners when rules are lax.

The possibility of robbery and assault is another danger that

Approximately 5,000 U.S. citizens die overseas each year: a recent analysis of the causes at the Johns Hopkins School of Public Health has shown that most are due to injuries, chronic diseases, suicides, and homicides, rather than infectious and tropical diseases. Wearing seat belts, and avoiding mopeds, motorcycles, and small (particularly nonscheduled) aircraft were identified as the most important preventive measures that could have been applied.

travelers all too easily forget. Tourists are prime targets for muggers, yet people who will not walk through their own city center for fear of attack are often happy to stroll unaccompanied through the more dangerous neighborhoods of cities they do not know, from Rio to Bangkok. Again, these risks are under your own control.

TRANSPORTATION RISKS

All forms of transportation pose some danger to the traveler—with road transportation at the top of the list. However, most hazards can be minimized with a little forethought and attention to detail.

ROAD TRANSPORTATION

Driving is by far the most dangerous form of transport. Of the 45,000 people killed on U.S. roads each year, more than 60 percent are below the age of 35; more than 3 million people are injured, and motor vehicle accidents are the major cause of injury to the brain and spinal cord resulting in permanent disability. On venturing abroad, motorists may find it difficult to keep their chances of injury down even to this appallingly high level.

The wisdom of wearing a seat belt and observing reasonable speed limits has already been mentioned. Other obvious precautions are to avoid driving when you are tired, when it is dark or conditions are poor, and above all not to drink and drive.

AIR TRANSPORTATION

Although air crashes and disasters hit the headlines from time to time and receive prominent coverage, the risk of injury on a scheduled airline is extremely small: the chances of being involved in an airplane accident in which there is at least one fatality are about one in a million.

Collisions between Australian drivers and kangaroos in rural areas have led to the widespread use of "Roo bars" on the front fender. A similar problem exists in Scandinavia, where there are frequent collisions with moose, and in Kentucky, where 11,648 people were involved in collisions with deer between 1987 and 1989 alone. Doctors from the United Arab Emirates have now reported a series of lethal and near-lethal injuries in drivers who have collided with camels. Camels weigh from 650 to 1,100 pounds, and often stray onto roads. The greatest risk is on unlit roads at night—when the temperature drops, camels like to lie on the warm blacktop. Accidents are frequent, and visitors need to be aware of the risk!

R.D.

Of course, certain airlines and airports have much worse safety records than others; the worst, according to a survey published in Condé Nast *Traveler* magazine, is Aeroflot, with a rate of nearly nineteen fatal accidents per one million flights, and as a rule of thumb, airlines of developing countries should generally be avoided. Magazines like *Flight International* regularly publish data on these risks: a little attention to such information can lead to a potentially safer routing for your trip (see also p. 225).

Certain aircraft also have a better safety record than others, although it is extremely difficult to base decisions about avoiding certain kinds of aircraft on such data. For example, a Lauda Air Boeing 767 was lost without survivors in Thailand in 1991; the accident was very unusual in that the aircraft was at cruising height and the cause was malfunction of the thrust reversers of the engines. The Boeing 767 aircraft is available with various types of engine and thrust reverser combinations, only one of which caused the accident.

Survivability of aircraft crashes is increasing: according to another Condé Nast *Traveler* survey, 68 percent of air crashes now have at least one survivor, and closer attention to in-flight safety is all the more important (see p. 235).

Your safety strategy should start at the airport. There have been several terrorist attacks on airport buildings—don't linger landside, but check in and go through customs and immigration to the much more secure airside.

Airlines are required by their regulating bodies to provide safety briefings on every flight. Listen carefully to the briefing, and read the safety instruction card. Even though you may have traveled by air hundreds of times before, this particular airliner might have a different configuration and different safety equipment. Not all oxygen masks fall out of the cabin roof on depressurization: on DC-10 aircraft they are in the head rest of the seat in front of you; the "brace position" has been changed to minimize injuries to the lower limbs, and is illustrated on the instruction cards. On flights with only short over-water sectors the crew may not brief you on the location of life vests; make sure you know where they are.

Turbulence occasionally causes injury, so move around the cabin as carefully as possible, and keep your seat belt fastened at all other times. Be particularly careful when hot drinks and meals are being served, because sudden movement can spill scalding fluid into your lap.

Baggage poses an additional hazard—both on and off the plane. Avoid traveling with more baggage than you can carry comfortably and beware of other travelers who cannot keep their luggage carts under control—this is a frequent cause of injury.

On boarding the plane, try to restrict your hand luggage to one small item: the more the cabin is cluttered, the greater the risk in an accident. Overhead racks are getting larger and larger, but resist the temptation to put heavy items on them; in an accident they may fall on top of you and may even prevent your escape.

Duty-free alcohol is a particular problem. A fully laden Boeing 747 may be carrying up to 90 gallons of flammable alcohol in its cabin: this not only creates an obstruction but also constitutes a considerable fire risk. The sooner customs authorities around the world rationalize the system and allow passengers to buy duty-free goods at the port of entry, the safer everyone will be.

Smoking on board aircraft is potentially hazardous—not only to your own health, but also to the safety of the aircraft. If you must smoke during a flight, be very careful to extinguish cigarettes and matches properly. Use only the ashtrays provided. Above all, do not smoke when moving around on the aircraft and never smoke in the washrooms. There is a recent example of a serious cabin fire caused by an unextinguished cigarette left in a washroom.

Hijacking is still a problem, so cooperate with security procedures. If it happens to you stay calm, do not do anything to single yourself out as a specially useful hostage, and try to form a bond of friendship with your captors (see pp. 277–78).

Once out of the realm of commercial airlines, the risks of accidents increase greatly. If you are thinking of traveling in a private

aircraft, try to form an impression of whether the operation is being
run professionally; if it is not, it is probably dangerous, and you
should make excuses and find another way of getting to your destination. "Fun flights" and helicopter rides are also more likely to
be dangerous, and should be avoided.

SEA TRANSPORTATION (see also pp. 252–54)

Accidents and injuries at sea to passengers on Western-owned
carriers are unusual, though the tragic loss of a car and passenger
ferry, the *Herald of Free Enterprise*, in 1987 highlighted problems
with ferries all over the world. There have been several horrific
accidents in the Far East and in Haiti, mostly due to overloading. If
a ferry is full, wait and catch the next one. On ships, always observe
simple safety measures. Make sure you know how all the safety
devices work, and where they are located. Where is your life preserver? Where is your muster station for the lifeboats? Where are
the emergency exits, and what signals will be used in case of an
emergency? Does someone at home know of your travel plans?

The loss of the *Oceanos* off South Africa in 1991 shows how
observance of safety procedures coupled with an efficient air-sea
rescue service *can* avoid loss of life even when the hull is a total
loss.

The risks of injury are greater from rough seas than from the
vessel foundering. Remain seated, make sure you are clear of any
loose fittings that may crash around, and if possible lie on your
bunk. If you have to move around, be very careful of wet floors and
in particular of steep stairways. Do as any professional sailor would
do and use both hands.

Finally we cannot leave the subject of sea travel without mentioning the possibility of piracy. In many areas of the world this is
still commonplace. In general, pirates are interested in robbery and
not in murder. If you are unfortunate enough to be the victim of
piracy, remain calm, obey instructions, give up your possessions as
required, and do not provoke an argument or a fight.

RAIL TRAVEL

Rail travel is remarkably safe; in Europe, where more people
travel by rail than in the USA, your chances of having an accident
are 125 times greater on a highway than on a train. In September
1993, 45 people died when an Amtrak train jumped the rails and
plunged into Bayou Canot in Alabama, after a barge struck a rail

bridge. Before this accident, there had only been 48 fatalities on Amtrak since 1971.

Many injuries are the result of being hit by open carriage doors, falling under the train on getting off, or from being hit by luggage falling from overhead racks. One cannot leave the subject of trains without mentioning the habit of riding on carriage roofs, and walking on the outside of carriages, which is almost the rule in some developing countries. It may be picturesque, and tempting in the heat, but don't do it—it is extremely unsafe.

RISKS AT YOUR DESTINATION

ROAD HAZARDS
The heavy toll of road accidents has already been mentioned. The risks of driving abroad may be compounded by bad roads with ill-maintained surfaces, and local traffic laws which are not enforced or are even dangerous (see also pp. 281–83). (Cities where traffic laws are generally ignored can be recognized by the constant sound of car horns—so familiar to many travelers—the last resort of drivers struggling to make their presence known.)

Unfamiliarity with road signs, local customs and driving habits, and especially driving on the "wrong side" of the road (see box, p. 269), are a hazard to drivers and pedestrians alike—most travelers are potentially at risk and should take particular care.

Moped accidents are very common among vacationers, and many island destinations have a particular problem with them: Bermuda, the Caribbean, Greece, and Bali have especially high accident rates. The problems are made worse by the fact that most people who rent mopeds abroad do not wear crash helmets or protective clothing, and that skilled medical care is often not available to treat the injuries incurred.

One recent survey of motorcycle and moped accidents abroad found that 60 percent were simply due to loss of control, and 20 percent involved collision with an animal. Other vehicles were involved in only 20 percent.

POLITICAL AND CULTURAL RISKS
Insurance policies exclude war risks and riots but unfortunately civil disturbances, bombings, or even invasion are liable to occur

COUNTRIES THAT DRIVE ON THE LEFT

Antigua/Barbuda	Indonesia	St. Vincent and Grenadines
Australia	Jamaica	Seychelles
Bahamas	Japan	Singapore
Bangladesh	Kenya	Solomon Islands
Barbados	Macau	Somalia
Bermuda	Malawi	South Africa
Bhutan	Malaysia	Sri Lanka
Botswana	Malta	Swaziland
British Virgin Islands	Mauritius	Tanzania
Brunei	Montserrat	Thailand
Cayman Islands	Mozambique	Togo
Cyprus	Namibia	Tonga
Dominica	Nauru	Trinidad and Tobago
Eire	Nepal	Turks and Caicos Islands
Fiji	New Zealand	Uganda
Grenada	Pakistan	UK
Guyana	Papua New Guinea	U.S. Virgin Islands
Hong Kong	St. Kitts and St. Nevis	Zambia
India	St. Lucia	Zimbabwe

virtually anywhere nowadays. Politically unstable areas (which vary from time to time) are obviously best avoided, although this may not be possible for the business traveler.

The State Department will advise intending visitors to trouble spots on request (see Appendix 8). If you are unfortunate enough to be caught up in a riot, *coup d'etat*, or invasion, keep in contact with your nearest consulate or embassy.

At a more personal level, most difficulties with the local population or authorities can be avoided by finding out how you are expected to behave at your destination. As a general rule avoid political discussions of any type, and avoid making political statements even in private. Don't use cameras or binoculars in aircraft, airports, government installations, or ports, however great the temptation to photograph an interesting item of local flora. In some societies women still have a very sheltered status; visitors to such countries are well advised to comply strictly with local customs.

THEFT

The risk of theft while shopping can be reduced by being discreet with large amounts of cash, and shopping only in areas which are known to be safe for visitors. If a bag, briefcase, or handbag is snatched, particularly by a motorcyclist, let it go. More people are seriously injured by being pulled over in this situation than in any other type of robbery.

HOTEL SAFETY

Fires Hotel fires are unfortunately all too common and smoke, reduced visibility, and panic are the most serious hazards. Some basic precautions include finding out where the fire exit is as soon as you arrive at a hotel, following it down to see exactly where it emerges, and if possible finding out what the fire alarms actually sound like. Keep a flashlight handy in your hotel room in case of an alarm at night, and in the event of a fire try above all to stay calm. Remember that smoke rises, and that it is safest to crawl on the floor in a smoke-filled room. In the ski resort hotel fire in Bulgaria in 1988, there were no burn or smoke injuries; all the casualties sustained broken limbs while jumping out of windows to escape from the smoke. See also p. 280.

Elevators Hotel elevators are a potential source of danger. If the elevator looks unsafe, it probably is; use the stairs instead. Elevator cages with only three sides (the fourth side being the wall of the elevator shaft) are common in some parts of Europe and pose a particular danger. Do not under any circumstances lean against the wall of the elevator shaft as it slides by; sadly, people have lost limbs when their clothes were trapped between the elevator cage and the shaft wall.

Balconies Finally, remember that hotel balconies and their balustrades are often designed to look nice rather than to be safe. Make sure the fixing of the balustrade is secure, and that the height of the balustrade is sufficient to stop you overbalancing and falling. There are numerous deaths among travelers each year as the result of falls from hotel balconies, often related to alcohol consumption.

CAMPSITES

Campsites in all countries pose particular risks: lack of security, leading to robbery and assault; and vulnerability to natural disasters such as fires, floods, sandstorms, and avalanches. In some countries there is also the risk of being attacked by dangerous animals or bitten all over by insects. Tents should be in groups, with someone always on the watch. If you choose to camp alone in a remote area, then you must accept that you are taking a serious risk.

SPORTS, HOBBIES, AND SPECIAL PURSUITS

Most sports and special pursuits involve a risk factor, which is often an important component of the sport's enjoyment and attraction. When accidents do occur, they can usually be traced to entirely avoidable factors—such as poorly maintained equipment, lack of training, or an inadequate level of fitness—rather than any intrinsic danger of the sport itself. Most serious skiing accidents, for example, are due either to inadequate mental and physical preparation or to badly adjusted ski bindings (see p. 342).

As a traveler intent on cramming the maximum amount of enjoyment into the time available, you may be tempted to cut corners, but this is unwise. Always make sure that the equipment you use is maintained to the highest standards—as the experts do—and if the sport you are interested in involves a high level of exertion, avoid "overdoing things" until you have built up an appropriate level of fitness and stamina.

Certain pursuits—for example scuba diving (pp. 333–39) and hang gliding—can be carried out safely only after a fairly long period of graduated instruction and training, including training in the avoidance of the specific risks involved. While abroad you may be offered an opportunity to indulge in such pursuits with only a minimal degree of instruction and supervision: offers of this type are best declined until you have undergone proper training, and preferably obtained a certificate of competence.

If your pursuit carries you far away from human habitation, make sure that a responsible person knows where you are going and when you expect to return to base. When you are injured on a crevasse on a mountain, or marooned in a boat at sea, nobody can help you unless they know where you are!

In our experience, however, it is not the esoteric pursuits on vacation that carry the biggest risk, but the simple ones. Fathers unaccustomed to exercise seem particularly prone to ligament and bone injuries, or even heart attacks from playing sports on the beach with their children. Every year, there is a terrible toll from diving into shallow water, with serious neck and spinal injury in young men leading to paralysis for life. This accounts for approximately one-tenth of all spinal cord injuries. *Do not under any circumstances dive into water of uncertain depth, or take running dives into the sea from a sloping beach.*

ALCOHOL

Travelers may use alcohol as an adjunct to enjoyment or in consolation for loneliness; it increases all other risks of injury and should be treated with great care. Alcohol and swimming make a particularly bad mix: almost half of all drownings are associated with alcohol consumption (pp. 330–31).

A recent study has shown that in traffic accidents involving pedestrians, the pedestrian is more likely to be intoxicated with alcohol than the driver of the car that hits him. Unfortunately, travelers are under great pressure to drink alcohol in excess, most of all on the airlines, where it is given out with reckless abandon, particularly in the first-class cabin.

CONSEQUENCES OF INJURY ABROAD

The consequences of any injury abroad are often more serious than they would be if the same injury was sustained at home. In many areas of the world no organized emergency medical services are available to provide care at the site of an accident, or even an ambulance service to take the casualty to the hospital. The more "unspoiled" and picturesque the location, the greater the probability of the local "hospital" being unworthy of such a title.

No medical help may be available at all. Small islands are always a risk. Usually, it requires a population of about a quarter of a million people to support a comprehensive medical service, and an island with a population smaller than this may well not have one (although better facilities may be available within reasonable range). If the island is many miles from the nearest mainland, even the simplest injury can cause problems. Similar risks apply to travelers visiting small, isolated communities anywhere—desert oases, for example.

If you or any of your companions have suffered injury, and you cannot speak the local language, you may not be able to summon help even when it is available. Find out how the local system works, and what the emergency telephone number is. Remember that however good the local emergency services, you have problems if you cannot contact them.

SUMMARY OF ADVICE FOR TRAVELERS

- All life's activities involve a balance between risk and benefit: we take risks in order to obtain benefit. Travelers who wish to avoid injury must examine the risks they run and decide whether they are justified. Everyone should have a strategy for safety, and wherever they are, whatever they are doing, travelers should know very clearly what their escape route will be and how to behave in an emergency. Above all, no one should expose himself to avoidable risks that he would never take in his normal environment.

PERSONAL SECURITY AND SAFETY ABROAD: AVOIDANCE IS THE KEY

Personal security abroad is an issue that is intimately related to health. Travelers may be extremely vulnerable, and must take precautions to avoid putting themselves at risk.

Edward L. Lee II was formerly Director of Security at the U.S. Agency for International Development and Associate Director of Security for Latin America at the U.S. State Department, and has spent the majority of his career abroad protecting diplomatic and business interests, principally in the Middle East, the Pacific Rim, and Latin America. He is on the faculty of George Washington University, Washington, D.C., and is the editor of The Latin American Advisor, a weekly faxed newsletter.

A gold necklace is ripped from a tourist's neck on a beach in Rio de Janeiro. A business traveler discovers his briefcase is stolen from his side as he skims magazines at an airport newsstand. An airline passenger waiting for a departing flight asks a fellow passenger to watch her bag while she is in the rest room—she returns to find both gone. A laptop computer is stolen from the hotel room of a freelance writer in Abidjan. A foreign motorist injures a local national only to discover that everyone involved in an accident in some countries is initially jailed and released only *after* the facts are known. And a business traveler is shot in the leg while resisting a "car-jacking" in front of his hotel in Caracas.

Each of these situations is based upon real incidents that have involved U.S. international travelers, largely because of their unfamiliarity with the culture and the criminal environment in which they have found themselves. The best way to learn about avoiding these kinds of situations is to attend country- or region-specific workshops, conducted by trainers experienced in dealing with security threats abroad, an approach used by many government agencies and corporations. However, the tips offered in this chapter provide a foundation for helping travelers reduce the risks they will face abroad.

THE FUNDAMENTAL PRINCIPLES

Keeping these important principles in mind significantly reduces the potential for becoming a victim:

Awareness Be alert to the fact that a security risk *always* exists in an unfamiliar environment—even when the locale is familiar: we can never know when criminals are likely to act.

Low profile Travelers should not draw attention to themselves by ostentatious dress, display of wealth, loud talking, or mannerisms that might attract the interest of either criminals or political radicals. In some countries, "wealth" may be considerably less than you think.

Unpredictability Although some routines simply cannot be avoided, travelers should realize that the plans of criminals and political extremists depend for success on being able to predict when their victim will be in a particular place at a particular time (hotel, office, walking/jogging route, etc.).

Adherence to a "buddy" system Few travelers become victims when they are in the company of others. Street criminals, for example, rarely target two or more persons.

PRE-DEPARTURE CONSIDERATIONS

Preparation for international travel is an opportunity to gather information about your destination that will not only result in making you aware of what the real concerns are, but should prepare you for virtually any personal dilemma.

Discuss the country you are planning to visit with those who know it well; obtain what information you can about any unique customs in the countries that you are visiting—failure to observe these can sometimes increase your potential as a target.

Ensure that your personal affairs are up-to-date. This is not a morbid thought, but one based upon responsible planning in an uncertain world. Take steps to make certain that proper power-of-attorney arrangements have been made. In one case, *a coup d'état* precluded a traveler from returning home for over 10 weeks. During that time, the traveler's spouse did not have access to necessary funding. Make certain that you leave details of how you can be contacted in each country, but inform only those who need to know.

Place a photocopy of your passport in your checked luggage. This will ease quick replacement of your passport if stolen or lost. Also carry extra passport photos. Remove from your wallet all items that are not necessary to your trip. Take only those credit cards with you that you plan to use abroad, and know how to cancel them. Keep copies of prescriptions for any medication that you are taking, and make sure that all medication is clearly labeled and identified (see p. 517). Obtain an International Driver's License—not all driving permits are recognized abroad.

Plan to dress casually when traveling so as not to draw attention to yourself. Leave expensive jewelry at home, especially if traveling to high-crime destinations.

Avoid travel on international airlines that have been known to handle terrorist incidents or hijackings imprudently and/or are known to have poor safety and maintenance records.

If you do not have a comprehensive medical and hospitalization plan that is applicable worldwide, you should consider enrolling in special international coverage programs which also includes medical evacuation features (see pp. 492–97).

LUGGAGE SECURITY

Do not place your home address on luggage tags; use your business address only, without giving the organization's name. A tag with a home address alerts others that you will be out of town for some time. Consider using tags that have closed faces.

Make sure that your homeowner's insurance policy covers personal effects stolen or lost while traveling. This can be important in the case of high-value items such as cameras, laptop computers, jewelry, camcorders, etc.

Use only sturdy luggage. Soft vinyl or leather bags can easily be cut open by dishonest baggage handlers during lengthy plane transfers. Use only lockable luggage. Unlocked luggage invites temptation and opportunity. Do not overpack: even the sturdiest bag with locks can be popped open if it contains more clothing than it was designed to hold. For added security, wrap strapping tape around your bag to prevent it from popping open if dropped. Never place valuables in checked luggage. Obtain an X-ray protected bag for photographic film.

Never leave your bags unattended. Luggage or carry-on bags have a way of disappearing when you are browsing at a newsstand or your attention is distracted.

AVIATION SECURITY

One consequence of the attack on Pan American Flight 103 over Scotland in 1988 was a renewed emphasis on aircraft and airport security throughout the world, and security has improved drastically in many countries. Yet there are still some inherent risks, and it is sensible to keep the following points in mind:

AIRLINE AND SEAT SELECTION

- Nonstop flights are preferable: fewer takeoffs and landings reduce the potential for problems.

- Select airlines that are known to have good safety records and extensive screening programs.

- If possible, route yourself through airports known to have consistent, high-standard security procedures and screening. Avoid those that do not.

- Fly wide-bodied aircraft. Hijackers don't like planes with large numbers of passengers.

Although first-class travel is a comfortable way of traveling, consider sitting in business or economy class when traveling on airlines or routes that have previously been targeted by hijackers, or during periods when a hijacking is possible. Keep in mind that the first-class section usually becomes the "command post" during a hijacking, and that anyone sitting in that cabin will be viewed as "important."

Although most travelers select an aisle seat on aircraft for the convenience of being able to get up and move around on long flights, window or center seats are preferable during a hijacking. Passengers in such seats will be less accessible to the questions and interests of hijackers, and during any attempt at rescue, those sitting in window and center seats will be less vulnerable to gunfire along the aisle.

AT THE AIRPORT

- Arrive at least two hours before an international flight.
- After checking your bags, proceed into the "passenger only" area. If security is an airport priority, only ticketed passengers will be allowed into this area.
- Be perceptive of people around you prior to boarding the aircraft. Suspicious persons should be discreetly reported to airline authorities.
- Do not ask strangers to watch your luggage or carry-on bag, in any part of the airport. They may be criminals.
- Do not leave your bags unattended, even in airline hospitality lounges.

WHAT TO DO IN THE EVENT OF A HIJACKING

While airplane hijackings are rare, they do occasionally occur. Unlike tourists, business travelers may not be able to avoid traveling at times of increased risk, or to trouble spots, and should take particular care to be prepared for that one chance in a million. Many travelers who have been hijacked have had experiences that have been far more traumatic and unsettling than necessary, simply because they were unprepared for such an incident, and had never given any thought to the possibility.

Even if your best efforts to reduce the probability of being involved in a hijacking are unsuccessful, remember that you have a 98 percent chance of surviving the incident. The first rule is to remain calm and obey the hijackers.

Hijackers often collect passengers' passports in order to determine their nationalities, and having your passport protected in a leather passport case or cover may make its identity less obvious; this may be helpful if persons from your country are likely to be singled out by hijackers from particular regions.

If a hijacking does occur, and you are wearing or carrying anything which could provoke or irritate the hijackers, discreetly remove it and get rid of it. If you are asked questions by the hijackers, respond simply. Avoid saying or doing anything that might give the hijackers a basis for taking more than a casual interest in you. Do not resist or attempt to aggravate the hijackers. Previous incidents have shown that those who react to the hijackers aggressively, challenge them, or cause them to lose face may be taking a risk that cannot be reversed.

Fear of death or injury is only natural. Recognizing that reaction may help you adapt to the incident more effectively. Try to regain composure as soon as possible after the hijacking occurs. Pause, take a deep breath, and attempt to organize your thoughts.

Try to make notes about the physical makeup of the hijackers: mannerisms, type of weapons carried, conversation, any names that they use, etc. This may be of great importance to law-enforcement agencies after the incident is over.

If you speak the hijackers' language, conceal it. Although it might be expected that using their language might enhance rapport, experience with previous hijackings indicates that travelers are better off speaking their native tongue, and acquiring what information they can by listening to the hijackers' conversation. This may provide you with vital information about what the hijackers plan to do next. During the incident, attempt to seem uninterested in what is going on. Read a book, sleep, or do whatever is possible to avoid attracting attention. When occupied in this way, you will be less influenced by the events around you; hijackers leave people alone who are not a threat to them. Cooperate and communicate. Becoming noncommunicative depersonalizes you in the eyes of the hijackers and could increase your risk.

If the hijacking lasts longer than a few hours, attempt to do isometric exercises in your seat, to enhance your circulation, to reduce muscle stiffness, and to keep your mind off the incident. If you believe a rescue attempt is imminent, slide down in your seat. Cover your head using both of your arms and a pillow to avoid being injured if gunfire takes place.

HOTEL SECURITY

Theft and the risk of a fire, in and near hotels, represent major risks to international travelers. Choose only reputable hotels that cater to foreign visitors. They generally provide good room security and offer newer buildings with good fire-safety features. If possible, select a hotel room in or near the locality in which your business will be conducted, unless of course that area has a high crime rate or is near government buildings in a politically unstable country.

CHECK YOUR ROOM FOR THE FOLLOWING FEATURES

In view of the recent increase in fires and crime in hotels, ensure that the following optimal features exist in the hotel where you are staying. If you see evidence of poor security and fire hazards in the lobby, consider moving to another hotel.

- A sprinkler system or smoke detectors, and preferably both.
- An external staircase for fire escape.
- Door locks that close securely.
- Room windows that can be locked securely and that are not accessible from other rooms.
- Your room should be between the third and sixth floors (out of reach of criminals, but within reach of fire ladders).

WHAT TO LOOK FOR AFTER YOU HAVE CHECKED IN

Make sure that you know:

- The location of all exits.
- The location of fire alarm boxes.
- The elevator and stairwell nearest to your room.
- The number of doors between yours and the nearest exit.

WHEN LEAVING YOUR ROOM

- Ask the maid to clean your room, in person or by phone. Do not display the "Please Clean Room" sign. Criminals can read, too.
- Display the "Do Not Disturb" sign at all times. It suggests that you may be in.
- Leave the television or radio on. It suggests that you are in.

- Do not tell the lobby clerk of your departure or the time of your expected return.
- Do not always turn in the key at the lobby desk.
- Do not leave important papers in your room that might generate the interest of others.

AROUND THE HOTEL

Be careful not to conduct sensitive or important discussions in your room or in areas where you can be overheard. Do not conduct sensitive conversations over hotel telephones; maintain a low profile when the hotel is used for business meetings.

The best place to safeguard small-sized valuables is the hotel safe deposit box; alternatively, use the safe of a business contact. Do not use lockable drawers or closets for valuables. Many keys may exist. However, hotels that offer containers with combinations set by the guest are normally acceptable.

IN CASE OF A HOTEL FIRE

- Respond to all fire alarms.
- Never use an elevator during a fire.
- If the fire is in your room, get out and close the door. Only then should you report the fire to hotel personnel.
- Leave your room if you can. Take your key with you. Feel the door. If it is cool, open it slowly and go to the nearest exit. Crawl on the floor if the hall is filled with smoke—there is more fresh air near the floor.
- If your door is hot, do not open it. Your room may be the safest place to be.
- Use the telephone to call for help, or signal from your room.
- Do not break a window. Open a window only if it can be closed again. An open window may draw smoke into your room.
- If you exit the floor during a fire and go down an emergency stairwell, ensure that you will be able to return to the floor— many exit doors to stairwells cannot be reopened.
- If you cannot leave your room during a fire, fill the bathtub with water, and seal all door cracks with wet towels, blankets, curtains, or clothing.

TRAVEL PRECAUTIONS

Upon arrival, invest in a good map of the city. Mark prominently such locations as your hotel, office, friendly embassies, police stations, and fire departments. Note any other significant buildings that might serve as a safe place if you encounter trouble. In particular, study the map and make a mental note of alternative routes from your hotel to your office. However, never consult a map in the street or in the car—do so before setting off.

Find out how to make a local telephone call. Specifically, know what type of coin is used (and always have a few on hand!), and what the procedures are for actually getting a call through. During an emergency is not the time to try to figure out how the phone works.

Make it a practice to automatically look up and down the street before you exit a building. If it looks suspicious or different, ask yourself why.

Do nothing at the same time every day. Vary your schedule and your route. Whether it be your destination, your arrival time at the office, shopping, or anything that is part of your regular routine at home. Avoid jogging in cities with which you are not familiar. If you must jog, vary your running schedule by at least 30 minutes and never use the same course. The best option, of course, is to ask a local contact for advice on the safest areas in which to jog. If they know of your interest they may even make a running area available to you.

DRIVING ABROAD

Although a majority of countries honor foreign driving permits, several countries require either an International Driver's License (IDL) or a temporary driver's license issued by local authorities. And some countries, such as Italy, Austria, and Germany, require drivers to carry a translation of their country's drivers' license with them.

To be on the safe side, no matter where you're going or where you might end up, obtain an IDL. Virtually every country recognizes them for short-term drivers. They must, however, be obtained before you leave your country of origin.

Before planning to drive on international business trips, be mindful of the following:

- IDLs can be issued to drivers over 18 years of age who hold a valid driver's license from their country of residence. You will be required to have two passport-type photographs and a completed application. There is also a fee. When driving abroad, carry both your IDL and your nation's drivers' license, to be safe.

- Some countries have both minimum and maximum driving ages. You should therefore verify age restrictions before making firm driving plans.

- Many countries provide stiff fines for violators who do not "buckle-up" while driving.

- When renting cars, don't take chances by not opting for liability and property damage insurance. Not doing so can cause financial disaster on your trip. Such coverage is available through the American Automobile Association.

- Traffic codes, laws, and regulations vary abroad: obtain a copy of the local driving regulations. Doing so will eliminate ignorance of the law.

Driving on the "left" (see p. 269) can be downright dangerous for those not used to it, particularly when making right-hand turns! It is suggested that you practice on a Sunday morning when few cars are on the streets before experimenting with the rush-hour traffic. In such countries, dangers also exist for pedestrians who look the wrong way when crossing the road.

Terrain can make a difference, too. If you drive in the mountains, always beep your horn before coming into a curve. In some countries, "flicking" your high-beams is considered a "civilized" approach to alerting others that you want to pass.

Some countries have many traffic circles, or "roundabouts"; find out what local practice is. In some countries, those in the circle have the right-of-way, whereas in other countries those entering the circle have the right-of-way.

PREVENTING CRIME ON THE ROAD

Eighty percent of crime and political violence takes place while the target is in his or her car, or is in proximity to it. Regardless of whether you are driving a vehicle, being chauffeured, or taking a taxi, there are prudent precautions that you should always take:

Even as a passenger, you should know the routes, and have a

good map of the city. When getting into a vehicle, notice what is going on around you. Always fasten your seat belt, keep doors locked and windows up.

Don't get into a vehicle if you have an uncomfortable feeling about the situation; or if you were expecting a particular driver, and another arrives whom you do not recognize. Advise drivers of your destination only after the car is in motion. Don't give him/her a copy of your daily schedule. If you must provide advance notice of the destination, describe it only in the vaguest of terms; avoid arrivals or departures that are essentially at the same time each day.

Attempt to establish rapport with your driver. Don't permit the driver to pick up unknown passengers or hitchhikers. Do not buy merchandise from street vendors, do not offer money to the poor when the vehicle is at a stoplight, and do not pay to have the car's windows washed. All of these situations can escalate into serious crime and increase your risk.

When traveling in a car as a passenger, always keep your purse or briefcase on the floor. If on one's lap, they are vulnerable to criminals who may come up to the vehicle at a traffic signal or when stopped.

Ensure that drivers do not leave the vehicle unattended at any time. If they must leave the vehicle, it should always be locked.

If you are confronted with a "car-jacking," keep your hands visible and surrender the car to the criminal. Do not argue with the criminal.

PUBLIC TRANSPORTATION

If you must use public transport, ensure you understand the metro, subway, underground, rail, or bus system for boarding, alighting, payment, and routes before setting out. Travel in daylight or in well-lit conditions, and stay with other passengers. Do not appear ignorant or nervous, and always remain alert. Carry as little cash as is reasonable; know and avoid dangerous areas.

PREVENTING STREET CRIME

Although many cities are exotic and exciting to walk in, street crime exists virtually everywhere and is inevitable where unemployment, poverty, inflation, overpopulation, or political instability are present.

Travelers should be cautious, and should constantly try to anticipate what might happen next. Being prepared includes having a good pedestrian map and knowing the area that you are walking in. Find out where the police stations are and where crimes generally occur in the city. A quick glimpse at local newspapers should alert you to where crime is occurring.

Think for a moment of naive travelers who wear gold Rolex watches, gold chains, and jewelry. They open wallets laced with credit cards, and flash a roll of local currency when bargaining with merchants on the street. Such persons can only be described as foolish, especially when they are exposed to people who are either out of money or out of luck.

- Leave your passport in your hotel safe deposit box and carry only a photocopy.

- Whenever possible, walk in the middle of the sidewalk. Walking too close to buildings or to the curb leaves you vulnerable to a would-be thief.

- Stand several feet back from curbs while waiting to cross the street. Motorcyclists have been known to grab purses or briefcases while pedestrians wait for the light to change.

- Do not wear expensive or *expensive-looking* jewelry, especially those of sentimental value, including wedding or engagement rings and dress watches.

- Carry small-denomination bills in one place for normal purchases and large denomination bills in another. This will prevent criminals from knowing how much money you have.

- Don't carry a large amount of cash, and don't carry credit cards you do not plan to use. Use traveler's checks wherever possible and ensure that you have signed them only once.

- For women, do not be careless with your purse. Carry it close to your body with the latch side facing in or the zipper closed. Some women find that it is safest to carry their money and identification in a small purse that they can safely place in a pocket. If necessary, a bag for sunglasses, cosmetics, and other inexpensive items can be carried that would be expendable in the event of a robbery. A money belt worn under clothes is ideal.

- Men should carry their wallets in front pockets to combat the threat of pickpockets.
- Avoid walking or jogging alone at night.
- If you are approached or followed by a suspicious person, cross the street or change direction. Seek areas where the presence of others will discourage personal threats.
- If a robbery does occur, don't resist! Street criminals are invariably armed! Your ego and any valuables you are carrying should not take precedence over your life and safety.

CON GAMES PLAYED ON INTERNATIONAL TRAVELERS

Even the most experienced traveler can be duped by confidence artists. Fatigue, unfamiliar surroundings and customs, and, occasionally, verbal misunderstandings result in travelers being victimized. Some examples to watch out for include:

Bogus porters An individual outside an airport terminal approaches you and claims to be a porter. He may even have a cap and a uniform. Be careful to whom you give your bags. Never place your hand-carried bag onto a porter's cart.

Faulty taxi meters Inoperative meters and exorbitant fares are commonplace, but particularly in countries where taxis are not rigidly regulated. Insist upon using the meter or, better yet, always agree on the fare in advance. In many countries, taxi fares are based on a barter system.

Hurried cash transactions This often leaves the buyer with marred, unserviceable, or faulty goods or change in local currency that is no longer in circulation.

Credit card exchanges The card returned to you after making a purchase is not yours, but an expired or stolen one that has outlived its usefulness. Always examine your card when it is returned to you to make sure it is yours. Destroy the carbons.

Obsolete currency exchanges This occurs where money exchangers offer you "a better deal" on currency conversion. The buyer often is given counterfeit local currency or currency that is no longer in circulation. Using authorized vendors solves this problem.

Remember, also, that local police often represent themselves as money exchangers in the hope of involving an international traveler in a currency violation, and demand a "gratuity" for their silence. In many cases, those purporting to be police are only money exchangers using a time-tested technique to elicit money from a nervous traveler. Again, the best advice is simply to exchange currency only through legitimate channels.

THE ONSET OF *MURPHY'S LAW*

Murphy's Law simply says, "If things can go wrong, they will," and it knows no boundaries. Just in case, here are some suggestions for situations that, while remote, could occur while traveling internationally:

YOUR PASSPORT IS LOST OR STOLEN

Lost or stolen passports are one of the most common problems encountered abroad. Report the loss to your embassy or consulate as soon as possible. Make sure that the loss or theft is reported to the local police and immigration authorities. Hopefully, your local contact or embassy can assist you with this.

No matter where your destination is, always carry with you a photocopy of your birth certificate, visa, the first two or three pages of your passport, and extra passport photos. Having these will reduce the time it will take to issue your new passport.

IF YOU ARE ROBBED

The most important thing to remember in a robbery situation is *don't resist.*

Immediately following the robbery, report the incident to local police: ask your local contact to assist you, or ask the staff of your hotel to help. Next to having an automobile accident, one of the most frustrating experiences you can have abroad is to have to report a theft or robbery to local police, who often do not speak your native tongue; you may have to wait hours while they attempt to locate an interpreter who speaks your language and who can prepare a report.

Obtain a copy of the police report, especially if your passport was among the stolen items. This is also true of the stolen items you may have declared on your customs declaration when you entered the country. In some countries, failure to take certain types of property back out of the country may result in heavy duties or fines. You may need a copy of the police report for any insurance claim later.

If you do not need a police report and the losses were insignificant, you may save considerable time by not even reporting the crime.

IF YOU ARE ARRESTED

Even though international travelers rarely encounter problems that might result in their arrest, it can and does happen. Frequently, such arrests are the result of language problems and misunderstandings. Infrequently, they are the result of "victimless crimes" or currency, customs, visa, or religious violations. Regardless of the cause, the experience of being arrested or detained in another country can be far different from what occurs in your home country.

If you are arrested, ask permission to notify your employer and your embassy. If you are turned down, keep asking. Be polite but persistent.

What your embassy or consulate can do for you:

- Provide you with lists of local attorneys. However, you are better off being referred to a lawyer that someone you trust is acquainted with.
- Visit you in jail.
- Advise you of your rights under local law.
- Arrange for the transfer of money, food, and clothing for your use from your family and friends to prison authorities.
- Advocate on your behalf if you are held under inhumane or unhealthful conditions, or if you are treated less favorably than others in the same situation.

What your embassy or consulate cannot do:

- Pay your legal fees or related expenses.
- Serve as attorneys or give legal advice.
- Guarantee the competence or integrity of the attorneys whose names they furnish you with.

IF YOU ARE DETAINED BY LOCAL INTELLIGENCE AUTHORITIES
The best advice is to do nothing that would give a local intelligence service reason to have an interest in you. However, if you are arrested or detained by an intelligence service, you should ask to contact your embassy or consulate immediately. Do not admit to any wrongdoing or sign anything, and try to report the incident to your organization's management as soon as possible.

CONCLUSION

Most foreign travelers have incident-free trips, but 20 percent of all international travelers run into problems of the type considered in this chapter. These arise when travelers fail to understand the local culture, and fail to recognize the likely problems and what can be done to avoid them.

Avoidance is the key to reducing the risks travelers face abroad. Failure to follow these precautions can seriously mar any business or pleasure trip.

HIGH ALTITUDE

Mountain sickness is a serious, but largely preventable illness, and travelers who are well informed and take sensible precautions should have little reason to fear it.

Dr. John Dickinson *was Medical Superintendent of Patan Hospital, Kathmandu. After serving as a Christian missionary in Nepal for 17 years he is now a consultant physician with the British Royal Army Medical Corps, and served in a field hospital during the Gulf War.*

The traveler who feels the effects of altitude follows in a long tradition. Plutarch refers to mountain sickness in his account of the crossing of Alexander's army into India in 326 B.C., and ancient Chinese sources refer to the dangers of the "Headache Mountains" of the Karakoram. The Inca civilization of the Andes (A.D. 1100–1532) suffered from "soroche," a word still used today for mountain sickness in South America.

Mountain sickness is still found in the Andes, where road, rail, and air routes can take the traveler quickly to 13,000 ft. (3,950 m.)

or more, the Himalaya, which in Nepal draws about 50,000 trekkers a year, Mount Kenya and Mount Kilimanjaro in East Africa, and the Rockies of Canada and the USA, where climbers, skiers, and even residents are frequently affected.

Although the first autopsy on a victim of mountain sickness was performed in France on a climber from Mont Blanc, severe mountain sickness is rare in the Alps because most climbers sleep in

TABLE 8.1. SOME ALTITUDES

Place	Feet	Meters
Mt. Everest	29,028	8,848
Mt. Kilimanjaro	19,340	5,895
Mt. Kenya	17,058	5,199
Everest base camp	16,900	5,150
Mont Blanc	15,771	4,807
Mt. Kinabalu	13,455	4,101
Mt. Cameroon	13,353	4,070
Potosí, Bolivia	13,045	3,976
Lhasa, Tibet, China	12,002	3,658
La Paz, Bolivia	11,736	3,577
Cuzco, Peru	11,152	3,399
Aspen, Colorado	7,908 to 11,212	2,410 to 3,417
Quito, Ecuador	9,249	2,819
South Pole Station (USA)	9,186	2,800
Sucre, Bolivia	9,154	2,790
Val d'Isère, France	6,609 to 11,480	1,850 to 3,499
Zermatt, Switzerland	5,315 to 12,533	1,620 to 3,820
Toluca, Mexico	8,793	2,680
Bogotá, Colombia	8,393	2,644
St. Moritz, Switzerland	6,089 to 10,837	1,856 to 3,303
Cochabamba, Bolivia	8,393	2,558
Pachuca de Soto, Mexico	7,960	2,426
Addis Ababa, Ethiopia	7,900	2,408
Asmara, Ethiopia	7,789	2,374
Arequipa, Peru	7,559	2,304
Mexico City, Mexico	7,546	2,300
Netzahualcoyotl, Mexico	7,474	2,278
Darjeeling, India	7,431	2,265
Sining, Tsinghai, China	7,363	2,244
Sana'a, North Yemen	7,260	2,242
Simla, India	7,225	2,202
Puebla, Mexico	7,094	2,162
Manizales, Colombia	7,021	2,140
Santa Fe, USA	6,996	2,132
Guanajuato, Mexico	6,726	2,050

villages and mountain huts, most of which are at relatively low altitudes.

Nowadays, in addition to travelers, soldiers, trekkers, and mountaineers, people who engage in a wide variety of other curious sports and activities may need to take account of the effects of altitude. There have been expeditions by canoe down Himalayan streams, and across mountain ranges by balloon, mountain bicycle, or hang glider; there have been expeditions to run mountain marathons, and diving expeditions to the bottom of deep lakes at high altitude (the main problem in the latter case proved to be the cold).

HOW HIGH IS HIGH ALTITUDE?

Where does the risk of mountain sickness begin? This is a hard question to answer, because people vary so much in their susceptibility. The disease is well known in skiers at 8,000 ft. (2,450 m.) in the USA and fatalities have occurred below 10,000 ft. (3,050 m.). I have seen a typical sufferer who insisted that he had not been above 7,000 ft. (2,150 m.). Generally, however, in Nepal most of our patients have become ill between 12,000 and 14,000 ft. (3,650–4,250 m.). That is not to say that we do not see cases from even higher: my "record" case was from 23,000 ft. (7,000 m.). Since Everest Base Camp at 16,900 ft. (5,150 m.) can be reached by simple (though strenuous) walking, it should be obvious that the high-altitude trekker is as much at risk as the mountaineer.

WHO IS AT RISK?

Table 8.2 gives an indication of the prevalence of mountain sickness in studies conducted at different altitudes. It is easily seen that the risk increases with increasing altitude, and the same studies also showed that the higher altitudes were associated with the worst problems.

Note that each study was conducted in a slightly different way and there were important differences in the rate at which the subjects reached the altitude at which they were studied. Mountain sickness was diagnosed when three or more significant symptoms were present. In general, risk increases with increasing altitude.

Speed of ascent is a greater risk factor than the absolute altitude reached. For this reason mountaineering groups seem less likely to

TABLE 8.2. PERCENT PREVALENCE OF ACUTE MOUNTAIN SICKNESS AT VARIOUS ALTITUDES

Feet	Meters	Maggiorini Swiss Alps 1990	Houston USA 1985	Montgomery USA 1989	Hackett Nepal 1976	Hackett Nepal 1979	Lassen USA 1982
6,500–9,190	2,000–2,800		12				
6,500	2,000			25			
9,350	2,850	9					
10,100	3,050	13					
11,980	3,650	34					
13,780	4,200				52.5	43	
14,410	4,392						67
15,090	4,599	53					

be troubled by mountain sickness than trekkers; they are usually better-informed and plan ascents to allow sufficient time for acclimatization.

Those who drive, ride, or fly to a high altitude are more at risk than those who walk, and those who climb rapidly are more at risk than those who take their time. People below the age of 20 and above the age of 40 have been more severely affected than the 20–40 age group in some studies, but it is hard to make allowances for differing rates of ascent between these studies. There is no significant difference in risk between males and females and there is no reason why anyone should not go to high altitude provided that reasonable care is taken. People who have previously suffered from acute mountain sickness, especially if it was at a relatively low altitude or after a slow ascent, are at particular risk, however, and should take extra precautions.

The risks of developing mountain sickness are to a large extent under the traveler's own control: mountain sickness is a preventable illness.

ALTITUDE AND THE HUMAN BODY

The important feature of high altitude, as far as the human body is concerned, is reduced atmospheric pressure. The result is that less oxygen is available to the body: although the *proportion* of oxygen remains the same anywhere in the atmosphere, the *pressure* of the atmosphere falls as we ascend from the surface of the earth. Atmospheric pressure at Everest Base Camp, for example, is about half that at sea level. It is *pressure* that drives oxygen from the atmosphere into our blood across the vast gas-exchanging surface of our lungs. Reduced pressure means less oxygen available to the tissues, a condition called *hypoxia* (see pp. 227 and 228).

Of course our bodies adapt to compensate for low oxygen pressure. There are increases in breathing and in the work of the heart. One effect of increased breathing, though, is to drive off more of the waste gas, carbon dioxide. This is not entirely a good thing because it causes the body to become more alkaline. Compensation for this can be carried out by the kidneys, but this takes a few days, and meanwhile increased alkalinity has a braking effect that limits the ability of the body to increase breathing. This is one aspect of the process of acclimatization.

Acclimatization also involves changes in the oxygen-carrying capacity of the blood and in the ability of the tissues to extract oxygen from the blood. There are also probably mechanisms that increase the efficiency of oxygen use at a cellular level.

Nitrogen is an inert atmospheric gas which is normally dissolved in blood and tissues to a small extent at sea level. On ascent to levels of lower pressure it is released from the tissues and may form small bubbles in the blood. This is similar to what happens when divers ascend from the depths (pp. 334–37). Although we do not develop "the bends" at altitude as incautious divers may, it is possible that these bubbles cause other problems such as increased coagulability of the blood.

Both cold and exercise have effects on the body that may summate with the effect of hypoxia and contribute to mountain sickness.

TYPES OF MOUNTAIN SICKNESS

Acute mountain sickness (AMS) is used here to refer to all the interrelated types of mountain sickness that occur after exposure to altitude, commonly within two to four days. In rare cases, AMS may be delayed by as long as three weeks. Chronic mountain sickness and the recently described subacute mountain sickness in infants and adults are seen in long-term residents at high altitude and, not being of importance to travelers, are not considered further here.

BENIGN AMS

Benign acute mountain sickness is called just "AMS" by some specialists. Sufferers experience loss of appetite, headache, nausea, vomiting, sleeplessness, and a sense of "fullness" in the chest, or some combination of these symptoms. As far as it goes, the condition is fairly harmless, but it may progress to a more serious form. It is therefore not only a nuisance, but also an *important warning* and should not be ignored.

MALIGNANT AMS

Malignant acute mountain sickness is so called because it may be fatal, and therefore must be handled correctly when it threatens. It may develop from benign AMS or it may begin with little or no warning.

There are two types of malignant AMS, which may occur independently, but the commonest pattern in Nepal is for both to occur together:

Pulmonary acute mountain sickness **(high-altitude pulmonary edema)** Fluid builds up in the lungs. This "waterlogging," together with other changes, leads to breathlessness which persists even at rest, cough, white sputum, and often blueness of the lips (cyanosis).

Cerebral acute mountain sickness **(high-altitude cerebral edema)** Sufferers develop headache, drowsiness, unsteadiness on the feet, abnormal behavior, impaired consciousness, and often coma. If the onset is gradual, the "drunken" walk and inability to sit upright may give clues to what is happening, but commonly the patient passes rapidly into coma, often overnight, so that he or she "wakes up unconscious" the next day.

CAUSES

It would be nice to be able to give a neat, convincing explanation of how AMS is caused. Unfortunately, although there are plenty of theories, there is no general agreement. Some studies have suggested that people with poor increases in ventilation (breathing) at altitude are more likely to develop symptoms, but a puzzling paradox is that elite climbers and Sherpas, who do supremely well at high altitude, tend to have poor, "blunted," ventilatory responses. Among probable factors that lead to edema of the lungs are patchy high blood flow and increased permeability of the small blood vessels to water. Similar mechanisms may operate in the brain, where fragile capillary vessels may be deprived of their usual protection from surges of blood pressure.

It has been known for years that people tend to pass more urine at high altitude and those who get mountain sickness pass less urine and retain more water in the body than those who do not. Hormone changes probably play a part in this, and there has been recent interest in a hormone called atrial natriuretic peptide. There is no definite evidence that the menstrual cycle alters women's susceptibility to AMS or that the use of oral contraceptives is harmful.

Small and even large blood clots are often found in the blood vessels of those who have died from AMS. These may be the result of the nitrogen bubbles discussed earlier, and they may affect the permeability of the capillaries to water. This theory is revived from time to time, with no conclusive evidence. Another factor may be that low levels of oxygen in the brain interfere with the ability of nerve cells to communicate with each other, a situation that must clearly alter brain function.

If it were possible to establish these or other underlying mechanisms as the definitive cause of mountain sickness, we might be in a position to identify people at risk before they went to high altitude, but this is beyond our present state of knowledge.

TREATMENT

BENIGN AMS

In the event of benign AMS, the rule is to remain at the same altitude until you have recovered. This often takes only one or two days, and you can then ascend cautiously if you wish. If you do not seem to be able to recover in three to four days, or if things get worse, you should go down.

MALIGNANT AMS

Malignant AMS sufferers are often in no condition to make decisions for themselves. Their judgment may be impaired as well as their physical capacity. *They should be brought down as a matter of urgency.* Sometimes they can walk, or stagger down; most sufferers will need to be carried by a porter, yak, or horse. Descent should not be delayed while a helicopter is summoned and it should start even at night if this is possible. An American physician once saved the life of his wife: he heard her groaning at about midnight and could not awaken her. Recognizing cerebral AMS, he insisted that his Sherpa guide arrange for her to be carried down at once. She eventually recovered, but it was touch and go; if he had delayed till morning, she would certainly have died.

When evacuating a cerebral AMS victim, it is important to prevent obstruction to breathing. Patients lying on a stretcher should be turned to one side. Pulmonary AMS patients are often more comfortable in the sitting position and may be brought down sitting on a yak or in a basket on a porter's back; the head should always be kept forward. If oxygen is available, give it, but this is much less important than descent.

Patients with pulmonary AMS often improve rapidly after a descent of 2,000–3,000 ft. However, patients with cerebral or mixed AMS may not regain consciousness for days or even weeks, though recovery, when it occurs, is usually complete.

DRUG TREATMENT

For practical purposes, drugs and oxygen have only a minor part to play in the emergency management of AMS, so that *a well-informed lay person can be as effective as a physician*. Among doctors, there is a lot of discussion about the place of drugs in treatment, and the right drugs to use in each situation. All drugs have side effects and risks, of course, so it is a matter of balancing many factors. It seems that both dexamethasone and acetazolamide (Diamox) can relieve the symptoms of benign AMS to a significant extent, but they are not necessary in most mild cases. It seems probable that dexamethasone can give some benefit in cerebral AMS, but it is always essential to bring the victim down and the drug is used only as an adjunct to this. Similar arguments apply to the calcium antagonist drug, nifedipine, in pulmonary AMS.

OXYGEN

It is not usually practicable to carry large amounts of oxygen on mountain trips, though major expeditions may do so. If it is to make any difference, high concentrations at high flow rates must be used.

Another approach to improving oxygenation is to recompress the victim to a pressure closer to that found at sea level. Large, static compression chambers have been tried at strategic points on main trekking routes, and a portable compression system, the Gamow Bag*, has been developed and used by expeditions to parts of the world where descent and rescue could prove very difficult. It is operated by a foot pump but is quite expensive and so is not recommended for routine mountain journeys. A more sophisticated version with a self-contained life-support system that eliminates the foot pumping is now available. DIY enthusiasts should not devise their own models from garbage bags and wire as provision for correct removal of waste gas is vital.

PREVENTION

I have said enough to make it clear that gradual ascent is the key to prevention. The schedule for any given journey has to depend on local details, but it is essential to avoid rapid ascents and to allow time to acclimatize above 8,000 feet.

Those who fly to high-altitude airfields must be prepared to spend time acclimatizing on arrival. In addition, I recommend "rest days" every 3,000 ft. above 9,000 ft. On the Everest trek, for example, it is advisable to stay two nights in the region of Namche Bazaar (11,300 ft., 3,450 m.) and another two at Pheriche (14,000 ft., 4,250 m.). During these "rest days," you can actually climb as high as you like, provided you return to sleep at the same altitude as the previous night. "Climb high, sleep low" is a useful motto. The Himalayan Rescue Association in Kathmandu provides advice on safe schedules for Nepal.

I am frequently asked about the use of drugs to prevent mountain sickness. The two that have been studied most are acetazolamide (Diamox) and dexamethasone, both of which have been mentioned under drug treatment, above. Both undoubtedly prevent or reduce symptoms of benign AMS, but people taking them have been known to develop malignant AMS, and we do not know definitely that they give protection against malignant AMS in anyone.

---

*   Gamow Bags can be purchased or rented from Altitude Technologies Inc, 100 Arapahoe Avenue, Suite 10, Boulder, CO 80302, USA; Tel: (303) 444-8683; Fax (303) 494-6994. The bag and accessories weigh 15 pounds and cost approximately $2,200; a two-person version is also available.

These drugs have their own side effects; in one study the benefits of acetazolamide were masked by the discomfort the drug itself produced, namely nausea, tiredness, and poor sleep. I can testify personally to the tingling discomfort it can cause in the arms and legs, disturbing sleep. Dexamethasone is a "steroid"; should it be used in mountaineering when it is banned in track and field?—a philosophical point to ponder, perhaps. It is safe for most people when taken only for short periods, but it could upset people with diabetes.

My personal advice is not to use prophylactic drugs unless rapid ascent is unavoidable, for example on a rescue attempt. Very susceptible people might also use them, but, more important, they should ascend with even greater caution than is necessary for others, and should not rely on the drugs to keep them safe.

The optimum doses of these drugs are uncertain, but if you decide to use one or the other, dexamethasone tablets 4 mg. twice or three times a day **or** acetazolamide tablets 250 mg. three times a day is probably about right.

It is always good to be physically fit for a walk or climb, but unfortunately this does not prevent AMS. In fact, some of the fittest have become victims for the obvious reason: they go up too fast.

As already mentioned, those who have previously suffered from AMS should ascend particularly cautiously. One experienced Alpine guide, unused to Himalayan altitudes, was evacuated with malignant AMS in two successive seasons. Others have also had multiple attacks, but some seem never to be affected and we await a good explanation for these differences in susceptibility.

OTHER PROBLEMS AT ALTITUDE

Some people develop swelling of the body at high altitude (high-altitude subcutaneous edema). Many of these are otherwise well, although some may show the features of benign AMS. The swelling should probably be regarded as a warning sign.

Bleeding at the back of the eye (high-altitude retinal hemorrhage) occurs in many people but most are not aware of it unless a doctor examines their eyes with an ophthalmoscope. Only rarely may vision be affected, and then usually only temporarily.

If you have significant disease of the heart, lungs, or blood, you will probably find it difficult to tolerate the extra strain placed on the body by high altitude, especially if you are planning to walk or climb. It is extremely important that you consult your physician for advice about going to high altitude.

Epilepsy and migraine are conditions that occur in attacks, and there may be more risk of an attack at high altitude. Many asthmatics, on the other hand, do not have attacks at altitude, unless precipitated by exertion or cold.

Careful studies have shown adverse changes of mood at high altitudes, and reaction times may increase. At very high altitudes, hallucinations may be experienced, such as the ghostly "Third Man" on Everest, but significant mental changes at high altitude are rare and most climbers like to think that they are transient.

People with sickle-cell disease or trait usually know that they have the condition but may not be aware that they may get "crises" at high altitude. These are painful and may be dangerous.

CONCLUSION

For many of us, there are few satisfactions greater than reaching the high and lonely places of the world. There is no reason for this to be spoiled by illness if we are aware of the risks and take simple precautions.

MALARIA

Malaria transmission does not take place at altitudes greater than 6,600–8,000 ft. (about 2,000–2,500 m.) WHO advises that travelers on a weekly dose of mefloquine (Lariam) should avoid the drug during ascent, extending the interval between doses by a few days if necessary, so as to take their next dose during or after descent. The reason is mainly theoretical, and other antimalarial regimens should not be interrupted in this way; mefloquine can cause side effects similar to symptoms of early AMS.

R.D.

EFFECTS OF CLIMATIC EXTREMES

Throughout history, sailors and soldiers, pioneers and prospectors, traders and trappers have traveled, worked, and fought in all climates. Men and women of every race and all ages have explored for the sake of adventure or personal gain; some braved the elements in search of peace of mind, and others sought respite from persecution. Not all survived.

Dr. James M. Adam *was a Consultant Physiologist with the British Army for nearly 30 years, responsible mainly for problems of maintaining combat effectiveness of British soldiers in all extremes. He served in Antarctica, Korea, Malaysia, and the deserts of the Middle East, and left the Army to help set up the Institute of Environmental and Offshore Medicine, Faculty of Medicine, University of Aberdeen.*

It is perhaps a sad reflection on human nature how often advances in the technology of living and surviving have followed fast on the heels of warfare: and this applies particularly to research into the problems of heat and cold. Cyrus the Great, for example, was worried about the possibility of heat illness in his troops when he was reorganizing the armies of the Medes and Persians in 539 B.C.—so he ordained that they be taken into the desert every day to work until they sweated. In similar vein, the potentially lethal effects of cold-water immersion seem to have first been noted during the naval wars between the Greeks and Persians in the fifth century B.C. Such lessons have had to be relearned again and again up to the intensive research that followed World War II.

The ease of high-speed air travel to distant climes, whether for business or leisure, has occasioned risks to many travelers. The fatigue of such flights, especially those with a large easterly or westerly component (causing the greatest "jet lag") will upset particularly the unfit person, the ill, the infirm, and the aging. On arrival, a hostile climatic environment may compound the stress.

SOME GENERAL CONSIDERATIONS

HEAT TRANSFER

Physicists have long since determined the rules that govern the exchange of heat from one object to another; the fundamental principles of such heat exchanges are of great relevance to an understanding of the effects on the human body of climatic extremes.

Net flow of heat energy is always from hotter to colder objects. Such heat flow can occur in three main ways:

Radiation All objects radiate heat energy in the form of electromagnetic waves of various wavelengths; the hotter an object, the more heat it radiates. Radiant energy can be absorbed by another, distant object, the amount absorbed depending on such factors as the color and texture of the receptive object's surface (light-colored surfaces tend to absorb less than dark-colored surfaces). Heat can pass by radiation even across a vacuum, as when the sun heats the earth across space.

Convection is the term given to the transport of heat by the motion of warmed fluid (or gases). A small amount of the fluid is in contact with the heat source and is heated by conduction (see below). As its temperature rises the fluid expands, becomes lighter, and so it rises away from the heat source. Further fluid replaces that which has floated away, is heated in turn, and so on. As the heated fluid cools elsewhere, it contracts, becomes denser, and sinks. In this way a convection current is set up.

Conduction is the transfer of heat from a heat source to a cooler object by direct contact and without demonstrable motion of the parts of the object such as described above in "convection current." Metals conduct heat away most readily, while still air is the most effective barrier to heat lost by this route.

BODY TEMPERATURE AND ITS CONTROL

The upper limit of the average normal temperature of the human body at rest is 98.4°F. (36.9°C.), although patients inactive in bed may register a normal value of 97.5°F. (36.4°C.). In very hot or very cold climates accurate temperature measurements cannot be made by means of a thermometer in the mouth, and instead the thermometer must be placed in the rectum.

The human body exchanges heat with its surroundings by the avenues mentioned above. Heat is gained by the body by the absorption of radiation from distant hot objects (such as the sun) and also by conduction and convection from the surrounding air or water if these are at a higher temperature than the body. Conversely, heat can be lost by radiation to distant cooler objects and also by conduction and convection to the surrounding air or water if these are at a lower temperature than the body.

In addition, two other processes have an important influence on the body's heat balance. First, the body is always *gaining* heat produced during the digestion of food and from working muscles. Second, heat is *lost* by the evaporation of sweat from the surface of the skin. Heat loss by sweat evaporation is at the rate of 550 kilocalories per pint of sweat (1,464 kilojoules per liter), which is a considerable but at times very necessary heat loss. In experiments with fit paratroopers working under severe desert conditions, I have measured sweat losses of more than 20 pints daily, providing a heat loss of about 6,000 kilocalories just to keep body temperature constant.

Our bodies function efficiently by means of a myriad of chemical changes that occur almost simultaneously. These have an optimum temperature of reaction for continued health of 98.4°F. (36.9°C.), with the slight variations described above.

Many of the vast number of reactions are centered in the main organs of the body, and of these, the brain is the most sensitive to temperature change. Indeed, a departure of just over 1°F. above or below the normal 98.4°F. central body (core) temperature, as measured in the rectum, can be demonstrated to produce malfunction of this organ and of the parts of the body that it governs. The further the departure from normal, the greater the degree of malfunction, so that a rise of core temperature of 3.6°F. to 102.0°F. (38.9°C.) is accompanied by signs and symptoms of definite illness. Equally, a fall of the same magnitude to 94.8°F. (34.9°C.) takes the person into the realms of hypothermia, which is defined as a core temperature of 95.0°F. (35.0°C.) or less.

All evidence available points to the existence of a heat-regulating center in the hypothalamus (an important area of the brain). The control mechanism is influenced not only by the temperature of the blood reaching the brain, but also by nerve impulses arising in the skin. The mechanisms by which the hypothalamus controls the body temperature are very complex and cannot be considered in detail here. Suffice it to state that in the fineness and speed of its control, the hypothalamus is a better thermostat than most of those available commercially.

CATEGORIES OF CLIMATIC EXTREME

A better understanding of the possible ills which may result from climatic variations requires a redefinition of some basic variable factors. Consideration of the extremes of temperature and humidity give four main climatic categories:

Hot/wet describes the environment of the rain forest, the jungle and secondary jungle in which the air or shade temperature is rarely above 100°F. (37.8°C.) in daytime and is more commonly 91–3°F. (33-4°C.). The combination of abundant moisture, tree canopy, and frequent cloud cover serves to maintain the temperature at a fairly constant level all the year round, with little variation between day and night. The humidity is high, varying between about 65 percent by day and 100 percent by night; air speeds are generally low.

Hot/dry describes the climate of the tropical and subtropical desert and semiarid tracts of land. The tropical deserts have low humidity, scarce or absent vegetation, cloudless skies, intense sunshine, air-speeds varying from low to violent with dust- and sandstorms, and scanty and erratic rainfall. At night, the clear skies permit rapid heat loss to space by radiation and convection, so there may be heavy dew and occasional frost. There is thus a high day-to-night variation in air (shade) temperature from as high as 131°F. (55°C.) by day (the record is 136.5°F. [58.05°C.]) to as low as 24°F. (−5.6°C.) in the Western Sahara or −43.6°F. (−42°C.) in the wintertime Gobi desert at night.

Cold/wet describes the climate of large areas of the world, including most of Western Europe north of the latitude of the Pyrenees. The term "temperate zone" is often applied to such regions, but is something of a misnomer since it may lead people to underestimate the speed with which changes in the climate can occur, as well as its hazards and severity. The air temperature ranges between about 50°F. and 28°F. (10°C. and −2°C.), with rain, hail, sleet, mud, puddles, and high winds as possible accompaniments.

Cold/dry is the environment in which the air (shade) temperature rarely if ever rises above the freezing point of water (32°F. or 0°C.) at any time of the day. The terrain is frozen, and there is no free still water (as in puddles and ponds). Snow and ice cover may be total, skies are often clear of clouds, and sunshine may be brilliant, especially in the absence of wind. However, movement and navigation can sometimes be hampered by "white-out" conditions, snow precipitation, and blizzards.

HOT CLIMATES

ACCLIMATIZATION

An oft-repeated statement is "Man is a tropical animal" but, one would suggest, the tense of the verb is wrong and should be "was," especially in the case of the temperate dweller who is heading for the tropics for the first time.

The body possesses the mechanisms necessary to survive in hostile, hot climates, but time is required to evoke them. The adaptive process takes one, two, or three weeks depending on the severity of the hot climate. Briefly, the strain on the body is shown by a high pulse rate and body temperature, and the condition will progress to one or other of the heat illnesses (see below) unless the stress is lessened or muscular activity reduced.

With graded exposure and gently increasing activity, the sweat glands are trained to produce more, start more quickly, continue longer without sweat-gland fatigue and to retain more salt in the body. The circulatory system (heart and arteries) learns to absorb water in much larger quantities from the stomach and intestines, and to transport it to the sweat glands in the skin, whence it emerges to be evaporated for cooling the body.

In circumstances where the air temperature is higher than body temperature, the body can no longer cool itself through radiation, convection, or conduction and must rely *solely* on the evaporation of sweat for continuing health. On first exposure to the stressful conditions there is a great deal of discomfort, which varies according to the amount of muscular activity. As adaptation or acclimatization progresses, this discomfort gradually diminishes and disappears after about two weeks.

Acclimatization is generally more difficult in the jungle climates than in hot/dry or desert environments. There are two main reasons for this:

1. The high humidity of the hot/wet environment is maintained by day and by night, and the higher this relative humidity the more difficult it becomes for sweat to evaporate from the body and cool it.
2. Nights in the desert vary from cool to cold, so the body's sweating mechanism has some rest. This is not so in the jungle.

A state of acclimatization to the jungle may be transferred to the desert without ill effect, but the reverse is more difficult, for the reasons already mentioned.

Heat acclimatization can be achieved to a considerable degree in the privacy of one's own home. Commencing three weeks before the intended journey, devote one hour daily to fitness training, and one and a half hours to lying in a bathtub with the water kept as hot as possible (108°F. or 42°C.). Staying in the tub for this long may be difficult for the first two days or so, but persevere. As much of the body should be immersed as possible, eyes, nose, and ears only out of the water. This is one of the simplest methods of "artificial acclimatization," but it should be attempted only if you are physically fit.

AGE AND BUILD

Children adapt to hot environments very quickly and happily, especially thin, wiry, active children who have a large surface area/weight ratio, which facilitates evaporative cooling. The same build is an advantage to adults, but the rule again is "the younger and fitter, the faster." Unfit, heavy, and obese people represent an increasing order of risk. The elderly and anyone with known heart or circulatory disorders such as high blood pressure and arteriosclerosis should either be dissuaded from facing the stress of a hot climate or, with medical advice, should take special precautions—absence of exertion, travel by sea rather than by air, and as much air-conditioning as possible.

THIRST, SALT, AND WATER

The human thirst sensation is defective where water requirements are concerned. It seems, in general, to account for only about 75 percent of the body's actual needs in the tropics. Despite a high degree of training in these matters, the British Army has had four times as many cases of kidney or urinary stones directly attributable to inadequate water consumption in the Middle and Far East as in home stations. The message for the newcomer is to drink water or watery drinks (beware alcohol, which dehydrates) *beyond* the point of thirst-quenching. *Alternatively, ensure enough intake by drinking sufficient water to produce urine that is consistently pale in color*: dark urine or a low urine output are both signs of developing dehydration.

Loss of salt from the body in the sweat has been mentioned above, and this chemical must be replaced if bodily function is to continue. Salt tablets are often used but can cause vomiting and stomach upsets. The author has put entire regiments onto pre-salted water with excellent effect, by treating all tea, coffee, cocoa, soup, lemonade (from crystals) as well as all water used in cooking. The required salt concentration is one quarter of a level teaspoonful (about one gram) per pint or two level teaspoonfuls to each gallon. This concentration is below the taste threshold and must be accompanied by a mixed diet.

CLOTHING AND SHELTER

The jungle Nudity is the ideal state for the jungle environment, as even the thinnest material can interfere with the required loss of heat by radiation and convection. But sweat can be evaporated from the clothes instead of the skin with the same amount of cooling by either route.

Clothing is usually required, however, not only to satisfy local customs and religions, but also to protect against thorns, cutting plants, and the onslaughts of biting insects. Protective leg- and footwear is essential for jungle trekking for these reasons as well as for protection against snakebite and parasitic diseases such as hookworm.

The desert The intensity of sun in the desert necessitates head and body protection to prevent sunburn, which apart from being extremely painful may hinder the function of sweat glands, thus causing serious illness. Again, the materials used must be the lightest possible, not only in weight but also in color. While color is not important for jungle clothing, in the desert a light or white color will aid the body's heat balance by reflecting radiant heat away.

Desert clothing comprises loose-fitting long-sleeved upper garments, preferably cotton, with long pants, to minimize the skin's exposure to intense solar radiation—until a good tan has developed after strictly graded sunbathing. Here the head requires a broad-brimmed floppy hat to protect forehead and neck before "tanning." The Arab headdress, the khaffieh (a three-foot square of muslin) is very useful in a variety of ways: it can be wrapped around the face for protection in sandstorms or used as a neckerchief to prevent sunburn under the chin in the vicinity of water (which reflects ultraviolet solar radiation upward). (See also the next chapter— "Sun and the Traveler.")

Footwear Footwear can be as diverse as there are people to have opinions. The author's preference has been quite simple—boots and puttees (leggings) for trekking in the jungle and "flip-flops" for rest periods to allow skin and footwear to dry out. The heavy tread of boots provides warning to jungle denizens such as snakes, who will, hopefully, go away.

Desert boots with thick crepe rubber soles and uppers mostly of reversed calf leather, but sometimes of canvas, are preferable to almost any other form of footwear for the desert. A word of caution, however, if you intend to clamber around the very sharp rocks characteristic of some deserts: these require much stouter boots. As in the jungle, desert footwear requires "time off" to dry out.

Shelter Shelter in the jungle environment, from the single-person poncho or bivouac to permanent buildings, requires a waterproof roof and little else, to take advantage of every slight breeze. Tents and houses should be surrounded by deep runoff systems for the frequent heavy downpours that occur. Sleeping platforms, well above ground level, must be surrounded by mosquito nets. Temporary or permanent shelter in the desert climate should preferably have a double roof (*not* corrugated-iron sheeting) to minimize heating of the interior by direct solar radiation.

Air-conditioning Sweat-soaked clothing will chill the wearer rapidly on entering an air-conditioned environment. Carry either a complete change or extra items for such eventualities. Air-conditioned offices are a mixed blessing for many, especially for newcomers to the Far East in Singapore, Bangkok, Hong Kong, and the like. They find that they can work intensively during the day but, on leaving the cool, fairly dry conditions for the "outside world," they are quite exhausted by early evening. Reliance on alcoholic refreshment is an unwise habit to develop in these circumstances.

HEAT ILLNESSES

HEAT HYPERPYREXIA (HEAT STROKE)

Hyperpyrexia means "high fever" and some specialists regard it as the first stage in the development of heat stroke, while others use the terms as alternatives. "Sunstroke" is a misnomer as the illness may occur without direct exposure to the sun.

This serious condition begins with impairment of the heat-regulating mechanisms of the body, although how this occurs is not yet fully understood. Sweating diminishes and the body temperature rises—a sufferer who is still sufficiently alert will complain that he or she is feeling peculiar and is not sweating very much. The body temperature will be in the region of 102°–106°F. (39°–41°C.), and the higher it rises, the worse the likely outcome: *this condition can result in death within two to four hours* of the first symptoms.

In the areas where sweating has ceased, the skin becomes flushed and red. Headache develops and soon becomes severe, often described as dull and pounding. Walking soon changes to staggering, and signs of mental confusion and perhaps unusual aggression appear. Unable to stand, the sufferer becomes delirious, develops stertorous breathing, and may convulse.

In the total absence of sweating, the temperature continues to rise until death occurs at about 109°–111°F. (43°– 44°C.). The only treatment is immediate cooling. Under shelter from the sun, remove all clothing and cover the patient with a wetted bedsheet, towel, or other lightweight material and start fanning to promote cooling by evaporation. Keep the coverings wet, and fanning and wetting must continue all the way to the hospital, where electrical fans and needle-spraying of cooled water will hopefully be available. Rehydration is also important, and is part of the cooling process.

Definitive prevention of the condition is difficult because the cause of the failure of the body's regulatory system is not yet fully understood. Factors that play a part in its occurrence are these:

• Continuous heat stress, day and night

• Lack of fitness, or obesity

• Overindulgence in alcohol

• Strenuous exercise (causing excessive internal heat production)

• Too much clothing for the conditions

• Certain kinds of medication, e.g., cold remedies and diuretics

• A premature return to activity after a previous episode of heat exhaustion, particularly in an unacclimatized person

• Any of the above in a person whose sweating ability is seriously impaired by a skin complaint or disorder

Do not forget that the patient may have a fever-producing illness in addition, which may not have been recognized. It is essential to treat hyperpyrexial patients for *cerebral malaria* as well as cooling them, if there is a danger of malaria in the area (see also Map 5.1, p. 123).

HEAT EXHAUSTION
Heat exhaustion may be one of the three types, namely water-deficiency, salt-deficiency, or anhidrotic heat exhaustion (anhidrotic means absent sweat). Each is serious and the first and third progress to heat stroke because of the implied interference with cooling by evaporation of sweat.

Water-deficiency heat exhaustion occurs when there is a restriction of water intake in a heat-stress situation. Extreme examples occur in people stranded in a desert or adrift in tropical seas without water. Remember that water requirements in a hot climate may be very high (10 quarts a day in the example cited above). The potential victim is thirsty and complains of vague discomforts, then lack of appetite, giddiness, restlessness, and tingling sensations. Any urine passed is in small quantity and deeply colored. Lips, mouth, and tongue become so dry that speaking is hardly possible. The temperature rises steadily, the pulse rate increases, breathing becomes faster, and the lips are blue. Hollow cheeks and sunken eyes complete the picture before the victim sinks into a coma and, if not treated, death.

The comatose patient requires cooling and fluids supplied intravenously, if possible, with medical assistance. The patient who can still understand and walk is quickly restored in cool surroundings with the following regime: 1 pint of water of any flavor to be drunk every 15 minutes for two hours or until a large quantity of pale urine is passed. Thereafter keep the patient cool for two days and advise on drinking past the point of thirst-quenching.

Salt-deficiency heat exhaustion commonly occurs in the inexperienced newcomer, after two or three days of heavy sweating and work, with plenty to drink but no salt replacement because of lack of appetite. Quite frequently, vomiting and/or diarrhea have hastened the onset. The body's salt "reserves" have vanished and the cells and tissues that require it are malfunctioning. Increasing fatigue is soon followed by lethargy, headache, giddiness, and extremely severe muscle cramps. Pallor of the face and around the lips is very typical as the patient collapses, still soaked with sweat.

Do not allow the casualty to sit up or move as this may precipitate a fatal collapse. Urgent treatment with bed rest in cool surroundings, and a high intake of salted drinks—1 level teaspoonful of salt per pint given every hour for six hours will supply some 15 g. of the daily requirement of 20 g. of salt. Thereafter, return to the presalted water regime mentioned above—had this been observed in the first place, the condition might not have occurred! The presalted water replaces one half of the salt lost in unacclimatized sweat, and the rest should come from the diet. Be prepared, however, to supervise your patient's eating habits and to insist on empty plates. A return to work should be gradual.

Anhidrotic heat exhaustion arises as a disorder of sweating in people who have been in a hot climate for several months. It may be defined as a state of exhaustion and heat intolerance. The skin, mainly of the trunk and upper arms, shows a rash of little vesicles (called *miliaria profunda*) and there is little or no sweat in these parts when all around are sweating freely. Fairly rare, it is worst in the heat of the day—symptoms include fatigue, unpleasant sensations of warmth, giddiness on standing up, frightening palpitations, and rapid, sometimes gasping breathing. The face sweats profusely, and there is a frequent and insistent urge to pass urine, sometimes in larger quantities than usual. The disorder is often preceded by an attack of prickly heat (see below). These seriously heat-intolerant individuals should be removed to a cool environment for one month's rest, and then be supervised carefully on return, because another attack may lead to heat stroke.

OTHER CONDITIONS CAUSED BY HEAT

Prickly heat or miliaria rubra (literally red millet seeds) consists of a vast number of vesicles or tiny blisters set in red, mildly inflamed skin, worst around the waist, upper trunk, armpits, front of the elbows, and even on the scalp. The rash is accompanied by intensely aggravating prickling sensations. The cause is not yet clear, but an important factor is the constant wetting of the skin by unevaporated sweat as occurs at times of high humidity in hot/wet climes. The skin becomes unhealthy and water-logged, sweat ducts are blocked with debris and infection starts, causing a large number of pimples. Sleep is almost always upset and is delayed until the coolest period of the night, around 4:00 to 5:00 a.m. As a result, bad temper and irritability are usual, with a diminution in working efficiency. The prickling can be relieved by taking a cool shower, gentle dab-drying of the skin to prevent further damage, then calamine lotion and zinc oxide dusting powder. The clothing should be starch-free and of loose fit. (See also p. 460).

Heat edema (heat swelling) of the ankles used to be called "deck ankles" and appeared in passengers when the ships first entered tropical waters. Now it is indistinguishable from the swollen ankles of long air journeys (p. 233), and is found to last for a few days in the unacclimatized newcomer to extreme heat. The condition requires no treatment and will disappear as acclimatization progresses.

Heat cramps may occur without the signs and symptoms of salt-deficiency heat exhaustion described above, and are due to the same problem—salt lack—from whatever cause. They are excruciatingly painful, and occur at random intervals in whichever muscle groups are used most. The treatment is the same as for salt-deficiency heat exhaustion.

Heat syncope (fainting) occurs typically in the unacclimatized on first exposure to the heat. Due to circulatory instability during the early days, it occurs after prolonged standing or on sudden change of posture. The "head-low" or lying position will return the blood to the brain. An hour or two of rest and graded exercise will soon banish the condition.

COLD CLIMATES

"Cold," in this context, simply denotes an immediate environment that is below body temperature and is likely to cause the body temperature to fall.

HYPOTHERMIA

As stated earlier, heat always flows from a hot source to one that is lower in temperature, and the human body can lose heat through conduction, convection, and radiation.

The requirement for a stable central or core temperature within 1°F. of 98.4°F. has already been stressed. If this temperature falls by a generalized chilling of the body to 95.0°F. (35.0°C.), the resulting condition is called hypothermia (deficient heat). A special low-reading clinical thermometer is necessary to record such low body temperatures. Hypothermia leads to deterioration of the function of organs and cells, and if not controlled and corrected, ultimately to death. The brain tolerates hypothermia badly, and the manifestations of its malfunction are virtually identical to those which occur under conditions of excessive heat—a point that has received little or no attention—possibly because few investigators have had the opportunity to study both.

COLD INJURY

Central or core temperature is maintained in two ways: first, and of greatest importance when the body is at rest, heat is generated by the use of the body's fuel reserves of fat and carbohydrates; second, any muscular activity generates further heat. In a fit person, muscular activity may increase heat production by a factor of 10 or 15. Heat is conveyed from the core of the body to the skin and extremities by the circulating blood. Heat is then lost to the environment, and the cooled blood returns, tending to lower the core temperature. In cold conditions, therefore, the body's heat can be lost through inadequate insulation of the skin and extremities in generalized chilling. If there is severe localized chilling, cold injury can occur even if the core temperature is not substantially altered—and such injury can be sufficiently serious to require hospital treatment.

Different forms of cold injury include the nonfreezing type called "immersion foot" ("trench foot" of World War I) from long exposure to cold, damp conditions, and frostbite, which follows freezing of the tissues of the extremities, especially the nose, cheeks, chin, ears, fingers, and feet in cold dry environments. Less serious injuries—though often annoying ones—include chapped skin of the lips, nose, and hands in cold windy weather; and sunburn (pp. 322–330) and windburn which, with snow-blindness (p. 382), typically occur in cold dry climates.

ACCLIMATIZATION

The human body has no mechanism for acclimatizing to cold which corresponds to the way it adapts to hot climates. Instead it must rely on insulation, provided not only by our layers of body fat, but also by modern clothing and shelter technology. Travelers generally have to rely on trapped still dry air in clothing and housing to keep them warm, and this remains the best insulant known.

Prevention of the effects of cold thus depends upon the maintenance of body heat by an adequate supply of energy (food and drink) for internal energy production; on blocking avenues of heat loss; and finally upon preservation of an insulating shell of still dry air.

It is pertinent at this point to discuss a source of possible confusion in terminology. The World Health Organization has decreed that hypothermia in this context should be known as "accidental hypothermia." Terms such as exposure, mountain hypothermia, and immersion hypothermia are no longer recognized.

WIND: AN ADDITIONAL RISK

Wind speed has an important effect on human heat balance in both cold/wet and cold/dry conditions. Much of the important research on this subject was carried out by the late Paul Siple and his colleague C. F. Passel, who in 1945 published a method of assessing the effects of wind, which has stood the test of time and is known as the Wind Chill Factor. A slight modification of the original is reproduced here (Figure 8.1, p. 317) as the Wind Chill Index. By measuring or assessing the present and possible trend of temperature and wind speed, the traveler can allocate the prevailing conditions to one of the zones A–G on the graph, and then decide whether it is safe to stray away from shelter.

When using this method, I recommend deeming the air temperature to be 11°F. (6°C.) *lower* than actual temperature if the clothing is soaked through with water. This adjustment is necessary because of the extra heat loss by conduction through waterlogged clothing.

Use of the method obviously requires some means of measuring air temperature and wind speed. Air temperature is simple to measure using inexpensive equipment such as the sling or whirling psychrometer. As the name implies, this apparatus is rotated rapidly like a British football rattle for a minimum of 30 seconds and the reading taken. Of great use in cold and hot climates, the instrument can be small enough to slip into the pocket.

If very cold conditions are expected, a thermometer containing colored alcohol that will not freeze is required. Measurement of wind speed requires an anemometer, which is generally a rather delicate and expensive instrument. The Beaufort table of wind-speed, shown in Table 8.3, p. 314, supplies an alternative to the use of an instrument, but does require some practice in its use.

COLD EFFECTS AND INJURIES (see also pp. 344–46)

The most important harmful effect of cold is that already referred to as accidental hypothermia, defined as a result of the generalized chilling of a person such that he or she has a core temperature of 95.0°F. (35°C.) or less.

In the field, the measurement of temperature in the mouth, arm-pit, or ear is useless. Placing the thermometer in the stream of urine as it is passed is reliable, but requires a full bladder, or a minimum of about half a pint of urine. Usually the only reliable method with simple apparatus is to place the thermometer in the rectum.

In practice, the onset of the condition may be fast or slow, and this is a convenient approach to its description as acute or chronic.

ACUTE ACCIDENTAL HYPOTHERMIA

This is most commonly due to immersion in cold water. Falling into water colder than 41°F. (5°C.) is a grave emergency with almost immediate effects. The victim gasps, shivers violently, curls up, inhales water, and is dead from drowning in about 5–15 minutes. It is doubtful whether even onlookers experienced in the first aid of drowning can act quickly enough. If the victim is wearing plenty of clothing that retards the loss of body heat, a life preserver that keeps the head out of the water, has face protection to prevent cold water from splashing on it (which stops the breathing, slows or stops the heart, and predisposes to drowning), and has been well enough trained to know to keep *perfectly still* in the water, he or she has well-established average chances of survival from the immersion. These expectations are: about 50 minutes in freezing water; around three hours in water at 50°F. (10°C.), some six hours at 59°F. (15°C.), and very many more hours at 70°F. (20°C.) and above.

Other factors that influence the onset of hypothermia in water are increasing age; lack of fitness; liability to panic; lack of recent food intake for internal heat production; and the recent drinking of alcohol, which without food causes a severe fall in blood sugar, with immediate confusion and clumsiness.

Any insulating material will protect against hypothermia. The protective influence of fat under the skin as an insulant against heat loss in the water led Professor Keatinge of the London Hospital to bring an old adage up to date by suggesting that, instead of "women and children first," it should read "thin boys and men first," and then "plump girls and women."

TABLE 8.3. A GUIDE TO ESTIMATING WIND SPEED (BEAUFORT SCALE OF WIND FORCE)

Wind speed (miles per hour)	Beaufort scale	Wind force	Effects
1	0	calm	smoke rises vertically
1–3	1	light air	wind direction shown by smoke; wind vane does not move
4–7	2	slight breeze	wind felt on face; leaves rustle; wind vane moves
8–12	3	gentle breeze	leaves and small twigs in constant motion; light flag lifts
13–18	4	moderate breeze	dust and loose paper raised; small branches move; snow begins to drift
19–24	5	fresh breeze	small trees begin to sway; wavelets created on inland waterways
25–31	6	strong breeze	large branches in motion; umbrellas difficut to use; high snow-drifts
32–38	7	high wind	whole trees in motion; visibility obscured by drifting snow
39–46	8	gale	twigs break off trees; walking increasingly difficult
47–54	9	strong gale	slight structural damage to buildings
55–63	10	whole gale	inland trees uprooted
64–72	11	storm	rare; widespread damage
73–82	12	hurricane	very rare; widespread severe damage

If the casualty is known to have collapsed in the water after some 5–15 minutes' immersion, then drowning is the most likely explanation. If he or she is conscious, can talk only clumsily, or is incoherent and cannot answer questions, then hypothermia is the diagnosis.

Do not constrict the chest with any harness or allow the victim to make any movement, especially climbing nets to board a ship or to clamber into a small boat—there have been many surprising deaths after rescue that are now thought to be due to sudden stress on a heart already grievously affected by the cold.

Ideally, the patient should be placed in the horizontal position, with the head slightly down, protected from further heat loss and taken immediately to a facility for rapid rewarming. Try to ascertain if water has been inhaled in however small a quantity, because hospital investigation is then urgent. In the meantime commence rapid rewarming in a bath (showers are not of any use) in which the water is kept at 107.5°F. (42°C.) or as hot as the *bare elbow* can tolerate.

If the rectal temperature is being monitored during this treatment, it will be found that it continues to fall for the first 15 minutes or so—the notorious "after-drop," the significance of which is not yet completely understood. Resuscitation facilities should ideally be available—collapse may occur at any time until the patient is out of danger. If rapid (bath) rewarming is not available the victim must be allowed to "come round" from his or her own internal heat production in a bed with quilt, "space blanket," or light blanket insulation only. The supply of external heat by electric lamp cradles, electric blankets, and the like requires a hospital environment, with intravenous fluids, oxygen, and injectable drug supplies ready to hand.

CHRONIC ACCIDENTAL HYPOTHERMIA

This is defined here as being much longer in its onset than acute hypothermia (which may require 20–30 minutes only, if the water is cold enough). The very young and the elderly are generally the most susceptible to hypothermia, but the accent here is on middle age groups engaged in hiking, exploring, biological surveys and observations, hill-walking, mountaineering, or stranded in a cold and hostile environment. Commonest in the cold/wet climate, it is usually the product of soaked garments and a wind chill factor in zone C or above in Figure 8.1. It is often complicated by overexertion, especially in those who are unprepared for sudden weather changes, who become lost and also have no reserve food or clothing, tent or sleeping bag. Mist, rain, sleet, hail, snow, and white-out may occur suddenly, and absence of map and compass, flashlight and whistle, help to compound the situation.

Early recognition of the condition is of the greatest importance, and this requires one or more companions in a group (beware the lone ranger) who know each other well and can adopt the "buddy system" to watch one another. Warning signs include complaints of feeling cold, tired, or listless; inability to keep the pace, progressing to stumbling and then repeated falls; unexpected, unreasonable, or uncharacteristic behavior with unusual aggression; and failure to understand or respond to repeated questions or commands.

Uncontrollable bouts of shivering, which then cease, and disturbances of vision herald collapse and unconsciousness with dilated pupils. The victim's pulse at wrist or neck will be irregular. In the unlikely event that temperature measurement has been possible, it will have been about 95°F. (35°C.) at the start of the above list of signs and symptoms, and about 90°F. (32°C.) by the time the shivering is diminishing. The risk to life is now increasing and death may occur suddenly below 82°F. (28°C.), with disturbance of the heart rhythm and eventual cardiac arrest. The sooner the following action starts, the better the outcome:

Fig. 8.1 Wind Chill Index. (Modified from: J. M. Adam (1969). *Community Health* 1, 39–46.)

The Wind Chill Index is indicated by the point at which the air temperature (vertical axis) and wind velocity (horizontal axis) cross; record it every hour to monitor deteriorating conditions.

Zone A: No danger.
Zone B: Little danger when wearing light clothing provided meals are regular and overexertion avoided. Beware of a sudden deterioration in the weather.
Zone C: Requires full clothing protection, waterproof shelter, hot food and drink, prevention of overexertion. In temperate climates, most deaths from hypothermia occur in this zone.
Zone D: Travel becomes dangerous on overcast days—sudden rain, sleet, hail, or snow can be hazardous.
Zone E: Temporary shelter is dangerous to live in, travel should be contemplated only in heated vehicles.
Zone F: Exposed flesh starts to freeze.
Zone G: Exposed flesh freezes in less than one minute, and survival efforts are required.

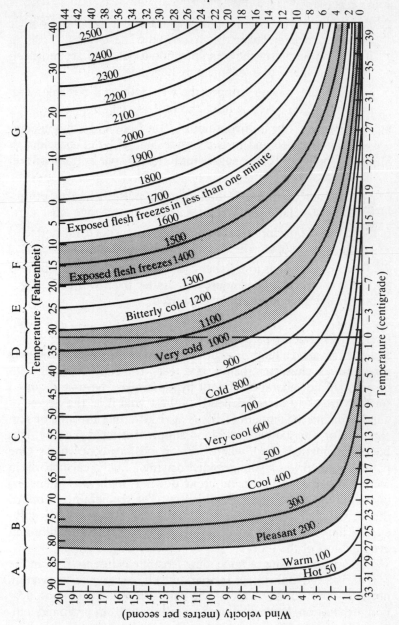

1. *Stop* activity.
2. *Protect* from wind, rain, etc., by rigging a tent, poncho, or other bivouac or shelter, laying the victim in the "head-down" position if he is conscious, or the coma position if not, on a groundsheet, "space blanket," or in a large polythene bag.
3. *Insulate* him, having stripped the wet clothing if possible, with sleeping bag(s) covering head and face as well.
4. *Rewarm* him if he is unconscious by the body warmth of a companion—stripped and in bed beside him. If he is conscious, a quick "brew-up" of hot sugary tea followed later by hot food will hasten recovery.
5. *Observe* for cessation of breathing or pulse, when mouth-to-mouth resuscitation and/or external cardiac massage must start.
6. *Send* two people for help, but first give them a hot drink and food in case they, too, are affected by the cold conditions.
7. *Treat* the patient as a stretcher case, no matter what may be said to the contrary. If he is injured, of course there will be no argument, and transport must be organized.

FROSTBITE

Local severe chilling of exposed or poorly insulated tissues— nose, cheeks, chin, ears, hands, and feet—can cause freezing with or without the general chilling of hypothermia. The time required for the "frost" to "bite" depends on how cold it is, the degree of wind chill and the amount of tissue at risk—either the area of skin exposed, or a tissue with its blood supply restricted (i.e., by tight boots and matted socks where feet or toes are concerned). One patient of mine was a young soldier driving a Euclid earthmover in wintertime Korea. His engine broke down as night was falling, so he curled up in the cab and fell asleep. The temperature dropped during the night, and the blood supply to his right foot was sufficiently impeded by his awkward posture to cause frostbite and eventual loss of the foot.

The initial warning of impending frostbite is intense pain in the part at risk, and at this stage the part must be rewarmed. The victim, however, may not be aware of the pain—from intense preoccupation, exhaustion, having suffered an injury, or from profound lethargy—and it eventually disappears. The part becomes numb, white, and hard to the touch because it is frostbitten. "Buddies" watch each other's faces for this.

Prevention of frostbite consists of being aware of the risk, keeping an eye on the wind chill index and discussing the conditions with local inhabitants, and wearing adequate protective clothing (see below).

Treatment At the painful stage of impending frostbite, the treatment follows the sequence set out above—stop, protect, insulate, and re-warm the part. Cover nose, cheeks, or ears until shelter is erected and warm; hands and fingers are slipped under the clothes to the opposite armpit or between the thighs. Feet require the heroic test of friendship—through the clothing onto the belly of a companion! Pain will disappear and normal color and sensation will indicate when danger is over. Take the opportunity to correct any other factors that may predispose to frostbite by changing wet clothing, producing a hot meal, or reminding one's companions of other dangers such as touching bare metal with bare hands—this can cause instantaneous freezing, as can slopping gasoline onto bare skin.

Established frostbite is a serious problem, particularly when it involves fingers and hands, or feet and toes, when lasting damage may affect the victim's employment and earning capacity. A speedy but gentle journey to the hospital is essential. Once frostbitten tissue has thawed, up to three months of skilled medical attention may be necessary; moreover, if tissue once thawed is even slightly chilled again, it is liable to much more extensive damage. In an emergency involving a frozen foot (the worst) far from any hospital, there are three options:

- If the journey must be completed and no patient transport is available, remember that it is possible to walk on a frozen foot, though most certainly not on one that has thawed. Ideally hot food and drink are necessary, together with correction of any clothing defects. Give a painkiller such as two tablets of aceta-minophen, with an oral antibiotic such as a penicillin or tetra-cycline, dosage 250 mg. every five to six hours day and night to combat any infection.

- If a stretcher with men to carry it, or alternatively a man or dog-drawn sledge is available, treat the victim in warm shelter as above, not omitting the painkillers and antibiotics. Remove the boot and sock as carefully as possible, cover the foot lightly with gauze, pad it with cotton wool, and wrap it up loosely. Make him or her comfortable and warm and immobilize the foot gently before setting off.

- If the patient is at a static base with medical advice available and the possibility of eventual evacuation, then the patient should stay put. Keep him or her in a room, where a high temperature can be maintained (about 70°F. or 21°C.). Elevate the part on a pillow with sterile precautions if available. Expose the foot to the warm air, wash it gently with an antiseptic solution such as warm 1 percent cetrimide, dab it dry, inspect carefully and report the findings by radio for medical advice. This is likely to include the administration of a course of antibiotics and painkillers as above.

If the fingers and/or hand are frostbitten, clean the skin area with the cetrimide solution and dab dry very gently. Separate the fingers with cotton wool after winding a sterile bandage around each, and place a thick sterile pad in the palm of the hand so that the fingers are in a "glass-holding" position. Bandage the whole lightly and elevate the forearm in a sling. Commence a course of antibiotics and painkillers as already outlined. Reassurance and gentle treatment are of the essence until the patient arrives at the hospital.

Never rub frostbite with snow or anything else, because the delicate tissues will suffer more damage.

IMMERSION FOOT

Immersion foot occurs when the lower limbs and feet have been kept in cold conditions for hours or days, as happened in the trenches of World War I and in the lifeboats after shipwreck during World War II. After the first sensation of cold passes off, the feet feel numb, and this continues for the long period of immobility and restriction of blood that is a prerequisite of the disorder. The patient may be unable to walk, or walks with difficulty, complaining that it feels like walking on cotton wool. Inadequate food, general chilling, lack of sleep, and exhaustion complete the typical picture.

On examination, the skin is blotchy-white, the ankles are swollen and marked deeply with pressure ridges from boots, etc. As the patient becomes warm, and the affected area is dried gently, the feet become hot, red, and more swollen, and there is intense pain. The victim must be taken to the hospital, and if this is likely to take time, should be treated with painkillers and antibiotics as for frostbite. The legs must be elevated, protected from further damage and exposed in a warm room. Blisters may form on the feet in the first two days or so, and must be kept scrupulously (but gently) clean. It may be many months before an established case is able to return to work.

CHILBLAINS

Chilblains are the mildest form of cold injury and are due to alternate exposure to wet/cold conditions and rapid rewarming. The disorder occurs frequently: in the UK, 50 percent of the inhabitants are said to have suffered from it at one time or another. Prevention is by keeping the extremities warm, heating the house, eradicating drafts, and avoiding long periods of standing without moving (see also p. 363).

CLOTHING FOR COLD CONDITIONS

Clothing should be well fitting and built up on the "layer" principle from the innermost air-trapping layers to the outermost windproof and/or waterproof coverings. Each layer must be larger than the one beneath it to prevent constrictions and to preserve the insulating air. Neck and wrist openings are recommended as they permit ventilation by "bellows action" so that water vapor from sweat can escape when one is working hard. Thus the inner layers do not become wet with condensed sweat, which might lead to chilling. Layers, too, may need to be removed or added for that same reason, as the work load dictates. I do not favor turtleneck sweaters because they cannot be ventilated.

Special requirements include protection of the head, which, in still air at 32°F. (0°C.), can lose one-quarter of the entire body's heat production per hour; and this rate increases with lower air temperatures and higher wind chill. The peculiar shape of the feet and ankles make their insulation a problem, and great care should be exercised in the selection and fitting of socks and boots. Socks that are worn for too long become a double hazard by becoming matted or developing holes so that they lose insulation value, and by shrinking so that the blood supply to the toes and feet is impeded. Ensure a good overlap of sleeves with gloves or mittens, because a strip of frostbite on the inner side of the wrist is extremely painful.

SUMMARY OF ADVICE FOR TRAVELERS

Hot climates
* Full acclimatization takes about three weeks.
* Thirst sensation is a poor guide to your true water requirements in a hot climate—always drink more than you think you need.
* Salt requirements are also high—you may need to consider adding salt to drinking water, as described on pp. 304–5.
* Guidelines for preventing and treating heat stroke and heat exhaustion are given on pp. 306–10.

Cold climates
* No acclimatization is possible, so it is vital to be adequately prepared for cold conditions, with suitable clothing and equipment.
* Cold injuries and emergencies are described on pp. 313–22.

SUN AND THE TRAVELER

A suntan is often considered attractive and socially desirable, but obtaining one can have harmful effects both in the short and long term. Understanding the circumstances likely to lead to sunburn— and avoiding them—can help improve your trip.

Dr. John Hawk is Head of the Photobiology Department at the St. John's Institute of Dermatology, London. His main research interests include the effects of sunlight upon the skin, and the skin disorders that follow exposure to sunlight.

The sun's rays have been this planet's energy source for the past 4,500 million years. They have initiated and maintained life, both by providing warmth and light and by fueling specific important biological processes such as photosynthesis in plants and the manufacture of vitamin D in human skin. In addition, moderate sunshine improves the quality of life, and has been claimed to improve a person's overall work performance.

Unfortunately, not all solar energy is used to advantage by living matter, and in many circumstances it may damage exposed tissues: well-recognized examples include effects on all human skin such as sunburning, aging, and cancer, and cataracts of the human eye.

Other skin reactions affecting only some exposed subjects may also occur. As many as 15 percent of people develop an irritating, spotty rash within a few hours of sun exposure lasting for up to a week. This is polymorphous light eruption, often mistakenly called prickly heat, a harmless condition usually kept in check by high-protection-factor sunscreens and avoidance of strong sunlight. Other relatively common abnormal reactions include excessive sunburning from photosensitivity caused by certain perfumes, cosmetics, sun-barrier creams, and medications taken by mouth or applied to the skin (see box, p. 363).

During man's evolution, protective responses have developed which tend to protect against these phenomena, namely tanning and thickening reactions of the exposed skin. These occur, however, only as a result of sun damage and not before: thus a tanned skin may give protection against further exposure, but unless already genetically present, its acquisition through sun exposure is always associated with skin injury.

If a tan is considered a social necessity, however, it should be acquired gradually, moderately, and carefully to minimize damage and its unpleasant consequences, namely sunburn in the short term and skin aging and cancer in the long term.

SUN EFFECTS ON THE SKIN

THE HARMFUL RAYS

The damaging rays in sunlight are called ultraviolet radiation (UVR). Short-wavelength UVR, or UVC, is the most damaging to living cells, but is completely absorbed by the oxygen and ozone in the atmosphere. Thus, if atmospheric ozone layer destruction should occur as a result of its continuing depletion by chlorofluorocarbons and similar chemicals from aerosols and other sources, some UVC radiation might conceivably penetrate the atmosphere and lead to increased sunburning and skin cancer (and perhaps more important, to death of much unicellular life with consequent disruption of vital ecosystems). Middle-wavelength UVR (called

UVB), strong in midday midsummer sunlight, also has a marked tendency to produce sunburn. This is generally followed by tanning in susceptible people, and by skin aging and cancer after chronically repeated exposure.

Long-wavelength UVR (called UVA) also burns, but at much higher radiation doses than for UVB and UVC, and tanning usually occurs before burning. Chronically repeated exposure to UVA also causes skin aging, and may accelerate or induce the onset of skin cancer. UVA rays are the main component of UVR in sunlight, causing about one tenth of its effect on skin around midday in summer, and in tanning salon radiation.

CIRCUMSTANCES LEADING TO DAMAGE

The stronger the UVR dose received from sunlight, the worse the skin damage induced. The amount of damage thus depends on the time, locality, and circumstances of the exposure.

UVR in sunlight is strongest when the sun is high in the sky, namely in the middle of the day in summer, particularly at low latitudes near the equator. If in addition one is at high altitude, or there are adjacent reflecting surfaces such as snow, metals, white materials, or rippling water, or there is lots of blue sky visible, exposure will be increased. Sunburning is therefore particularly likely on beaches, at sea, in the desert, and on ski slopes.

Furthermore, cool winds, haze, light cloud, swimming in water, and thin, close-fitting, or loose-weave clothing do not much reduce UVR intensity.

SUSCEPTIBILITY TO SKIN DAMAGE

The damage caused by sunlight at times of high UVR intensity also depends on the type of exposed skin. Genetically black-skinned people are well protected against all the effects of the sun, and brown and yellow-skinned people are several times better off than white people, though they do burn if outdoors for long enough. Most white people burn relatively easily, particularly those with red hair and freckles. Others tan readily, sometimes with a little burning.

Most people know from experience how they react in strong summer sunlight and should protect themselves accordingly. If their skin is completely unable to tan, as in albinos, or unable in patches, as in the disease vitiligo, particular care is needed—although some protection still develops from superficial skin thickening.

While the short-term effects of sunlight are mainly a problem for sunbathers and watersports or skiing enthusiasts, the chronic effects such as aging or cancer of the skin may occur in any outdoor enthusiast or tropical dweller, particularly if fair-skinned.

THE EFFECTS OF UVR EXPOSURE

UVR penetrates the skin surface well, often better when the skin is wet or oily, and damages the nuclei and membranes of cells. Chemicals released as a result, associated with damage to the surrounding tissues, lead to short-term and long-term changes:

EARLY

1. Sunburn, i.e., pinkness, redness, soreness, or sometimes in severe cases, swelling, blistering, or weeping of sun-exposed skin.

2. Tanning, i.e., formation of brown melanin pigmentation in the skin.

3. Hyperplasia, i.e., thickening of all skin layers, but particularly of the superficial dead horny layer.

LATE

1. Aging, i.e., degenerative changes of chronically exposed skin, apparent as loss of substance, dryness, coarseness, brown blotchiness, yellowing, wrinkling, and laxity, sometimes with blackheads, whiteheads, or spidery dilated blood vessels.

2. Precancers and cancers, i.e., persistent rough patches or irregular slowly growing lumps or sores, sometimes colored brownish or reddish.

All these changes are responses to injury, but the tanning and hyperplasia are also useful protective responses against further damage. These act by partly absorbing subsequent UVR before it reaches vulnerable skin targets. However, acquisition and maintenance of skin tanning and hyperplasia always result in a degree of permanent injury that is never fully repaired.

The only definitely beneficial result of skin UV exposure is the production of vitamin D in the skin, but since adequate amounts are also available in the normal diet, UVR exposure for this reason alone is not justifiable. It has further been claimed that UVR exposure from sunlight may improve one's mood and work rate. However any such improvement seems unlikely to result from the UVR content of sunlight, but rather from the visible component acting through the eye, and skin UVR exposure for this purpose is thus also inappropriate.

The only other arguably useful effect of UVR exposure is the purely cosmetic, subjective, and psychological one of having a tan. It should be understood, however, that this has no known direct health-giving effect whatsoever!

PREPARATION FOR A SUNNY VACATION

You need do very little, apart from obtaining a good supply of a high-protection sunscreen of a type that suits you cosmetically. If possible, find a preparation that also claims to give good UVA protection.

EFFECTS OF TANNING SALONS

Although courses of tanning salon treatment have also been advocated to give a preliminary tan and consequent protection against later sun exposure, the protection obtained is usually minimal and the advantages of this are therefore extremely questionable. The only real reason for using sunlamps or tanning salons is essentially a cosmetic one, and as for sunlight UVR exposure, their use is not a healthy pastime: a small amount of skin damage always inevitably occurs. Often there are also other annoying side effects such as itching, dryness, redness, freckling, and occasionally drug rash, polymorphic light eruption, and a tendency to skin blistering and lessened resistance to minor injury.

If you are still desperate for a pre-vacation tan, exposure three times weekly (e.g., Monday, Wednesday, Friday) for two to three weeks until the vacation should give some color, but regular use of a sunscreen when you arrive at your destination is still necessary.

ON VACATION

Your intention on vacation should be to take full advantage of the enjoyable aspects of sun exposure while avoiding the harmful ones. So if you don't care about a tan, cover up, and wear loose-fitting but tightly woven, airy clothes, preferably cotton, and apply a highly protective sunscreen (see below) to any remaining exposed areas every hour or so when you are outside.*

If, however, you insist on a tan, you should start for the first day or two by exposing unacclimatized skin for no more than about 10–20 minutes per day when UVR intensity is high; in addition apply a highly protective sunscreen every hour or so, particularly after swimming or exercise. Over the next few days, gradually increase your exposure if you want to, and if your skin feels comfortable, apply the sunscreen a little less frequently or change to a preparation with a somewhat lower protection factor. At the end of a day in the sun, it is also worth using a moisturizing cream from time to time to help minimize skin dryness and irritation.

If you tan readily, you should be fairly brown after about a week to 10 days, although increasing tanning may gradually continue over a few more weeks. If you know that you burn easily on any particular areas of the body such as the nose, lips, or white patches, you will have to take extra care with these areas. Conventional high-protection sunscreens are generally pretty effective, but zinc oxide or titanium dioxide–containing creams and pastes are particularly good for such areas. However, these are often cosmetically unsuitable for widespread use on the skin because of their white or brown color, and newer preparations containing very fine (so-called microfined) titanium dioxide particles are generally preferable for all-over maximal protection.

If you decide to wear very little or to go topless, you will need to be very careful with any pale, previously unexposed areas of skin, especially when the UVR intensity of the sunlight is high, so once more use a particularly high protection factor cream, preferably one containing microfined titanium dioxide. If you ever start feeling uncomfortable and weatherbeaten, cover up.

In general, with a little thought and care, and with today's strong sunscreens, you should have no problems, and you should get your tan as well, unless you are using the very high protection creams containing microfined titanium dioxide to give high UVA protection, or you don't tan well anyway. However, carelessness and over-

---

* Typical summer clothing is said to provide protection equivalent to an SPF of around 5-9. A range of high SPF clothing is available from Sun Precautions Inc., 168 Denny Way, Seattle, WA 98109.   Tel: (800) 882-7860, (206) 441-6688.

doing it on the first few days will very likely result in painful burning, swelling, blistering, and peeling, a poor or patchy tan, and a legacy of permanently damaged skin to increase your chances of later wrinkling and even skin cancer.

SUNSCREENS AND TANNING LOTIONS

Use of sunscreens (also known as sun-barrier preparations, sun-block sun creams, and suntan oils or lotions) is a very effective way of protecting against many of the effects of UVR in sunlight, particularly since very high protection factor preparations are now available. There are two main types of these preparations: absorbent and reflectant.

Absorbent sunscreens are the well-known, conspicuously packaged, and pleasantly perfumed oils, creams, and lotions available at drugstores and pharmacies. They act by absorbing many of the potentially harmful UV rays before they reach the skin surface and then dissipating them as relatively innocuous minor quantities of heat. The advantages of the absorbent sunscreens are their cosmetic acceptability and their efficacy in protecting against UVB. Their disadvantages are the ease with which many dry or wash off (most people thus need repeated applications), their tendency to produce allergic rashes on occasion, their tendency to irritate the skin immediately after application, and their relative inefficiency against UVA rays, although many newer preparations do stay on well and give reasonable UVA protection.

Reflectant sunscreens, usually containing zinc oxide or titanium dioxide, are reserved mainly for occasional medical use, but may be applied thickly to limited areas such as lips and nose which are particularly liable to sunburning. Newer preparations containing microfined titanium dioxide are much more cosmetically acceptable; however they are still a little messier than many of the absorbent products.

The efficacy of sunscreens can be gauged to a large extent from their experimentally estimated sun protection factor (SPF), a rough guide to the amount of protection they give against sunburning. Thus the SPF tells approximately how much longer you may stay in the sun if you apply the product regularly every hour or so during the day. For example, a product with an SPF 12 means you can stay exposed for about 12 times longer before you burn. Attempts are also being made to give an indication of the UVA protection provided by a sunscreen, but no method has yet been universally agreed. Some general indication, however, is given on many product packages.

SPF values are approximate, so do not assume that a preparation of SPF 10 is necessarily much different from one of SPF 9 or 11. Cost is no guide whatsoever, so choose the cheapest product that suits you. If you find a sunscreen causes you unpleasant effects, change it. If you burn easily, you should start with a preparation of SPF greater than 15 that also gives UVA protection. If you burn initially but later tan a little, look for an SPF 10–15. If you burn a little and tan well, choose an SPF of 5–10. If you do not burn, you need only an emollient or a cream of SPF less than 5. However, there is never any harm in choosing a higher SPF than you need or using a cream that also provides UVA protection.

Tablets to protect against the sun, for example, those containing vitamin A, beta-carotene, or canthaxanthin, have never been shown to work effectively, and the added possibility of adverse side effects on eyes or elsewhere means you should best avoid them except for very occasional short courses.

Pre-tanning agents are virtually useless, although artificial or fake tanning preparations which stain the skin brownish for a few days are harmless and do often provide a reasonable color. However, they provide no protection against later sun exposure.

If you get a spotty red, itchy rash when using your sunscreen, it is usually not because of the sunscreen but because of polymorphic light eruption, the annoying but harmless condition mentioned earlier. Use a higher SPF sunscreen and cover up for a few days. If the trouble persists or recurs, you may need to see a doctor on your return home. Herpes blisters (cold sores) may also occur with sun exposure (see p. 366).

TREATMENT

Too much sun exposure is harmful. It causes pain, redness, swelling, blistering, and occasionally scarring of the skin, and very rarely with extreme exposure fever, coma, or even death in the short term; in the long term dryness, thinning, yellowing, wrinkling, coarseness, looseness, freckling, spidery vessels, or cancers of the skin are possible.

The delayed effects of constant sun exposure cannot be reversed, except perhaps a little by plastic surgical techniques and to a lesser extent by the use of moisturizers. Recently, long-term application to the skin of tretinoin (Retin-A) has also been advocated to improve skin aging changes, but its effects are at best mild to moderate and continue only as long as the preparation is used; in addition, it may irritate the skin, while its other side effects have not yet been fully evaluated.

The short-term effects of sun exposure can be only partially reversed as well, although of course they resolve spontaneously within hours or days. Calamine cream or lotion may soothe burned areas, and mild painkillers such as aspirin and acetaminophen will also somewhat relieve pain and inflammation. Indomethacin 25 mg. tablets taken three times a day have been shown to help a little if started very soon after exposure. Steroid creams may also be slightly helpful. In addition, to minimize damage, do not sunbathe the day after any burn, but allow full healing to take place first.

Treat patches of severe sunburn in the same way as an ordinary heat burn, by protecting the area and keeping it clean to avoid infection. Widespread severe sunburn may need to be treated with painkillers, drinking plenty, and resting in bed; steroid tablets and antibiotics may also be required (see also p. 361).

SUMMARY OF ADVICE FOR TRAVELERS

- Excessive sun exposure causes skin damage.
- Acute episodes of sunburn or repeated sun exposure over the years increases the risk of certain kinds of skin cancer.
- The best way of minimizing problems is to avoid excessive sun exposure in the first place rather than trying to treat the symptoms once they have occurred.
- Understanding the circumstances that lead to high UVR exposure, plus the use of suitable clothing and appropriate sunscreens where necessary should enable you to have a pleasant burn-free tanning vacation while still enjoying the sunshine.

WATER AND WATERSPORTS

Travelers should prescribe themselves a large dose of caution to go with their sea- and lakeside adventures on vacation—and should make sure that activities like scuba diving take place only in a safe, well-supervised setting.

Surgeon Commander Simon Ridout is Principal Medical Officer at Royal Naval Air Station Culdrose, UK. He has been diving for the Royal Navy and for sport for more than 15 years.

Many people consider water and watersports an essential part of their vacation, but unfortunately most activities involving water—from swimming to snorkeling, scuba diving, sailing, windsurfing, and waterskiing—also involve some element of risk. Water in any form, from hotel swimming pool to river, lake, lagoon, or open sea, demands respect.

The old adage not to swim with a full stomach is correct, and alcohol is its most dangerous filling: as many as half of all drownings in the 20-to-30-year-old age group take place after drinking. People drink more on vacation, but should bear in mind that mixing alcohol with watersports too often results in tragedy.

SWIMMING

Swimming pools, whether freshwater or saltwater, require filtration and cleansing unless the water is frequently changed. If this is not done, eye and ear infections are a hazard. If the general cleanliness and hygiene standards of a hotel are satisfactory, its swimming pool is likely to be safe.

Freshwater lakes, dams, and slow-flowing rivers are all infected in countries where schistosomiasis (bilharzia) is endemic (Map 4.1, p. 96). Do not be influenced by the attitude of local kids. They frequently have a low-grade chronic infection which gives rise to a partial immunity.

Seawater is safe from schistosomiasis. Other aspects of seawater and disease are discussed on p. 79 and pp. 81–83. The open sea does pose the danger of tidal streams and currents: local advice should be sought if in doubt as to the strength of the tide. Few people can swim against a current of one knot (one nautical mile per hour) and even the strongest swimmer cannot swim against half a knot for very long. Swimming along the shore rather than out to sea is always safer, and reduces the danger of overestimating how far one can swim.

- Leptospirosis (also sometimes called Weil's disease) is another hazard that faces people who swim in fresh and brackish water. Leptospires are spirochetal bacteria shed in the urine of many wild and domestic animals. These organisms can enter the body through small breaks in the skin, particularly after a period of immersion in the water, or through the mucous membranes of the conjunctiva and nasal passages. After about 10 days, illness begins abruptly with high fever, headache, chills, vomiting, diarrhea, muscle aching, and marked reddening of the conjunctiva. The illness can be quite serious, with a fatality rate of about 1 percent overall. Penicillin and doxycycline are effective for treatment. A brief period of renal dialysis may be necessary in some patients.

- Leptospirosis can be a significant hazard for travelers to resort areas such as Hawaii and the Caribbean islands. Recreational swimming, as well as canoeing, rafting, and caving, are recognized as significant risk factors for leptospirosis in these areas. A recent study has shown that doxycycline is an effective prophylactic agent against infection while swimming. A dose of 200 mg. of doxycycline is taken on the first day of exposure, and then once weekly through the period of potential risk. This regime is not recommended for long-term use.

Dr. Arnold Kaufmann, CDC

Sharks, sea snakes, and other dangerous marine animals are another reason for caution. Local advice and custom should be sought: for example, some areas are safe by day but not by night. (See section on animal bites and stings, p. 194.)

SNORKELING

Snorkeling is an easy, cheap, and pleasant method of bridging the gap between the sea surface and its floor. It enables the swimmer to see the underwater world of fish and coral reefs. Snorkeling is safe provided a few simple rules are obeyed.

First, the right sort of equipment should be used. A mask is essential because, unlike those of fish, our eyes are not designed for use underwater: we require air in contact with the eyes in order to see clearly. As well as shielding the eyes, the mask *must cover the nose*: during descent, the increasing pressure pushes the mask painfully against the face, but this can be counteracted by blowing some air through the nose into the interior of the mask. Snorkelers who use goggles without a nosepiece are liable to end up with black or bloodshot eyes: goggles should therefore be avoided.

The snorkel should be a simple J- or L-shaped tube about 0.75 inch in diameter and 13 inches long. Too long or too narrow a snorkel should be avoided as it will increase breathing resistance. Modern snorkels have purge valves that make them easier to use.

Do not take more than one deep breath prior to a dive. The urge to surface for another breath derives from the buildup of waste carbon dioxide in the blood rather than from the falling level of oxygen. Taking several deep breaths, or "hyperventilating" before a dive delays the buildup of carbon dioxide, so that the snorkeler may use up all his oxygen and lose consciousness before the urge to surface and breathe again is felt. Hyperventilating prior to a dive in an attempt to stay underwater longer has led to many deaths by drowning.

Beware of sunburn: use a water-resistant sunscreen on your back, or wear a T-shirt, when the sun is strong.

SCUBA DIVING

Scuba is an acronym for Self-Contained Underwater Breathing Apparatus—also known as an aqualung. Scuba or aqualung diving can be a fascinating pastime, but it is also potentially dangerous unless carried out with proper training beforehand and an appreciation of the risks involved and methods of avoidance. Some of the main medical and physiological hazards are described below, but newcomers to the sport should realize that these are not the *only* hazards (or necessarily the most common ones) and would be well advised to undergo a full training course before attempting even a supervised dive in open water.

MEDICAL FITNESS

Anyone intending to take up scuba diving should have a medical checkup if there is any doubt about fitness; dive centers in some countries may require a medical certificate, possibly including a chest X-ray report—check before you go, because obtaining a certificate abroad can be difficult and expensive.

A medical history of chronic ear and sinus disease, severe head injury or cranial surgery, asthma, bronchitis, pneumothorax, heart disease, or chest surgery is sufficient to make you unfit to dive, as your body will be unable to cope with the stresses imposed underwater. A history of epilepsy means a complete ban on diving, and diabetics should not dive because of the risk of hypoglycemia and a probable increased tendency to decompression sickness (the "bends").

A number of physical handicaps do not, however, cause much difficulty under water, and scuba diving is growing in popularity with handicapped people (see box, p. 474).

EFFECTS OF PRESSURE

On land, our bodies are subject to atmospheric pressure—the pressure exerted by the column of air that extends for 10 miles or so above our heads. Underwater, pressure increases rapidly: in fact, with every 30 feet of depth, the pressure increases by an additional one atmosphere (14.7 pounds per square inch or p.s.i.). Thus at 30 feet depth, the total pressure is twice the surface pressure, and at 90 feet it is four times the surface pressure.

Fluid-filled parts of the body are not affected by the increase in pressure but air-filled parts, such as lungs, ears, and sinuses, are noticeably affected. Unless the pressures inside and outside the body are equalized, the higher pressure squeezes the lower pressure and causes tissue damage and pain.

LUNGS

Charged aqualung cylinders contain air at high pressure (up to 3,000–3,700 p.s.i.); the aqualung regulator (which delivers the air to the diver's mouth) is designed to reduce this pressure and supply air to the diver at the same pressure as that being exerted externally on his or her chest, irrespective of depth. Thus at 30 feet, air is supplied to the diver at a pressure of 29.4 p.s.i., and at 90 feet at a pressure of 58.8 p.s.i. In this way, the pressure of air in the diver's mouth is equalized to the external pressure, and breathing is just as easy as at the surface, apart from a slight resistance to the airflow caused by the regulator. During ascent, however, the air in the lungs expands as the external pressure drops *and if the diver makes the mistake of holding his or her breath, the lungs will overinflate with the risk of a "burst lung"* (p. 337).

EARS AND SINUSES

During descent, some discomfort or pain is usually experienced in the region of the eardrums and less obviously over the forehead,

SCUBA DIVING ABROAD

- A basic aqualung-training course should include instruction and practice in the use of diving equipment (including buoyancy control and life preservers); safety and emergency procedures including lifesaving; lectures on the theory and practice of diving, the various hazards involved and their avoidance; and the supervised acquisition of experience, beginning in a swimming pool or shallow water and gradually progressing to deeper dives in open water. A full-time course covering the above could be expected to take around two weeks.

- In addition to physiological hazards caused by pressure changes, divers have to learn to deal with all sorts of other stresses, which range from mask-flooding to air-supply failure, from buoyancy problems to zero underwater visibility. While a trained diver will be able to cope with such eventualities, a succession of such mishaps can rapidly reduce the novice to a state of helplessness or panic, with disastrous results.

- Travelers thinking of taking up diving on vacation should undergo some basic training—for example at any diving school run by instructors certified by the Professional Association of Diving Instructors (PADI) or National Association of Underwater Instructors (NAUI). Alternatively, a number of diving centers abroad offer formal instruction in courses lasting around two weeks.

- Most diving centers abroad apply stringent safety procedures and will not hire out equipment or organize dives except for those who can produce a recognized certificate of competence (such as the PADI "open water diver" qualification) or have undergone the center's own training course. In some places however, a beginner may be offered a "try-out" dive with little or no instruction or supervision, while at the same time being asked to sign an insurance disclaimer absolving the diving center of any responsibility in the event of an accident. *This arrangement is best avoided unless you are unconcerned about your safety*: beginners should insist on several hours' instruction in the basic techniques, and on their first few dives, the accompaniment and *undivided attention* of an experienced instructor.

due to the difference between the external pressure of air in the ears and the sinuses. This discomfort is easily relieved by pinching the nose and (by means of a little expiratory effort as though you were sneezing) forcing some additional air up into the sinuses and middle ear, via natural passages connecting these structures to the back of the nose (see pp. 232–33).

During ascent, this additional air escapes back out again without any action on the part of the diver. Problems are rarely encountered except when injury or illness has caused damage to the air passages, or during a heavy cold when the passages may be blocked by mucus: diving with a heavy or even moderate cold is inadvisable.

DIVING ILLNESSES

Decompression sickness, also known as the "bends," can always be avoided by diving within the rules of well-tried diving tables. Under pressure, more nitrogen is dissolved in the body tissues. The amount dissolved depends upon the depth (pressure) and time spent under pressure. If the pressure is released quickly, bubbles of nitrogen come out of solution into the body tissues (just like gas bubbles appearing in a bottle of soda when the top is released) and cause the symptoms of decompression sickness.

The symptoms depend upon where the bubbles are released. Joint pains are the most common, but more serious symptoms are caused if the bubbles affect either the spinal cord or the brain. Weakness or numbness of the limbs, difficulty in passing urine, disturbance of vision or balance are all symptoms of decompression sickness. Decompression sickness symptoms usually appear within three hours of a dive but may be delayed for up to 24 hours.

Treatment of decompression sickness requires recompression of the diver in a recompression chamber (commonly but mistakenly called a decompression chamber) to force the offending bubbles of nitrogen back into solution. Oxygen is also breathed to speed the elimination of nitrogen from the body. The chamber operator then follows a schedule, called a therapeutic table, for bringing the recompressed diver safely back to the surface pressure.

In the absence of a recompression chamber the diver should be given oxygen to breathe while transport is arranged to the nearest chamber, if necessary by low-level flight in an aircraft or helicopter. (Water and aspirin are also a useful emergency treatment to reduce blood viscosity.) Never try to treat decompression sickness by diving again. This will make the diver worse rather than better.

Decompression sickness can be avoided by always ascending slowly from a dive (no faster than 50 feet per minute) and diving within the rules of a set of diving tables. These indicate what "stops," if any, the diver should carry out during the ascent to release the nitrogen safely from the body tissues.

Any aqualung training course should include instruction in the use of diving tables, which cannot be described in detail here. Remember always to err on the side of safety when calculating safe dive times, depths, and decompression stops. If diving in a locality remote from a recompression chamber, it is wise to add a safety factor to further reduce the risk of decompression sickness.

Decompression computers are now widely used in many diving areas. They appear attractive because divers are given greater time underwater when diving a variable depth profile in which there is gradual ascent throughout the dive, compared to traditional dive tables which assume a rectangular dive profile. While diving computers are based on the same mathematical algorithms as dive tables, they have not been tested on human dives to the same extent. A safety factor should always be added, rather than diving to get every possible minute under water. Problems can occur if only one diver of a pair has a computer, for example, if the other goes deeper (even by two to three feet, for one or two minutes), or if partners are swapped for a second dive. Possibly because of such reasons, the introduction of dive computers in the UK was associated with a marked increase in the prevalence of decompression sickness. While this has now been reduced, it is still not known if the return to previous levels is due to improved familiarity with dive computers, or to a reduction in the number of dives taking place on account of factors like economic recession.

Burst lung While ascending from a dive, the air in the lungs expands as the pressure reduces. Normal breathing allows this excess air to be dispersed. If, however, divers either hold their breath, or have a preexisting lung disease that causes air to be trapped in the lungs, problems can occur. As trapped air expands it can cause the lung to burst. The medical term for this is pulmonary barotrauma. The air escapes from the lungs, may enter the bloodstream, and may reach the brain via the heart. A bubble of air in the brain can cause a blockage of blood flow and dramatic symptoms. This is known as arterial gas embolism.

The symptoms of pulmonary barotrauma and arterial gas embolism always occur either on surfacing or within the first 10 minutes after surfacing. The symptoms include coughing up blood, chest pain, shortness of breath, confusion, visual disturbances, weakness or paralysis, convulsions, or unconsciousness. The need for treatment is urgent—recompression in a chamber is required.

Burst lung is unlikely with correct training, which teaches divers to avoid holding their breath while ascending, and thorough medical screening, which prevents those with past or present chest disease from diving.

NITROGEN NARCOSIS

A further important physiological hazard of diving is nitrogen narcosis. Although also caused by the presence of nitrogen in the body, this is quite different from decompression sickness in that the symptoms appear *at depth* rather than during or after the ascent.

Below a depth of around 100–130 feet, nitrogen builds up in the bloodstream to a level at which it may have toxic effects on the brain quite similar to the effects of alcohol or drug intoxication. Although nitrogen narcosis has been described as "rapture of the depths," the symptoms are not necessarily pleasant, with a feeling of detachment from reality, possibly fear or apprehension, and, most dangerously, a loss of concentration and slowing of thought processes. The symptoms become more acute the deeper the diver descends below 130 feet. Fortunately, nitrogen narcosis is fairly easily dealt with by ascending 15–30 feet, when the symptoms will clear.

On occasion, nitrogen narcosis combined with apprehension may induce a state of panic. This is particularly dangerous under water as it may lead to either drowning or a pulmonary barotrauma if the response is to initiate a rapid ascent, for instance by inflating the life preserver. Diving in pairs, with each member of a team alert to the possibility of nitrogen narcosis in the other and ready to step in with pre-taught emergency drills is the only solution. The dangers of nitrogen narcosis can be reduced if the maximum depth of the dive is built up gradually over a series of dives, e.g., 85, 100, 115, 130 feet on successive days.

One hundred and sixty feet should be considered as the absolute maximum depth for sports diving, below which it becomes unacceptably dangerous. This is for three reasons. First, mental coordination and thought processes are slowed due to nitrogen narcosis, limiting the diver's ability to act correctly in an emergency. Secondly, the high density of the air that is being breathed under pressure increases the diver's work of breathing, limiting physical performance. And finally, decompression tables have not been well tested and are less reliable below this depth.

OTHER DIVING PROBLEMS
Other problems are more minor but far more frequent.

Ear infections The ears are a frequent cause of trouble. In either polluted or warm tropical water, infection of the outer ear canal (*otitis externa*) may occur. This leads to a painful ear. As a preventive measure, otic Domeboro or 8 percent aluminum acetate eardrops may be used. The drops should be instilled two to three times a day after diving or washing. Other measures include showering in fresh water after the dive, and drying the ear canal by shaking the head. Do not try to dry the ear canal with a towel, cotton wool, or a finger.

Antibiotic eardrops should be used only to treat established infections and should preferably include an antifungal drug, because fungal infection is a frequent cause of otitis externa. Eardrops containing alcohol should not be used, because this dissolves part of the cerumen (ear wax), reducing its naturally protective effect.

Infection of the middle ear (*otitis media*) is caused by bacteria from the nose or throat entering the ear while diving. This is another reason for not diving with a cold, sore throat, or chest infection.

Cuts and grazes sustained while diving in tropical waters may take up to three months to heal if nematocysts (pp. 217–18) or other microorganisms have entered the wound. Wounds are easily prevented by wearing a wetsuit, or a Lycra or Darlexx "skin" if the water is very warm. Underwater photographers are particularly at risk, as they concentrate on looking through their camera viewfinders and may miss seeing a coral outcrop.

DIVING AND AIR TRAVEL
Finally, at the end of a diving vacation, it is not safe to fly home immediately after a dive. The decreased pressure, even in a pressurized aircraft, can bring on an attack of the bends. No dive requiring decompression stops (or, for complete safety, no dive to a depth greater than 30 feet) should be undertaken in the 24 hours prior to a flight.

INSURANCE AND MEDICAL SUPPORT
Divers' Alert Network provides a 24-hour emergency telephone advice service for divers with medical problems, and is based at Duke University Medical Center. Tel. (919) 684-8111. DAN also sells inexpensive insurance coverage.

SAILING AND WINDSURFING

Sailing and windsurfing pose few medical problems. A sense of balance is needed for windsurfing. Always sail upwind first, not downwind, or along a coast rather than out to sea. This lessens the dangers if the wind strength increases while sailing. Windsurfers can quickly tire in a strong wind and become exhausted, particularly in cold water. There are many types of protective clothing available. These are either wetsuits or drysuits, both of which if correctly fitted will retain body heat without causing overheating during the often strenuous activity. Do not overestimate your abilities and sail into dangerous waters. Wearing a life preserver or other buoyancy device is always advisable, however experienced you are.

WATERSKIING

Waterskiing is quickly learned by anyone with a sense of balance and timing. Unless high-speed or competition waterskiing is tried, the risks are few. Always wear a life preserver in case you are stunned when falling into the water. Women should prevent a high-speed vaginal douche and serious internal injury by wearing an adequate bikini or swimsuit which provides protection. For competition or high-speed waterskiing, a wetsuit should be used to help cushion the blow when falling onto water at high speed.

SKIING AND SKI INJURIES

Most ski injuries can be prevented by preparation, instruction, care on the slopes, and awareness of the potential hazards.

Basil Helal is a Consultant Orthopedic Surgeon at the London Hospital and the Royal National Orthopedic Hospital. He is a medical adviser to the British Olympic Association.

Skiing is an exhilarating experience, and provides exercise in an environment that is often majestic. It is one of the fastest-growing sports: there are now more than 17 million American skiers, and increasing numbers now travel overseas to ski, often to Europe.

There are three main forms: downhill skiing; Nordic (cross country) skiing; and ski mountaineering. "Hot-dogging" is a form of acrobatics on skis, and ski jumping or "flying" is for the few who dare. "Figling" is done on boot-length Figl skis and generally used to ski over fresh avalanched snow. For the very expert, there is also the monoski, with platforms for both feet, and the surfboard.

Each has its advocates. Perhaps ski mountaineering provides the purist with the most attractive elements that this form of sport can offer.

However, unless skiers are aware of the possible hazards they face, and take careful steps to protect themselves, skiing can also be a most dangerous pastime.

PREPARATION

SELECTION OF CLOTHING

Skiwear should be warm, waterproof, and windproof. The ski outfit should in addition be easily visible against the snow and should not be so smooth as to allow frictionless descent down a mountain after a fall.

Hats and helmets Around 20 percent of body heat loss can take place through the head—so an adequate, warm, waterproof head covering that will also protect the ears is essential. Children can easily damage the skull in falls and collisions; a child's skull is not as strong as an adult's and crash helmets are strongly advised.

A face mask to protect from high wind and driving snow is also a valuable asset.

Goggles or glasses should either have photosensitive lenses or should have exchangeable lenses for varying conditions. They should protect against driving snow and high wind, and against strong sunlight. They should also provide side cover for the eyes, and this is especially important for ski mountaineering.

Mittens are warmer than gloves. A thin pair of warm gloves, cotton or silk, worn inside mittens allows one to handle metal bindings without getting a "cold burn" in very low temperatures.

Socks A dry spare pair is always worth carrying, especially if ski mountaineering or touring is envisaged.

Ski leggings should be worn by anyone planning to ski in deep snow, to prevent snow from entering the boots.

Undergarments should be light and allow freedom of movement. Two thin layers provide more insulation than one thick layer.

A small backpack or knapsack does not interfere with skiing and can be used to carry clothes that are not needed—weather conditions change rapidly and in any case it is much cooler toward the end of the day—as well as any extra items that may prove useful, such as bandages, and a screwdriver and pliers for running repairs.

SELECTION OF SKIS, BOOTS, BINDINGS, AND POLES

Ski boots should be comfortable and allow some toe movement. Boots that are adjustable for heel grip and midfoot grip as well as for ankle grip are preferred.

A different, softer boot is required for climbing on skis, and for Nordic skiing a special shoe with a toe extension is necessary.

Bindings anchor the boot to the ski and are designed to release if an undue force is applied in a rotational or forward pitch direction. They should be adjusted according to the weight, bone thickness, and strength of the subject, and this is best done by an expert. The bindings require some momentum to release easily, so the most dangerous fall is a "slow" one.

Special bindings which allow the heel to rise when climbing but anchor for skiing are necessary for the ski mountaineer, and quite different bindings, which provide only a toe grip, are used in Nordic or cross-country skiing.

Skis should be selected with care. They should not be too long, as this makes turning more difficult. The short, wide "Scorpian" ski (or ski skate) is ideal for the beginner, who can graduate to longer skis with an increase in expertise. Longer skis increase leverage on the leg in a fall.

Ski poles These should be of correct length, and the loops should break away on a strong tug.

GENERAL FITNESS

A high degree of general fitness is desirable: skiing is an energetic pastime and is carried out at altitudes where the pressure of oxygen may be lower than most skiers are accustomed to in their home environment; exercise is an essential part of preparation.

Running is most suitable for those who are accustomed to it, but can cause stress injuries in people who take it up suddenly and intensively in a last-minute attempt to get fit for a skiing vacation. It should preferably be carried out on grass or forest floor rather than on concrete or asphalt.

Cycling is much less traumatic and besides improving fitness, will also serve to strengthen the muscles that are used in skiing.

Leg strength Exercise specifically intended to strengthen the quadriceps muscles should be dynamic and not static; otherwise patellar chondromalacia (softening of the articular surfaces of the knee cap) may ensue.

Practicing ski skills on dry slopes Dry slopes are sensible places for beginners to become familiar with ski equipment and basic skills, but dry-slope skiing carries its own hazards. Most artificial ski surfaces consist of nylon brush squares; falls can be abrasive, and if the thumb is caught in this surface its ligaments are easily torn.

SPECIAL EQUIPMENT
Ski mountaineers need other special equipment, such as avalanche detectors, harnesses (e.g., Whillan's), and rope, and extra clothing protection.

ENVIRONMENTAL HAZARDS

ALTITUDE (see also pp. 288–298)
Skiing generally involves ascent to altitudes of 10,000–12,000 feet or over, where the atmospheric pressure is lower and the air is drier. Oxygen transfer to the lungs is less easy.

Altitude or mountain sickness can be very dangerous, and can cause both pulmonary and cerebral edema; diuretic treatment and oxygen may be of some help, but descent to a higher-pressure zone is the safest answer if there is no response to other forms of treatment. An early diuresis (passage of a large volume of urine) on ascent seems to indicate good adaptation to altitude. Minor symptoms are relatively common, especially at some of the higher ski resorts.

More evaporation occurs at altitude, and the nasal passages dry more easily, especially during sleep, when this is often exacerbated by central heating. It is best to increase fluid intake—have an extra drink of water before you go to bed, even if you don't feel especially thirsty. Try also to keep the humidity in the bedroom high—a bowl of water or wet towels on the radiators can be very helpful in preventing a dry sore throat.

COLD (see also pp. 310–322)

Skiing requires snow—except on artificial surfaces, of course. Unless you're unlucky with conditions, you are likely to be skiing at temperatures around 32°F. (0°C.) or lower.

Skiing also requires muscular effort and this is optimal at body temperature or slightly above 104°F. (40°C.). Getting yourself chilled is at best uncomfortable and at worst can be fatal, so it is wise to be prepared.

Insulation Several layers of clothing will trap air at body temperature efficiently (pp. 321–22). Generally speaking, clothes made from cellular materials, especially natural fibers, are best, and animal fur is the warmest. As mentioned previously the outermost layer should be windproof and not too slippery.

Wind The chill factor in wind can lower the effective air temperature rapidly and substantially. Thus with a wind speed of 45 miles per hour, 32°F. (0°C.) will feel the same as −58°F. (−50°C.) on a windless day (pp. 316–17).

Damp Insulation is rapidly degraded if clothing becomes wet. Wise skiers therefore carry a dry pair of woolen socks in a plastic bag, for feet can easily get wet when skiing in deep powder snow.

Heat conservation If cooled, the body tries to preserve its central core temperature. Heat loss is reduced by reflex constriction of the skin blood vessels. Heat is produced by muscle activity and this is the reason for the shivering reaction. Anything that reduces activity such as being stranded on a chair lift or on a drag lift can result in a rapid fall in temperature, and it is best to try to maintain some movement of the limbs under these circumstances. Similarly, concussion or any injury that results in immobilization will cause a rapid fall in temperature.

Alcohol Heat loss is increased by dilatation of the blood vessels of the skin; alcohol is a vasodilator—so beware. (Like drinking and driving, drinking and skiing do not mix; drinking increases the risk of an accident on the slopes.)

Cold injury The skin itself is at risk from injury, and the skier should carry a face mask to protect the nose and cheeks, and warm headgear that can come over the ears. The lips are also vulnerable. Frost "nips"—white, numb patches on the skin—should have external warmth applied rapidly. Rubbing is dangerous, however, and can further damage the skin. Frostbite involves freezing of the deeper tissues and starts at the tips of the fingers and toes. Rapid and careful rewarming is essential.

Hand protection In practice the hands are better protected by a mitten than a glove for this allows better movement of the fingers. Chemical hand warmers that can be inserted into gloves and mittens are available at sporting goods stores. Remember that for handling of metal portions of equipment at very low temperatures a light cotton glove worn inside the mitten will protect against a cold burn. On no account should metal at temperatures below 14°F. (– 10°C.) be handled even with warm hands as skin will blister or adhere to the metal.

Children Children are particularly susceptible to cold injury and even frost-nipped hands and feet can suffer permanent damage with subsequent distortion of or stunting of growth. Make sure that children stay warm, and inspect them repeatedly if they are playing in snow, snowballing, etc.

Cigarettes Among the many harmful effects of cigarettes is vasoconstriction, or clamping down of blood vessels at the extremities. This has been well established by thermographic and doppler tests. So please do not give injured skiers a "steadying" smoke—it may quite literally result in loss of their fingertips and toes.

Cold collapse is a response to a falling core temperature and to a reduction in the blood sugar level. Brain function fails if the core temperature falls below 95°F. (35°C.). Early signs include weakness with frequent falls, followed by a stage of aggressive behavior which goes on to apathy, and then collapse and loss of consciousness.

Rewarming Rapid warming is essential and a fit person's body heat is perhaps the best emergency solution. If both victim and rescuer huddle together in a thermal blanket (which is made of light foil, can fold to the size of a handkerchief and can be carried in a skier's pocket) or a sleeping bag if one is available, there is an excellent chance of raising core temperature to a safe level—particularly if the partner is of the opposite sex!

If the limbs are frostbitten do not thaw them if there is a likelihood of refreezing and do not rub the frozen part as this will further damage the skin.

Back in civilization the accepted method of restoring the core temperature is by immersion in a warm bath 104°–111°F. (40°–44°C.) until flushing of fingertips occurs. Blisters should be kept intact if possible and antibiotics given to prevent infection of any damaged tissue; use open dressings to allow easy inspection.

SURVIVAL IN THE COLD

Failing visibility, perhaps due to mist or fog, may cause a delayed return. At nightfall, there is usually a marked drop in temperature. If there is no hope or even some doubt of reaching shelter, construct an igloo or a substantial snow hole and huddle if there are a number of you or curl up tight to reduce the surface area from which heat loss can occur if you are alone. This will give you the best chance of survival.

People with certain medical conditions should take particular care to avoid chilling or placing themselves at this risk: they include sufferers from previous heart attacks, chronic bronchitics, people with poor circulation, and some people in whom low temperature causes their red blood cells to break down (this is a form of allergy to cold).

SUN

Sunburn is a real hazard in the clear mountain atmosphere and barrier creams should always be worn, particularly by the fair skinned (see p. 328).

Reflected glare from expanses of white snow can cause severe eye damage—conjunctival burns and even *uveitis* leading to so-called snowblindness (see also p. 382). This is best prevented by wearing adequate sunglasses, possibly with side protectors.

VISIBILITY

Conditions may change very rapidly and in certain flat light conditions it is impossible to identify hollows, drops, and rises; skiing "blind" is very difficult and can be most dangerous.

Even worse are conditions of heavy mist or driving blizzards. Often under such circumstances it is better to ski where there are trees as these provide light contrast and visibility is much improved.

TERRAIN

Cliffs are especially dangerous in poor visibility. Crevasses are fissures in the earth that are often concealed by a bridge of snow. Some are large and deep, and there is danger of injury or death from the fall. Others are narrower and a skier may be trapped a few feet down, be unable to move, and die from hypothermia if rescue is not rapidly to hand.

Collision can produce serious injury; obstacles include trees, buried rocks, and other skiers. If a skier wishes to stop he or she should do so off the piste or track, and away from the bottom of a run.

AVALANCHE

Avalanches normally occur on steep slopes where there is already a substantial depth of snow, and the risk is usually greatest when the weather changes and there is a sudden rise in temperature. They can be triggered by noise or by skiers, and also occur spontaneously. In most ski resorts automatic devices are placed to set them off before they can cause harm; they are precipitated by small grenade explosions.

There are two types of avalanche—the soft snow avalanche which forms a wave, and the slab avalanche in which heavy blocks of snow and ice come away.

Two types of injury occur—crushing and drowning.

AVALANCHE SURVIVAL

If an avalanche starts above you, try to ski away from its line of fall. If you have time, take off your skis, and hyperventilate so as to be able to hold your breath for as long as possible if you are covered. Curl up and protect your head, and hang on to your ski poles.

Once you have been covered, try to create an air space. Do not panic, but push the ski poles up to see if you can create a breathing hole, then gradually move snow down from the roof to the floor of your hole, packing it below as you go.

If you are caught high up by the avalanche, spreadeagle, and try to ride the surface and swim as you would surf-ride a wave.

HAZARDS FROM LIFT EQUIPMENT

Cable cars Cable cars have been known to crash from a height, but such accidents are exceptionally uncommon.

Chair lifts Poor coordination when joining or leaving a chair lift can result in injury. The chair can give the unwary skier a sharp knock. People have also been injured by falling out of chairs and by having articles of their clothing hooked or trapped by the chair as they alight. Failure of the lift system, leaving the unfortunate skier trapped, suspended, and very cold, can provide a powerful temptation to try and jump off. Don't—even mild frostbite is preferable to severe injury or death.

Drag lifts T-bars and tow bars can entangle with clothing, or if released at the wrong moment can recoil against other skiers and cause injury.

ACCLIMATIZATION AND ORIENTATION

On arrival at the ski resort, allow yourself time to acclimatize. The higher the resort, the longer this may take.

Check that your clothing and equipment are suitable and in good order. Obtain a map of the ski area and select runs that are appropriate for your experience and ability.

It is important to obtain adequate insurance for yourself and your equipment as well as third-party insurance (see pp. 492–97). In isolated mountain resorts, medical costs are high and facilities and standards are sometimes poor; medical insurance should be sufficient to cover the cost of bringing you home by air ambulance, if necessary.

SKI INJURIES

The average overall injury rate is 4 per 1,000 "skier days."

In a recent survey, 58 percent of injuries were in beginners, with 36 percent in intermediate skiers, and 6 percent in expert skiers.

Not surprisingly, leg injuries are most common—and in another survey, accounted for 86 percent of all injuries. Of these, 45 percent were knee injuries, and 43 percent were tibial (shin) fractures. Eight percent of injuries involved the arms—mainly wrist fractures—and 4 percent were shoulder dislocations. Ski surfing tends to produce knee contusions and effusions (fluid in the joint) from falling forward onto the knee.

EQUIPMENT FACTORS

There are three important ways that the ski itself can produce injury. Firstly, it acts as a lever on the leg; a torque of as little as 15 pounds at the tip of a ski can produce a fracture of the tibia (shin bone). Modern rigid ski boots protect the foot, ankle, and lower tibia from this kind of injury, but in doing so, inevitably transfer stress to the knee, making ligamentous injuries at the knee joint an increasingly common hazard.

Secondly, if the bindings release a ski during a fall, and the ski is tethered to the ankle by a safety strap, the tethered ski may recoil against its owner; ski edges are sharp, and can produce severe lacerations. "Ski stoppers"—a pair of prongs which project below the undersurface of the ski when the boot has been released from the binding are preferable to safety straps. (Some skiers reduce the risk of losing skis without safety straps in deep snow by trailing ribbons from their bindings when skiing in deep powder.)

Thirdly, a "rogue" ski—released during a fall—can become a dangerous projectile if it accelerates unchecked down a slope. It may strike or impale other skiers in its path. Ski stoppers reduce the likelihood of this occurrence.

Check that your bindings release under reasonable force. They should have been adjusted professionally according to the size of your bones, your general muscularity, and your experience, but you should always test them yourself. Do not handle the bindings or any other metal with your bare hands when temperatures are below freezing, or a cold burn will result.

Boots must be comfortable and hold the foot firmly so that movement is transmitted instantly to the ski, thereby protecting the ankle from injury.

Ski poles can cause injury, especially to the thumb; the strap and ski-pole handle should never be held in such a way that the thumb may become trapped.

VICTIMS OF FASHION

The pattern of ski injuries changes slightly each season. Sometimes it is the weather: scant snow in Europe for a couple of seasons caused a significant increase in injuries from collisions and falls as frustrated skiers crowded onto a few icy slopes. Sometimes it is due to fashion. The skier's fanny pack is now a well-established fashion accessory, with the pouch often worn in front. In a fall, the pouch and its contents (especially cameras) can cause severe internal abdominal injuries: rupture of the spleen, liver, and small intestine have all occurred. When skiing, the correct position for the pouch is behind.

R.D./R.F.

You should always be able to see both hands in front of you when you are skiing. Holding the poles close in to one's side can be dangerous, especially upon reaching the bottom of a slope, where a sudden rise uphill can drive the pole handle up and into the eye; I have seen an eye enucleated by this form of accident. One other important point about the ski pole is that its loop should break loose with a strong tug. If its basket catches, on trees or brush, for instance, a severe injury to the shoulder can occur if the loop does not release. Such an injury can commonly result in a dislocation of the shoulder, but can also cause a less common but more serious injury—a traction injury on the *brachial plexus*, damaging the main nerves that enter the arm from the neck to supply the muscles and sensation of the upper limb; permanent paralysis may ensue.

OTHER CONTRIBUTORY FACTORS

Many important factors that contribute to the risk of injury are under a considerable degree of individual control:

- *Fatigue* The majority of ski injuries occur on the first day of a ski vacation, especially toward the end of the morning or afternoon session. Make sure you stop skiing well before the stage when you are feeling tired and your legs ache.

- *Inexperience* There is no substitute for skilled, *professional* ski instruction, so don't try to get by without lessons.

- *Poor technique* Having attained a basic level of proficiency, don't become complacent about the need to improve your technique further. Lessons are not just for beginners.

- *Excessive speed*, especially dangerous on crowded slopes, often causes collisions with other skiers, accounting for up to 10 percent of accidents.
- *Poor surface and conditions* Avoid them.

If you need to rest, do this off a run. The worst possible places to stop are near the bottom of a run and in the center of the trail. This invites a collision.

LIGAMENTS

While skiing, the body's weight is borne by one or other leg unless one is traveling directly downhill. Unlike the straight knee, the *flexed* knee permits a degree of rotation without damage to ligaments. An important principle to remember is that in an unstable or uncontrolled situation, totally unloading the inactive ski (usually the uphill one) and further flexing the knee bearing your weight will protect the ligaments from damage; sitting down may be undignified on skis, but ignominy is preferable to any sort of injury.

FIRST AID

In the event of an injury, first-aid treatment is most important in order to avoid compounding any damage that may have occurred. No skier who feels even moderate pain or the least instability on standing should ever attempt to continue skiing. A further fall may result in a much more serious injury. Any doubt about the integrity of joints, ligaments, or bone must be treated seriously and the part protected by splinting until an expert opinion can be obtained. The vast majority of doctors practicing in ski resorts are very experienced and generally give wise counsel. Local orthopedic surgeons usually give an extremely good service. There is, however, in some places, a tendency to resort to surgery when perhaps a conservative line of treatment would suffice, and this certainly happens in some European resorts. An injured skier can always request immobilization of the injured part in a cast and return home for treatment by a surgeon of his or her choice.

CONCLUSION

Despite its many hazards skiing is an enjoyable and popular activity. With care and attention to simple safety precautions, the small risk of injury can be reduced even further.

"Après ski" activity has its pleasures and its hazards, but that is another story.

PSYCHOTROPIC DRUGS

The use and acceptability of mind-altering drugs varies from one country to another. Travelers who use such drugs do so at their own risk, but should realize that locally produced substances may have unexpectedly potent and possibly dangerous effects and that the penalties for illegal possession are frequently severe.

Dr. Martin Mitcheson is the Clinical Director of the South West Regional Drug Advisory Service and the Avon Drug Problem Team, UK.

Roger Lewis is a research specialist in international drug traffic and is the author of a number of studies of illicit drug makers in Britain, Italy, and elsewhere.

In almost every society in the world, mind-altering, or *psychotropic,* substances are used for recreational, ritual, and medical purposes. Just as different nations favor different pharmaceutical, homeopathic, and folk preparations, they also display preferences for different types of social and recreational drug use. These preferences are influenced by such factors as the plant life indigenous to the region, traditional familiarity with particular drug effects, the impact of aggressive colonial marketing, and the solace and oblivion that some drugs may provide for individuals suffering from boredom, poverty, and privation, or ethnic groups threatened with extinction or assimilation.

PATTERNS OF PSYCHOTROPIC DRUG USE WORLDWIDE

TOBACCO AND ALCOHOL
Tobacco and alcohol are, broadly speaking, available throughout the world, although some Islamic countries such as Saudi Arabia impose severe penalties upon individuals who consume or traffic in the latter.

CANNABIS
Cannabis, known in its various preparations as hashish, ganja, marijuana, bush, grass, and countless other names, grows or can be

cultivated in most parts of the world. Since the 1960s one of the attractions of countries such as India, Pakistan, and (until recently) Afghanistan to young European travelers has been the quality and quantity of cannabis preparations readily available to them. In Africa and the Americas the drug usually comes in herbal form and, despite the denials of many governments who view alcohol as "civilized" and cannabis as "primitive," cannabis is consumed in a controlled and considered fashion by large sections of the world's population.

THE OPIUM POPPY

The opium poppy, from which morphine and heroin are derived, grows within a geographical band running from Vietnam's Gulf of Tonkin to Turkey's Anatolian plain. Some tribal peoples have successfully integrated the poppy into their daily lives, although addiction has emerged as a problem in Iran, Pakistan, and parts of Southeast Asia.

Once refined and converted into heroin, opiates present a particular threat to the young, semi-Westernized populations of Bangkok, Karachi, Tehran, and Singapore—as well as an increasing problem of addiction, with associated severe physical and psychological difficulty, among young people in developed countries.

COCAINE

Cocaine is derived from the coca leaf, which originates in Latin America. The Indian peoples of Colombia, Bolivia, and Peru chew the leaf or drink an infusion as a source of nutrition and energy for work and relaxation. Problems have arisen associated with "gringo" entrepreneurs intent on profiting from the sale of the plant's chemical derivative, cocaine, to North America and Europe. Like "crack" in North America, cocaine-base smoking has become an increasing problem in South America.

OTHER DRUGS

Apart from the major psychotropics, travelers may come across other drugs that may create legal, medical, and psychological problems. The peyote cactus, for example, may be found in the Southwestern USA and northern Mexico, the psilocybin mushroom in Western Europe and North and Central America, and "fly-agaric," the white-spotted mushroom of fairy tale, in North America,

Northern Europe, and North Africa. They all have strong hallucinogenic properties and are treated with respect by those folk cultures that employ them for such properties.

DRUG PROBLEMS INVOLVING TRAVELERS

Travelers may experience unforeseen physical problems from the consumption of psychotropic drugs abroad; and legal problems with the possibility of arrest and imprisonment, as a result of illegal possession (including inadvertent possession).

PHYSICAL PROBLEMS

If drugs are used in situations where there is uncertainty about the strength of preparations, and if drugs are injected when sterile equipment is not available, the potential hazards of drug taking are increased considerably.

Problems include: overdose of drugs, either accidental or deliberate; intoxication produced by sedative tranquilizers; panic reactions resulting from consumption of a variety of drugs, including potent preparations of cannabis and psychedelic drugs such as lysergide or mescaline; and acute paranoid states from cocaine and amphetamines. Regular daily consumption of drugs of the sedative tranquillizer group, or of the opioid group, followed by abrupt cessation, can produce an unpleasant and potentially dangerous withdrawal illness, particularly when coinciding with physical illness of the type that may easily occur abroad. Physical complications may arise as a result of the mode of administration, particularly injection, or where a drug-centered existence leads to the neglect of nutrition and personal hygiene.

Overdose The distinction between overdose and other acute reactions is partly dependent on the type of drug consumed and partly on the relative dose level. Broadly, opioids and sedative tranquilizers depress cerebral function and decrease the sensitivity of the brain's respiratory center. When sedation is profound, reflexes that normally protect the airway by coughing when foreign material is present, are suppressed. A sedated person may be lying in a position where simple mechanical obstruction to an airway can occur.

When someone is believed to have taken an overdose of this kind of drug, hospital treatment is always recommended; while waiting for assistance, turn the affected person into the semiprone position. This is achieved by laying him on his side, with the upper leg bent, his face at an angle toward the floor, and his neck gently extended, with the lower jaw pulled forward to maintain an airway. In this position, regurgitated food from the stomach is much less likely to be inhaled into the lungs. If breathing is so depressed that mouth-to-mouth ventilation is necessary, it is important to remember to clean any food debris from the mouth before inflating the lungs. These techniques are clearly explained and demonstrated in first-aid books. The specific medical antidote for opioid overdose is an injection of the pure antagonist, nalorphine.

Other acute reactions Acute anxiety or fleeting hallucinatory experiences can occur under the influence of alcohol, other sedative tranquilizers and volatile inhalants, as well as psychedelic drugs. Acute panic reactions, popularly referred to as "bad trips," occur most frequently among novice consumers, those taking the drug in anxiety-provoking situations, older people experimenting with an unusual experience, and any consumer who unexpectedly encounters an unaccustomedly large dose. These factors are more likely to occur in a foreign country.

Adverse reactions are uncommon from the relatively weak psychedelic drug cannabis, particularly when this is consumed with some care by inhalation; but they are more likely to occur when cannabis is consumed by mouth with less control over the dose. The predominant symptom and sign of an adverse reaction is acute anxiety, which may be related to subjective perceptual disturbance, or to external anxiety-provoking events. In a severe reaction, true hallucinations may be experienced. These perceptions may lead the sufferer to believe he is experiencing a severe psychiatric illness, and a simultaneous increased heart rate may lead to fears of imminent death. The management of these acute reactions is reassurance, which will need to be repeated often since short-term memory is usually also affected. A companion should endeavor to relate the sufferer's current experience to the fact that he has consumed a drug. The use of tranquilizers plays a small part in the management of acute reactions. Admission to a psychiatric institution is generally counterproductive.

Persecutory delusions (paranoia) are the principle serious adverse reaction to both amphetamines and cocaine. Individual dose response can vary widely. The acute episode is indistinguishable from acute schizophrenia. Disorder is generally self-limiting within a period of two or three days if the person ceases drug use. Administration of major (phenothiazine) tranquilizers may confuse the diagnosis.

DRUG-WITHDRAWAL REACTIONS
Withdrawal from the sedative tranquilizer group of drugs is potentially medically hazardous since epileptic convulsions and a confused state with hallucinations can occur (the syndrome known as delirium tremens—DTs—in alcohol withdrawal). The immediate management of severe withdrawals is to administer any convenient drug of this group such as alcohol, phenobarbital, or benzodiazepines such as diazepam (Valium). It is highly probable that the alcohol-withdrawal syndrome is exacerbated by poor nutrition, which is common in chronic alcoholics, and it is important to ensure adequate vitamin supplements, particularly B_6, to avoid the risk of permanent brain damage.

DISEASE IN DRUG USERS
Hepatitis occurs commonly among heavy drug users and is broadly of two types: hepatitis A, otherwise known as infectious hepatitis, occurs in association with poor hygiene, and is common where food products may be contaminated by excreta used as fertilizer or infection carried by flies from latrines to food preparation areas. The onset usually occurs within four weeks following infection. Hepatitis B, C, and D, otherwise referred to as serum hepatitis, are usually transmitted by blood products or other body fluids (see p. 54). In relation to drug use, this occurs as a result of using a needle or syringe contaminated by blood from an infected person. It should be noted that it is extremely difficult to adequately resterilize the disposable syringes now almost invariably used in industrialized societies. In an emergency, when sterile syringes and needles are not available, it is of some benefit to use the following cleaning method, draw up clean (boiled but cool) water, and flush the equipment twice; discard the water and repeat twice with fresh household bleach (not disinfectant); rinse twice with clean water. The relative poverty of medical services in the developing countries often results in needles and syringes being reused, with a high risk

of *any* infection as a result of any injection. Serum hepatitis has a longer incubation period than hepatitis A, of the order of two to three months from the time of infection.

HIV, though less contagious then hepatitis B, is transmitted in a similar way and is particularly common in Central and East Africa and areas where intravenous drug use is common or which are frequented for commercialized sex, including Thailand and India. It should be noted that in some areas blood transfusion is one means by which impoverished people can raise money and therefore blood transfusion products are more likely to be a source of infection.

Any form of hepatitis can be a debilitating and potentially serious illness requiring medical care and in severe cases medical repatriation is needed. Active immunization is available to protect against hepatitis A and B; but not as yet to confer protection against C and D hepatitis or against HIV infection. Hepatitis is discussed in greater detail on pp. 49–60 and HIV on pp. 419–30.

LEGAL PROBLEMS

Young travelers in particular may be quite frequently offered psychotropic drugs in foreign countries. Such drugs may be widely used by the local population, but are formally illegal. Some countries like Turkey and Thailand conduct the specific policy of applying the full force of their laws against foreign nationals, who are highly visible as well as being more vulnerable. This particularly applies to countries that have reputations as centers of illicit traffic and have attracted the censure of importing countries.

It always pays to do one's homework about the countries one intends to visit. Travelers in sunny places tend to forget that things are rarely as easygoing as they seem. A single cannabis cigarette in Greece means prison for one year plus one day, minimum. In some countries second-class passengers often ask first-class passengers to assist with their luggage allowance. There may be no ulterior motive to such a request, but even inadvertent smuggling still means severe penalties.

If taken into custody, never sign anything unless it can be read and understood. Remember this even under intense physical and psychological pressure. The only friend left in such circumstances may be your consul. Consular officials may not be able to do a great deal but should be able to recommend a local English-speaking lawyer (fellow-prisoners may also have some ideas). Different countries have different regulations regarding legal aid, if it exists at all. It makes sense to discover the details as soon as possible.

Your consulate will inform your family about your situation unless you wish otherwise. Generally, the consul is expected to visit you as soon as possible after your arrest, to ensure you are legally represented and to make sure that your treatment is *no worse* than that of the local population.

PRESCRIBED DRUGS

Many drugs such as heroin and other opioids, cocaine, and cannabis, are subject to international treaty agreements governing the international trade in these substances. At present the majority of stimulants and sedative tranquilizers, including barbiturates, are not so strictly controlled but may be restricted under local regulations. In many countries the importation of any potential drug of abuse may be regarded as a criminal offense.

Patients who need to take regular medication for the treatment of physical or psychological disease should of course have consulted their usual physician before undertaking foreign travel. Because of the laws regarding importation of psychoactive drugs, anyone requiring a continued supply should arrange with his physician to receive a local legal prescription from a doctor in the country he intends to visit.

Note that an open letter to "any doctor whom it might concern" will usually be insufficient to obtain immediate treatment because (a) any drug mentioned in the letter may not be legally available in the destination country and (b) even if it is, many doctors are not prepared to take on patients at short notice, nor are they prepared to take on nationals of another country.

On the other hand, specialists working in the field of drug dependence often do have knowledge of similar colleagues in other countries and may be able to organize medical care by prior arrangement, particularly if it is only to cover a short visit or to attend to family affairs, and in particular, bereavements. These particular precautions refer primarily to opiate drugs and amphetamines.

Minor tranquilizers and barbiturate sedatives prescribed in small amounts should be declared to customs officials and may or may not be accepted for importation. Major tranquilizers (phenothiazines such as chlorpromazine) and tricyclic antidepressants are almost always permitted, although problems could arise if a customs official was uncertain of the status or content of the tablets: in some cases, tablets may be confiscated for analysis.

SUMMARY OF INFORMATION FOR TRAVELERS

- Consumption of psychotropic drugs in a situation without the support of friends or in unfamiliar surroundings is more likely to result in an anxiety reaction.

- The strength of preparations available in producing countries is likely to be greater than that of preparations which are available at home, where the product may have been diluted to increase the seller's profit margin and where the active principle may have been reduced in potency due to the time taken in transit.

- The consumption of unaccustomed powerful drugs increases the risk of adverse reactions.

- The risk of physical complications from self-injection of drugs is considerably higher in countries where injecting equipment is expensive and imported.

9 SOME COMMON TROUBLES

SKIN PROBLEMS

Skin problems typically account for one third of all health problems in travelers. This chapter explains how to recognize, treat, and prevent the most likely problems.

Dr. Stanley Schwartz is a dermatologist in private practice in Fort Myers, Florida. He has a special interest in aquatic dermatology.

The main function of the skin is to provide protection from the external environment; it is therefore highly vulnerable during travel, especially when environmental conditions are drastically different from those at home: humidity, temperature, exposure to sunlight, unfamiliar plants, animals, foods, cosmetic products, infectious diseases, and unaccustomed recreational activities may all take their toll. Some of the conditions that result are not normally seen in the home environment, and may require specialist care.

This chapter provides a guide to preventing and coping with some of the most likely problems. If a condition fails to improve with the measures outlined here, you should seek advice from a qualified physician or dermatologist as soon as you can.

EXPOSURE TO SUNLIGHT

Problems resulting from exposure to sunlight are not restricted to people who travel to warm climates and go sunbathing; all kinds of outdoor activities, in hot or cold climates and at high altitude, can lead to significant sun exposure. This subject is considered in detail on pp. 322–30, and some aspects of it are also considered below.

SUNBURN

Acute overexposure to the sun results in the familiar, reddened appearance of the skin and a painful, burning sensation. Severe sunburn can also lead to blistering reactions sometimes called sun poisoning. These severe sunburns can be serious and may become infected if not properly cared for. A single blistering sunburn increases the risk of developing skin cancer by at least two or three times, and may also cause scarring and pigment changes. Particular care is necessary to protect children.

Travelers who try to get as much sun as possible during the early days of their vacation are likely to be left with severe sunburn and not much tanning. These individuals go home red and peeling and do the most damage to their skin.

Treatment Cold compresses, twice or three times daily, can be quite helpful in relieving the burning symptoms. Aspirin can help relieve the pain and inflammation of a sunburn. A variety of products (gels and lotions) containing aloe vera, or an Aveeno oatmeal bath, can also be quite soothing. Hydrocortisone 1 percent cream can be applied twice daily to help give relief. Severe blistering sunburns or sun poisoning should be treated by qualified medical personnel if possible.

Prevention Avoid long periods of direct exposure, especially during the middle of the day: stay out of the sun. During outdoor activities, use a broad-spectrum sunscreen with an SPF of at least 15. Choose

SOME PLANTS THAT CAN CAUSE PHOTOSENSITIVITY

Agrimony	Cow parsley, wild	Mustard
Angelica	chervil	Parsnip
Bergamot	Dill	Persian lime
Bindweed	Fennel	Red quebracho
Buttercup	Figs	St. John's wort
Celery	Giant hogweed	Wild carrot
Citrus plants	Milfoil	

a product that does not irritate your skin. Use an oil-free formula if your skin is prone to acne; use a water-resistant or waterproof type if you are swimming, waterskiing, or scuba diving, and use a PABA-free product if your skin is sensitive. Apply sunscreens early in the morning, preferably at least a half hour before sun exposure, and reapply them during the day. Also use a factor-15 lip protectant, and wear a hat that shades the ears and neck, and long-sleeved, shady clothing. Eye protection is discussed on p. 382.

POLYMORPHIC LIGHT ERUPTION
This is a raised, itchy rash that develops following exposure to strong sunlight. It is probably the commonest rash in travelers and is discussed on p. 323.

PHOTOSENSITIVITY
The sap and juices of many plants can cause a sun-sensitivity reaction rather like an exaggerated sunburn, with severe blistering and later pigmentation changes. These reactions tend to occur only on skin that has been in contact with the plants, often resulting in a strange distribution. If you handle plants, you may transfer sap to other parts of your body—your face and eyes, for example. The reaction may not occur until much later, by which time its cause may no longer be obvious. Some of the plants known to have this effect are listed above. Avoid squeezing limes or touching unfamiliar plants before sun exposure.

Many prescription medications can also sensitize the skin to the sun, and some of the products most likely to do this are listed opposite; the list includes several products that are commonly pre-

DRUGS AND MEDICINES THAT CAN CAUSE PHOTO-SENSITIVITY

Chlorothiazide (Diuril)	Nalidixic acid (NeGram)
Chlorpromazine (Thorazine, Largactil)	Oral contraceptives
Chlorpropamide (Diabinese)	PABA
Ciprofloxacin (Cipro)	Piroxicam (Feldene)
Coal tar	Promethazine (Phenergan)
Diphenhydramine (Benadryl)	Sulfa drugs
Furosemide (Lasix)	Tetracyclines (including doxycycline)
Hexachlorophene	

scribed for travelers, and if excessive sun exposure is likely, discuss the problem with your physician or pharmacist.

If you suspect that you are developing a photosensitive-type reaction while traveling, you should avoid any further sun exposure; use hydrocortisone 1 percent cream, and consult a physician as soon as possible regarding treatment of the reaction and alternative medication.

PRICKLY HEAT

Prickly heat, or heat rash, most often occurs in hot, humid environments. It usually appears as small red bumps on the skin, usually in covered areas, and is itchy and uncomfortable (see also p. 309).

Treatment Stay in a cool environment and apply cool compresses to the skin three times daily. Aveeno baths can be helpful and hydrocortisone 1 percent cream can be soothing. Antihistamine tablets may be taken for itching. Cool, loose clothing and avoidance of overexertion are helpful for prevention and during recovery.

COLD CLIMATES

Cold injury and frostbite are discussed on pp. 310–21. Some individuals are particularly sensitive to the cold and can develop painful reactions including color changes in the skin, such as chilblains and Raynaud's phenomenon. Gentle re-warming relieves symptoms in these cases, and the prescription medicine Nifedipine can help prevent episodes of Raynaud's phenomenon.

SKIN INFECTIONS

The most common types of skin infection in travelers are:

BACTERIAL INFECTIONS

Impetigo appears as yellowish, honey-colored crusted areas with underlying redness, and may occur in any location on the body, particularly the areas around the nose and face. It tends to occur when traveling under conditions of extremely poor hygiene.

Folliculitis is an infection of the hair follicles and appears as numerous red bumps or pimples on the skin surface, often in areas covered by clothing. The face and scalp are also frequently affected. The buttocks and back are commonly affected after sitting or lying down for extended periods on vinyl or other nonporous surfaces.

These types of infection can be prevented by paying particular attention to cleanliness and personal hygiene while traveling. Regular bathing with soap and water is helpful. Consider taking your own cushion if you will be traveling on extended bus journeys, or spread a towel over your seat.

Antibiotic treatment may be necessary. Bactroban ointment is effective in treating impetigo. Over-the-counter antibiotic ointments such as Polysporin, Neosporin, or Triple Antibiotic ointment are also effective. If impetigo or folliculitis do not respond to these medications, consult a physician for further recommendations.

FUNGAL INFECTION

These include ringworm, tinea cruris (jock itch or dhobie itch), and tinea pedis (or athlete's foot), and are often precipitated by travel to hot, humid areas (though sometimes also by travel to cold climates when warm, heavy clothing has to be worn). They can usually be recognized by redness and scaling of the skin, often in a ringlike pattern, and often scaliest at the border or edges. They can be prevented by keeping skin areas clean, cool, and dry. An antifungal powder such as Zeasorb AF powder should be applied daily in the morning to help prevent fungal infections of the feet and groin. Walking barefoot outdoors should always be avoided. Vaginal yeast infections are discussed on p. 394.

Clotrimazole (Lotrimin AF) cream is currently the best available over-the-counter antifungal agent, and should be applied twice daily to the affected areas. If fungal infections fail to clear within a reasonable time, seek medical advice.

Pityriasis versicolor is a fungal infection that causes small, scaly, red or brown skin patches. In dark-skinned people, the patches are lighter than normal skin, but in light-skinned people the patches are darker. They do not itch, but may be unsightly. For treatment, apply Selsun shampoo to the skin, covering as much of the body as possible, and leaving it for four hours; repeat this after a three-day interval.

VIRAL INFECTION

Herpes simplex virus is the most common problem, and causes cold sores (see p. 366) that may be triggered by exposure to sunlight, and genital herpes (see p. 408).

Varicella infections takes two forms. Chicken pox occurs in individuals who have not previously been exposed, and results in crops of small red blisters on the face, trunk, and extremities. The patient often develops a sore throat, headache, muscle weakness, and general malaise. It is common in industrialized countries, and most adults in the USA and Europe are immune. It is much less common in developing countries: only 30 percent of Singapore residents are immune, for example, and travelers *from* developing countries may be highly susceptible.

Varicella also causes shingles, which is characterized by numerous small blisters appearing in an area of skin in the distribution of a particular spinal nerve, often in a band at the side of the chest or abdomen, or sometimes on the face. It is not related to travel, but prompt antiviral treatment reduces complications and may not be easily obtainable in some countries; on the other hand, steroid creams are often dispensed freely without prescription in many countries and may be harmful.

PARASITIC SKIN INFECTIONS

Creeping eruption (cutaneous larva migrans) is caused by a worm that crawls into the skin and causes severe itching and a snakelike red, patterned rash (see pp. 107–8). Antihistamine tablets and hydrocortisone 1 percent cream can be helpful in relieving the itching, and topical thiabendazole solution is the best treatment.

COLD SORES

The herpes virus that causes cold sores predominantly affects the inside of the mouth, lips, and the areas of skin around the mouth, nose, and eyes. Initial infection usually passes unnoticed, though it can occasionally cause malaise, sore throat, enlarged lymph glands, and widespread ulceration of the mouth—the whole of the oral mucosa may be bright red and sore; this is most commonly seen in children, and is called herpetic stomatitis. A slow recovery takes place over a period of about 10 days. However, the virus is not completely eliminated from the body, and remains in a latent form which, when reactivated, is responsible for the production of cold sores.

Cold sores are caused by a complex reaction involving herpes simplex virus Type I, and the body's own defense system. Some individuals find that the condition may be triggered by exposure of the face to strong sunlight, although other factors such as cold temperatures, stress, menstruation, and any debilitating condition may also be important. The most common location for a cold sore is on the lip.

If an association between sunlight and cold sores has been observed, then the most sensible precaution is to keep out of the sun, and to wear a hat or sun shade; sun-blocking preparations on the lips and face are essential.

Typically, arrival of the lesion is preceded by a period of itching and irritation over the affected area. Within a few hours, blisters appear and these then burst and form a scab. Healing takes place over a period of about 10 days.

Be particularly careful not to touch the cold sore with the fingers and then rub the eyes. An infection of the finger end around the nails is possible, or worse, a serious infection of the surface of the eye. Do not kiss while you have a cold sore and especially avoid kissing children who may as a result develop herpetic stomatitis (see above). Obviously it is antisocial to go to the dentist with an active cold sore except in an emergency! Expect the dentist to protect himself and other patients by wearing rubber gloves.

Frequent sufferers should consider obtaining a prescription for the antiviral agent acyclovir (Zovirax) to take away with them. The cream should be applied to the affected area, and can shorten the duration of an outbreak considerably, especially when used immediately the first symptoms are recognized.   A. D.

Leishmaniasis is a parasitic disease that may result from the bite of a sandfly (see p. 150). Leishmaniasis of the skin is characterized by a nonhealing bump, boil, or sore that occurs at the site of a previous insect bite. Any nonhealing sores that persist after a trip to an endemic area should be suspected. Treatment of leishmaniasis is complicated, and specialist advice should be obtained.

Other infections and infestations include: tunga flea infestations of the skin of the feet (see p. 174); the tumbu fly (see p. 172); and a variety of other tropical diseases that also cause skin problems. Any traveler who returns home with an unusual rash, sore, or lump should be examined by a physician who has a specialist knowledge of these diseases.

SEXUALLY TRANSMITTED DISEASES

Sexually transmitted diseases (STDs) are considered in detail on pp. 404–19. Travelers are at increased risk, and many STDs that occur in the tropics are uncommon in the USA. They often cause skin manifestations and rashes that may be transient in nature; seeking skilled medical attention while these signs are still present may improve the chances of an accurate diagnosis and correct treatment.

LICE

These tiny, insect-like organisms are barely visible to the naked eye, and survive on blood obtained from biting humans and other hosts. Infestation with lice is itchy and uncomfortable (see also pp. 174–75).

Head lice are usually transmitted directly from person to person, but may also be transmitted by sharing hairbrushes and combs. Small concretions or sacs attached to the hair shafts can usually be detected; they are known as nits, and represent the egg cases of the lice.

Body lice may be acquired from infested clothing or bedclothes, or close physical contact. Itchy sores that resemble insect bites appear especially on covered areas of the body.

Pubic lice are often acquired as a sexually transmitted disease, or by sleeping in the bed of someone who has lice. Symptoms include itching and sores in the genital area.

Treatment with an over-the-counter preparation known as Nix cream rinse is quite effective for all forms of lice.

SCABIES

Scabies is a microscopic, insect-like organism. It causes small itchy bumps especially between the finger webs, on the umbilical area (navel), elbows, groin, breasts, and buttocks. The head is almost never involved except in infants and very small children. At times, the scabies lesions appear somewhat linear or elongated in their configuration. Each lesion represents the site where a small scabies mite has burrowed into the skin. It can be transmitted from person to person during physical contact, and also occasionally from contact with clothing and other articles (see also p. 176).

Elimite cream or Kwell lotion provides effective treatment. Itching often persists for some time, requiring antihistamines for relief, or sometimes more powerful steroid medication.

SKIN INJURIES

BLISTERS

Blisters from poorly fitting footwear ruin many trips, and avoiding badly fitting footwear is the best prevention: always make sure that you travel with at least one pair of comfortable, well-worn shoes, especially if you will be hiking or climbing (break in new boots at home, not while traveling).

If a blister does occur, do not pop it unless necessary: the blister fluid is usually sterile and will allow the underlying skin to heal better than any dressing you can provide. If a blister must be lanced, be sure to use a sterilized needle and carefully squeeze out all of the fluid. After this, some Polysporin ointment can be applied, and a Band-Aid type dressing can be placed over the area. This dressing should then be changed daily or after any bath or shower. If signs of infection occur, such as excessive redness, swelling, or pain, obtain medical attention. Blisters generally heal well provided that the source of the pressure trauma is removed; do not continue walking in the shoes that caused them.

Blisters can also occur on the hands, from carrying heavy luggage. It is better to carry two smaller bags than one larger bag. Shoulder straps can be helpful, but heavy items may also cause blisters on the shoulders.

CUTS AND ABRASIONS

Minor injury is extremely common in travelers: the most important rule is to keep cuts clean and dry: infection is much more likely under tropical conditions. Deep cuts should ideally be examined by a physician to see if suturing is required. Dirty wounds, such as those from animal bites, should not be sutured unless absolutely necessary. Wounds should be cleaned with hydrogen peroxide or alcohol, as well as soap and water. Any foreign debris should be removed by scrubbing gently with a towel or brush. The area should be completely dried with a clean towel. An antibiotic ointment such as Polysporin or Bactroban should then be applied and the area protected with a clean dressing such as a Band-Aid or Telfa gauze with paper tape.

If signs of infection occur, obtain medical advice as soon as possible. Infected wounds can require surgical debridement as well as antibiotic treatment in order to heal. A tetanus booster shot may be necessary (see box, p. 94), and you may also need to consider rabies protection (see p. 200).

FISHHOOKS

Injuries from fishhooks are common on vacation, and can be quite difficult to manage. Techniques for removal include depressing the hook to allow the barb to slide back through the skin where the puncture was made—using a piece of fishing line or string to apply the downward traction can sometimes be helpful. If this does not work, the skin may need to be repunctured and the hook clipped off with a wirecutter. During either procedure, keep the area clean by using soap and water or alcohol.

CONTACT DERMATITIS

Allergic reactions following skin contact are a frequent problem in travelers.*

Poison ivy, poison oak, and poison sumac may all cause dermatitis when the skin comes into contact with the oils and sap produced by these plants during hiking, walking, and other outdoor activities in areas where these plants are found. The rash may occur hours or days after contact.

Mango dermatitis can result from contact with sap in the skin of the

---

* The following free booklets may be helpful: *Poison Ivy* and *Allergic Contact Rashes,* American Academy of Dermatology, P.O. Box 1661, Evanston, IL 60204; and *Allergic Contact Dermatitis,* American Academy of Allergy and Immunology, 611 E. Wells St., Milwaukee, WI 53202; send an s.a.s.e.

fruit, while sucking off the flesh. A rash occurs, consisting of numerous small, itchy, red papules and blisters that may coalesce to form large red areas on the skin.

Cosmetics and toiletries A common cause of contact dermatitis is the use of new cosmetics or toiletries while traveling, especially small complimentary samples provided by hotels or airlines. Persons with particularly sensitive skin or a tendency to develop skin allergies, should travel with their own supply and should avoid using unfamiliar complimentary products on trips.

Treatment If plant oils remain on the skin surface, they may easily be spread to other areas, so wash the affected area thoroughly with soap and warm water. (If this is done soon enough after contact with poisonous plants is suspected, it may sufficient to prevent dermatitis from occurring.) Mild cases of dermatitis may be treated with cool compresses, and Aveeno bath or Domeboro compound may help relieve itching. Hydrocortisone 1 percent cream and antihistamine tablets can also help reduce itching and inflammation. Severe cases may require treatment with steroid cream or tablets, and antibiotics if infection occurs; skilled medical care may be necessary.

HIVES

Hives or urticaria (small red bumps or welts that occur in various areas on the body) occasionally occurs in travelers as a result of food allergy or an allergic reaction to an insect bite, though other causes should be sought if the problem does not clear up within a few hours or days. If swelling occurs around the face or head, urgent medical attention should be sought: swelling in the mouth and throat can interfere with breathing.

Antihistamine tablets are helpful, but severe cases may require treatment with prescription cortiscosteroids.

INSECT BITES AND STINGS

Insect bites are discussed in detail in other areas of this book.

Stings from wasps, hornets, bees or yellow jackets, and fire ants may produce significant pain and swelling if not properly treated. Fire ants can also cause uncomfortable, painful, and itchy bites.

SKIN CARE ITEMS TO PACK:

- Sunscreen, SPF 15 or higher.
- Lip protectant or balm.
- Polysporin or Bactroban antibiotic ointment.
- Steroid cream (hydrocortisone 1 percent is available over the counter, stronger preparations require a prescription).
- Clotrimazole (Lotrimin cream).
- Antihistamine tablets: diphenhydramine 25 mg. (Benadryl) is the most suitable over-the-counter antihistamine; alternatives include chlorpheniramine (Chlor-Trimeton, Atarax, and Hismanal); hydroxyzine and astemizole require a prescription; with the exception of astemizole, these may cause drowsiness and should not be used if you are driving or operating machinery (see also pp. 527–28).
- Assorted Band-Aids, paper tape, Telfa gauze, and cling wrap.
- Moisturizer or Vaseline petroleum jelly.
- Antifungal powder such as Zeasorb AF.
- Aveeno bath packets.
- Domeboro compound packets.
- Hydrogen peroxide or alcohol for cleaning abrasions or wounds.

Ice packs or ice-cold compresses can provide relief, and antihistamine tablets can be helpful in relieving swelling and itching. Severe reactions, resulting in difficulty in breathing, require urgent skilled medical care.

SPIDER BITES

A variety of spiders can produce painful or itchy skin eruptions when they occur; these are discussed on p. 220.

SEA BATHERS' ERUPTION AND SWIMMERS' ITCH

Sea bathers' eruption occurs in several distinct forms. Most cases are reported in tropical or subtropical areas such as Hawaii, Florida, and the Caribbean. Various organisms can cause these eruptions including algae (see p. 82), larvae, and perhaps other microscopic organisms. Prevention is the best approach, and local advice should be sought prior to swimming. If cases of sea bathers' eruption are being reported locally, it is safer just to swim in a pool. Immediate removal of bathing or diving apparel, and rinsing off immediately in fresh water, may prevent some cases, and wearing wet clothing for long periods of time seems to result in the worst outbreaks. The rash is itchy, and relief may be obtained with antihistamine tablets as well as hydrocortisone 1 percent cream. An Aveeno bath may also be soothing.

Swimmers' itch is caused by the larvae of small organisms that crawl under the person's skin and produce severe itching and bumps. These lesions most often occur on exposed areas and again might be prevented by immediate washing with fresh water after swimming (see p. 99).

PREEXISTING SKIN PROBLEMS

Acne and psoriasis improve with exposure to sunlight, though acne may become worse when conditions are humid. Eczema usually gets worse in a humid climate, and sufferers should avoid extremely humid conditions.

SUMMARY OF PREVENTIVE ADVICE:

- Avoid excessive sun exposure.
- Wear comfortable shoes.
- Don't touch unfamiliar plants.
- Avoid using unfamiliar personal hygiene or cosmetic items.
- Avoid exposure to conditions of extreme cold or heat.
- Wear clothing appropriate for the climate.
- Keep skin clean and dry.
- Dry your feet well after bathing or swimming.
- Use insect repellents (see pp. 182–88).
- Avoid casual sex, or at least use a condom.
- Avoid swimming where sea bathers' eruption or swimmers' itch is common (seek local advice).

DENTAL PROBLEMS

A thorough checkup prior to departure and adequate arrangements to cover the possible expense of emergency treatment are the main precautions to consider.

Dr. Gordon Seward is Emeritus Professor of Oral and Maxillo-Facial Surgery in the University of London. His profession has taken him to Europe, Africa, Australia, and the U.S., and he has acted as an Examiner in Nigeria, Malaysia, and Singapore. **Andrew Dawood** is a dentist in private practice in central London and also at Guy's Hospital, where he conducts research. He shares a family passion for travel and has worked in the jungles of South America and in teaching hospitals in South America and Asia.

Dental problems arising while traveling abroad are generally given little thought and consideration by prospective travelers and by those responsible for emergency treatment. If a dental emergency occurs, travelers may experience more difficulty obtaining help and are more likely to have to pay for it out of their own pocket than if they have a medical problem.

BEFORE DEPARTURE

Travelers on short trips or on vacation abroad are unlikely to face a dental emergency (other than an accidental one) if they have had a careful examination by their own dentist, including "bitewing" radiographs, within a few months of their journey, and any necessary treatment has been completed. However the examination is not a guessing game, and the dentist should be told about current symptoms or problems. Furthermore, the initial appointment should be booked a sufficient time before departure to permit treatment to be completed without haste. People with heavily restored mouths or large, complex restorations should seek advice from their dentist on coping with any particular problems that might arise.

Travelers intending to spend a long time abroad should consider treatment for any conditions likely to cause trouble in the future—for example currently symptomless impacted teeth or the replacement of a just adequate but ancient denture. Dental problems in long-term expatriates are surprisingly common: in Peace Corps volunteers (who each spend two years overseas), they consistently represent the third or fourth most frequently reported of all health problems. The cost of specialist care abroad can be considerable.

DENTAL PROBLEMS ASSOCIATED WITH TRAVEL

Few dental problems are directly a hazard of traveling. Seasick passengers, if they vomit over the side of the ship, may lose their dentures! Swimmers may also lose dentures or orthodontic plates. Ex-aircrew from World War II may recall that pressure changes could produce pain in filled teeth (a similar phenomenon may also occur with deep-sea divers), but as modern aircraft are fully pressurized, this does not happen to civilian passengers. Some people suffer pain and locking of the jaw joints, and an awkward posture on a long flight that induces lateral pressure on the jaw has been known to exacerbate this complaint. Too much alcohol can precipitate an attack of "periodic facial migraine" (Horton's syndrome), an uncommon cause of a recurrent severe throbbing pain in one cheek. For various reasons some people drink more alcohol when they fly, and sufferers may come to associate such attacks with flying.

DENTAL EMERGENCIES

Emergencies tend to fall into three categories: pain; lost or broken fillings and other restorations; and more serious emergencies (infection or traumatic injury).

TOOTHACHE

A relatively trivial dental problem can give rise to a totally disproportionate amount of pain, and can make life quite miserable. Extreme sensitivity to hot and cold may be the first sign of trouble; if treated at this stage, the tooth may settle down. If left untreated, the pain may become spontaneous and long-lasting; the nerve in the tooth may eventually die, and act as a focus for infection and abscess formation.

A dental abscess can cause severe, persistent pain, exacerbated by pressure on the tooth. In all cases, a swollen face should be taken seriously; it is wise to seek treatment early as there is a small but significant risk of life-threatening spread of infection if this is neglected.

The usual treatment for an abscessed tooth in many countries would be extraction; however if the abscess is caused by death of the nerve, it is often possible to perform root canal treatment to save the tooth—the nerve chamber is opened with a drill, and the infection drained. Later, the nerve chamber is filled with an inert or antiseptic material. Where a high standard of dental treatment is available, baby teeth may be treated in a similar fashion; otherwise it may well be more sensible to accept loss of a baby tooth rather than risk a spreading infection. If treatment is unavailable antibiotics should be taken, although every effort must be made to see a dentist as soon as possible.

Another type of abscess may develop where teeth are badly affected by gum disease. Such an abscess may sometimes be treated by deep cleaning of the tooth to remove infected deposits under the gum. However, once again, the only treatment offered in some countries may be extraction of the tooth. A similar abscess may develop around the crown of an impacted tooth, usually a lower wisdom tooth, and this is quite common in young adults. Extraction of the impacted tooth will eventually be necessary, although antibiotics, hot saline mouth washes, and good tooth brushing may help control the infection until the traveler returns home.

It is sensible for individuals who have suffered any kind of dental abscess in the past to discuss the management of such problems with their own dentist, who may well recommend traveling with a supply of antibiotics.

Occasionally, two to three days after a tooth has been extracted, the clot may liquefy and be lost from the socket, exposing bone. This allows food debris to accumulate in the socket, which may become infected. Warm water pumped by the cheeks in and out of the socket may be sufficient to keep it clean and relieve pain, but in more severe cases expert irrigation and a medicated dressing may be needed.

FILLINGS, CROWNS, BRIDGES, AND DENTURES

Though often a source of great inconvenience, the loss or breakage of a dental restoration cannot be considered to be a true emergency; the freshly exposed tooth surface is often sensitive to hot or cold, and jagged edges may irritate the soft tissues of the mouth. It is not, however, absolutely essential to seek immediate treatment unless there is considerable discomfort. The survival and fate of a tooth are unlikely to be affected by a delay even of a few weeks; this means that it is almost always possible to wait until you can see your own dentist, or can find a dentist on personal recommendation. Be careful not to damage the tooth with hard food as it may have been weakened by loss of the restoration.

If extreme sensitivity or a toothless smile necessitate treatment in the absence of adequate facilities, it is wise to seek provisional treatment only. It is often a simple matter for a dentist to insert a temporary filling, or temporarily recement a crown or bridge, but in many countries even the most basic dental materials may prove to be unobtainable.

"Do-it-yourself" repairs and temporary repair kits are not to be recommended unless you are reasonably dextrous or have a handy friend or traveling companion who can help. Even then, dental restorations are usually lost only as a result of underlying problems such as decay, breakage, or poor dentistry. Typically kits may contain a dental mirror, a mixing spatula, a cleaning and plugging instrument, and tubes of a dental dressing and temporary cement. One tube contains the paste, the other the catalyst to make it set. The cement will form a temporary filling for a tooth cavity, or can be used to recement a crown or bridge until expert help is available. It is essential that any debris inside the crown or bridge, which may prevent it from seating fully, is completely removed before the restoration is temporarily cemented in place. It is a good idea to check that the cleaned restoration can be properly inserted before mixing the cement. If the cemented restoration is loose, it should be removed as there is a risk that it may be inhaled or swallowed.

MORE SERIOUS EMERGENCIES

Fractured jaws and spreading infections need hospital dental treatment by an appropriate dentist (an oral and maxillo-facial surgeon). Standards of skill in treating jaw and facial bone fractures probably vary more from country to country than for any other injury. If it becomes clear that skilled treatment is not available locally, and if after emergency care the patient is deemed fit enough to travel and is not at risk from obstruction of the airway, it may be best to return home for further treatment.

A front tooth that has been broken as a result of a blow—particularly in a child—may not always seem to need urgent care: in fact, expert treatment within a matter of hours may make all the difference between conserving the tooth or losing it.

Americans knock out an estimated 5 million teeth every year. If a permanent front tooth is knocked out, it may be possible to reimplant it. The roots of some reimplanted teeth are subsequently eaten away by the body, like those of baby teeth, and the tooth is lost again; but others survive and give good service. If there is to be a chance of success, the tooth must be reasonably clean when picked up and it must be washed in cold water or milk. Hold the tooth only by the crown, and do not touch, rub, or scrub the root. The root must be kept moist, so put the tooth in a clean container, in cold drinking water to which salt has been added (one teaspoon to a glass), or some milk. If the tooth has been thoroughly washed it should be pushed back fully into its socket, straightaway. Be sure that the crown is the right way round! The procedure will not be too painful. The patient should bite on a handkerchief to retain the tooth in place, and get to a dentist as soon as possible. Baby teeth should not be reimplanted.

The dentist should splint the reimplanted tooth in place, give antibiotics, and arrange for a tetanus booster injection. If a dentist is not immediately available a temporary splint may be improvised using softened chewing gum (preferably sugar-free), pressed around the tooth and its neighbors, and covered with aluminum foil. It is best not to reimplant a tooth that has fallen onto pasture grazed by animals, because of the increased risk of tetanus infection.

Teeth successfully replaced within 20 minutes are most likely to reattach normally. If the tooth is kept moist there is a reasonable chance of success for up to two hours. Beyond two hours the results are poor. The splint should normally remain in place for about two weeks. In all cases the tooth should be checked by a dentist upon returning home, and subsequently at regular intervals.

CHOOSING A DENTIST ABROAD

Nonsterile instruments and needles may be a source of hepatitis B (see pp. 53–56) and HIV infection (see pp. 419–30). You should satisfy yourself that any dentist you consult uses instruments that have been adequately cleaned and sterilized. Instruments contaminated with traces of blood or injection syringes used on more than one patient are dangerous. "Cartridge" syringes are the safest for giving local anesthetic. These are made of metal, and a fresh glass tube, closed with a bung at each end and filled with sterile local anesthetic solution by the manufacturer, slides into the barrel for each patient. A fresh needle from an intact plastic capsule should be used for each patient. The syringe itself should be washed and sterilized between patients—autoclaving is preferable, but boiling of the cleaned metal part is acceptable. Absolute sterility of the metal part is less critical than with syringes in which the solution has to be drawn up into the barrel itself.

"Push-on" needles and plastic syringes should come from intact original packages, and should be discarded after each patient.

Beware of needles resterilized by soaking in antiseptics or by boiling. Beware particularly of plastic syringes that have been "resterilized" by soaking in antiseptic. Watch out for bottles of solution from which doses for other patients have been withdrawn. If needles which have been used on other patients are used to withdraw a further dose they can easily contaminate the contents.

The dentist should wear rubber gloves. They protect the hands and are more easily washed clean than bare hands. They do not have to be sterile surgeon's gloves. The dentist should wash them before and after touching the patient's mouth. They should be changed between patients if any bleeding has resulted from treatment.

Bear in mind that high-speed drills use water as a coolant, and this water (and any other water used in your mouth) is likely to be only as clean as the local supply.

Personal recommendation is usually the best basis for choosing a dentist.

IMPORTANT POINTS TO MENTION

If you have had rheumatic fever, chorea, have a heart-valve defect or disease, or a hole in the heart, a heart murmur, or have had heart-valve surgery, then you should have antibiotic cover for any extraction and should make this plain to any dentist you see. Antibiotic cover is also advisable for extractions if you have an artificial joint or a heart pacemaker.

You should also tell the dentist about any steroid treatment that you have had, even many months before, as it may be necessary for you to have additional steroid treatment at the time of a tooth extraction or similar surgery.

Patients who are taking anticoagulant drugs or who have had trouble with excessive bleeding from cuts, etc., or who suffer from hemophilia should make sure that the dentist understands the situation.

Naturally you should tell the dentist about any serious illnesses you have had and any medicines, injections, or tablets that you take as a routine. If you are allergic to any drugs (e.g., penicillin or aspirin), or dressings it is essential that the dentist or pharmacist know about this. Language problems may make this difficult.

Remember also that not all cultures attach a great deal of importance to saving teeth. You must make your own feelings on this subject quite clear!

FINANCIAL MATTERS

A few travel insurance policies include a specific section on emergency dental treatment, either as part of the package or as an optional extra. Many do not. If there is such a section, inquire beforehand about what it covers. While a spreading dental infection may need urgent hospital admission, insurance companies may not consider this to be included under the heading of emergency hospital treatment (perhaps because treatment is given by a dental specialist). Travelers at special risk of accidental injury (e.g., on skiing vacations) are advised to ensure that they are fully covered by appropriate insurance.

The cost of such emergency treatment may be very high; and so will be the cost of any crown, bridge, or denture work. In some countries with socialized medical systems, however, emergency care is sometimes provided free of charge.

LOOKING AFTER YOUR TEETH

When traveling in a hot country, it is sometimes tempting, and often necessary—when safe drinking water is unobtainable—to drink large amounts of canned or bottled sugary drinks. In some countries it may also be customary to serve guests with heavily sweetened tea or coffee. Frequent consumption of sugary food or drink is especially damaging to the teeth. It may take only a few months for early decay to develop in a previously unaffected tooth; small quiescent or reversing lesions may become active and irreversible.

Tooth cleaning becomes even more important when sugar consumption is high. Using dental floss or an interdental brush every day will help to prevent decay on otherwise inaccessible surfaces. Dental floss has been found to be a versatile and indispensable traveling companion by one of the authors, who has had cause to use it on occasion as a clothes line, for repairing a tent, and for hanging a hammock. The possibilities are limitless!

FLUORIDE AND LIVING ABROAD

A small amount of fluoride (1 part per million in temperate climates) in drinking water undoubtedly reduces the likelihood of tooth decay, particularly in children; however, an excessive fluoride intake (greater than 2 parts per million in a temperate climate), can lead to mottling and discoloration of developing teeth. In countries that have a well-developed piped drinking water supply, the fluoride content is carefully controlled to the proper level. Not only is the appropriate small amount added where it is required, but a natural excess of fluoride is removed.

Unless it is known for certain that fluoride is absent from the local water supply or is present only in a very low concentration (much less than 1 part per million), the use of fluoride supplements for children is unwise. In any case, supplements should be used only when prescribed by a knowledgeable dentist or physician. Where fluoride levels are high, it may be wise to use bottled water for babies and small children, bearing in mind that water intake and thus total fluoride intake is higher in hot countries. The fluoride content of bottled water is frequently stated on the label.

Young children often swallow a significant amount of toothpaste when they brush their teeth. If the toothpaste contains fluoride, and fluoride levels in the drinking water are already on the high side, this may result in an excessive total fluoride intake. Only under these circumstances is it better for babies and young children to use a fluoride-free toothpaste.

EYE PROBLEMS

Exposure to strong sunlight, dust, dry or polluted atmospheres, and infection, with limited access to skilled care if problems occur, are the main difficulties facing the traveler. Simple precautions will prevent most problems.

Peter Fison is a Consultant Ophthalmologist at Sutton Hospital in South London. **Timothy ffytche** is a Consultant Ophthalmologist at St. Thomas's Hospital, Moor-fields Eye Hospital, and at the Hospital for Tropical Diseases, London.

Because we rely constantly on our eyesight to orient ourselves in our surroundings, as travelers we should take particular care of our eyes. We take our eyesight so much for granted that it is only when things go wrong that we realize quite how much we depend on them. Fortunately, serious eye problems are unusual. A little common sense and some simple precautions will ensure that most damage to the eyes can be anticipated and avoided.

A particular problem for travelers is that in many parts of the world it is extremely difficult to find eye care of an acceptable standard when it is needed. Standards and methods of treatment vary considerably, and in many developing countries the number of trained ophthalmologists is very small; in several African states, for example, there is not even one trained ophthalmologist per million population. Some local doctors and pharmacists may have considerable skill in diagnosing and treating eye problems, particularly where specific diseases are common, but the traveler must not rely on this, and should beware of the risks of inappropriate therapy, harmful patent medicines, and folk cures.

The aim of this chapter is to provide information about the most likely hazards, especially in places where good health care is not readily available.

SUNLIGHT

The effects of strong sunlight range from acute damage to the front surface of the eye (conjunctiva and cornea) by ultraviolet rays, to the more long-term effects of various wavelengths on the skin of the eyelids and on the internal structures of the eye, particularly the lens and the retina.

SHORT-TERM EFFECTS

The eyebrows and eyelashes throw a shadow across our eyes, filtering the light, and a reflex action usually makes us screw up our eyes in strong sunlight. This reduces the amount of light reaching the two particularly sensitive areas, the cornea and the conjunctiva. Acute overexposure of the eye to ultraviolet light can temporarily damage the cornea. In mild doses, this causes discomfort, redness, inflammation and excessive lacrimation; when it is more severe, the pain becomes intense with extreme sensitivity to light, spasm of the lids, and blurred vision. This type of situation is most likely to occur at high altitude, over water, and particularly over snow, where the condition is often referred to as snowblindness. The excessive radiation causes edema and loss of epithelial cells on the surface of the cornea, which is extremely painful. As with all UV overexposure, the ocular effects have a delayed response time of several hours.

Treatment consists of applying an eye ointment to lubricate the corneal surface, and keeping the eyes closed, using an eye pad. This is usually sufficient to provide relief within a few hours from all but the severest episodes. Milder conditions can be treated with simple lubricant eyedrops, such as artificial tears. The best approach, however, is to avoid trouble in the first place—by wearing the appropriate protection such as a sun hat, ski goggles, or sunglasses that screen UV light.

While sunglasses are effective under most conditions, skiers and mountaineers will know from bitter experience that goggles are often necessary. At higher altitudes the concentration of ultraviolet light is greater, because it has not been filtered out by the atmosphere. Goggles are also helpful if weather conditions change, since they help prevent the reflex watering of the eyes induced by cold wind and snow that may blur your vision and endanger your safety. Remember, too, that harmful ultraviolet rays can penetrate apparently dense cloud cover at high altitude: cloudy conditions are often deceptive.

LONG-TERM EFFECTS

Although everyone is susceptible to acute damage from ultraviolet exposure, it is the fair-skinned, blue-eyed individual who is most at risk from long-term exposure. Skin cancers are more common in people with a history of long-term exposure to sunlight. Cancers may occur on the eyelids and can be particularly difficult to deal with at this site. Protection with sunscreens and sunglasses are the sensible way to avoid problems.

There is a strong link between long-term exposure to ultraviolet light and effects on the lens and retina—it dramatically increases the likelihood of developing cataracts and retinal degeneration. Retinal degeneration is a common cause of poor vision in elderly people; other factors that predispose to it are: known existing macular disease, a family history of the condition, and having fair skin and blue eyes. People who have had cataract surgery are also at risk—their lens, a valuable natural filter to the damaging wavelengths, is no longer able to provide protection. Even if this has been replaced with an intraocular lens implant containing UV screens, these may not be sufficient.

To prevent these complications, always protect your eyes when the sun is strong: wear a hat, and use good-quality sunglasses; don't forget that babies and small children also need good protection.

ENVIRONMENTAL CONDITIONS AND POLLUTION

Our eyes have efficient mechanisms for protection. These include both the voluntary and involuntary blink reflexes, the tear film over the corneal surface of the eye, and the extreme sensitivity of the cornea. Stimulation of the cornea by something like a particle of grit provokes violent reflexes of watering and blinking in order to wash away the foreign body; where the stimulus is less intense the eyes may just become red and feel sore and uncomfortable, particularly if the condition persists. Tears contain an enzyme (lysozyme) that functions as an antibacterial agent.

There are many irritants in the atmosphere. Dust, pollen, smoke, chemicals, water pollutants, and many more can all cause chronic discomfort, and there are certain localities in the world where these may be excessive. A further common source of discomfort is the drying effect that modern air-conditioning or central heating in buildings, aircraft, and cars may have on eyes and contact lenses.

All these things conspire to upset the natural lubrication of the eyes and can give rise to considerable discomfort, and sometimes cause long-term problems. Certain individuals are more susceptible than others, including those with known histories of allergies and those with naturally dry eyes. Treatment includes avoidance, if possible, of provocative atmospheres, and the liberal use of lubricating eyedrops or antiallergic medication if appropriate. A simple artificial teardrop or proprietary eye lotion is usually all that is necessary to help wash out the irritants or replace deficient tear secretion. Drops which whiten eyes have less logic since they act by temporarily constricting superficial blood vessels in the conjunctiva. This can reduce the eyes' response to the irritation and when the effects of the drops wear off there may be a rebound effect leading to a return of the redness; they mask the symptoms rather than treating the cause.

The combined effect of prolonged heat, dust, and wind in desert conditions may give rise to permanent changes in the eye. A condition known as pterygium can occur in people after prolonged exposure to this sort of environment. A slowly growing wedge of white, fatty tissue can extend from the conjunctiva across the cornea in the exposed part of the eye. Although benign, it may need to be excised if it becomes cosmetically unacceptable or causes visual problems by growing into the pupillary zone. Its exact cause is unknown but it is heavily associated with exposure to UV light, and occurs commonly in residents of developing countries; appropriate use of good-quality sunglasses will help prevent this condition.

INFECTION

Eye infections occur more frequently in hot climates, where a wide variety of germs may be present in the atmosphere, rivers, lakes, swimming pools, and the sea.

Conjunctivitis ("pink eye") Bacterial conjunctivitis is the commonest infection, often producing a crust or sticky discharge that is likely to gum your eyelids together when you sleep. The affected eye is usually red, and feels gritty or itchy. Although rubbing provides temporary relief, it can make the situation worse and cause the infection to be transferred from one eye to the other.

Bacterial infection usually responds within a few days to treatment with antibiotics, such as gentamicin, sulfacetamide, or neomycin eyedrops every two hours. Avoid using antibiotic preparations that also contain steroids; steroids may be widely available without a prescription in many developing countries, but may harm your eyes in the presence of a virus infection, which has identical symptoms.

Viral conjunctivitis does not respond to simple antibiotics; more specific treatment may be necessary. It should be suspected in any conjunctivitis that does not settle in a few days with antibiotics, and expert attention should be obtained. Patients with a past history of eye infections with herpes should be aware that attacks can be provoked by exposure to strong sunlight, and should therefore wear protective sunglasses; where possible, travel with appropriate medication that could be used at the first sign of a fresh attack.

During an infection, the eyes can be kept clean by frequent warm saline washes with an eye bath or by wiping the lids with moistened cotton wool. A simple irrigating solution can be easily made by adding a teaspoon of ordinary salt to a pint of *boiled* water and allowing it to cool before applying it to the eye.

Remember that many forms of conjunctivitis are very infectious and can be easily transmitted to others. Make sure that such items as handkerchiefs, towels, facecloths, eye baths, and eyedrops are not shared, and it is probably best to avoid swimming until the infection has subsided.

Trachoma One infection that gives rise to particular anxiety is trachoma. In hot, dry countries where this disease is endemic, it can lead to progressive blindness, and worldwide, more than 100 million children have active trachoma infection. However, travelers who contract trachoma conjunctivitis experience only mild symptoms of redness and irritation, with a sticky but rather watery discharge from the eyes. Blindness occurs only with recurrent infections over many years among people who are already debilitated through chronic malnutrition, primitive sanitary conditions, and overcrowding. The infective agent is spread by close contact with infected individuals, their fingers and their clothes, and by flies. Trachoma of the eye is caused by the same organism as the sexually transmitted disease chlamydia (see p. 406), and it is possible to have both infections at the same time. If you think you have trachomatous conjunctivitis, a three-week course of tetracycline eyedrops, with ointment at night, will cure the condition. Antibiotics (tetracycline or erythromycin) should also be taken orally to ensure complete eradication of the infection. If you remain in an area where trachoma is endemic, reinfection may occur, and a further course of treatment would then be necessary.

There are several forms of more severe eye infection that may occur in certain parts of the world; they may be transmitted sexually or by flies and other insects, and include parasites and worm infestations such as onchocerciasis, filariasis, and some rarer conditions. If there is any suspicion of such a condition, such as any eye problem that fails to respond readily to treatment, an expert opinion should be sought as soon as possible. Antibiotic drops and ointment, although unlikely to cure the condition, will at least prevent secondary infection until the correct therapy can be commenced.

TRAUMA

Major or even moderate trauma to the eye and lids requires speedy medical or ophthalmic attention. When chemicals or sprays get into the eyes the immediate treatment consists of trying to wash out the irritant by copious irrigation either with an eye bath, or under a running tap, or even, in extreme circumstances, by immersing the head in a bucket of water with the eyes open! No attempt need be made in this type of emergency to find an antidote to the chemical since this may waste valuable time.

Minor trauma consists mainly of abrasions caused by foreign bodies that sometimes become embedded in the eye. When this occurs the cause is usually obvious and if the reflex watering or the simple maneuver of pulling the upper lid down over the lower lid does not seem to wash away or dislodge the particles, then the likelihood is that there is a residual scratch, or that something is embedded on the cornea or under the upper lid. Impacted corneal foreign bodies are often visible and need to be removed by an expert in order to avoid damage, and antibiotic ointment should be instilled until the proper attention can be obtained. This may make the eye more comfortable and will help prevent secondary infection and allow an abrasion to heal.

DUST PARTICLES UNDER THE EYELID

In dusty conditions, whether you wear contact lenses or not, particles of grit may get stuck under the top eyelid. There are some fairly obvious ways to avoid this. Do not put your head out of the window while traveling. Keep your eyes closed in dust storms. Use protective eyewear whenever necessary. Dust particles under the eyelid are quite common, and should be suspected if nothing can be seen on the surface of the eye but the eye still feels as though a foreign body is present.

Removing a foreign body from under someone else's upper eyelid is a simple procedure, and gives immediate relief from severe discomfort. Sit down in front of the affected person (who should also be seated), and ask him or her to look down and to keep looking down. Gently pull the eyelid away from the eye by holding the lashes firmly between the index finger and thumb of your left hand. While your patient continues to look down (this relaxes the muscles of the lid), gently press the center of the eyelid about a quarter of an inch from the lid margin, where you can see a shallow groove in the skin. Press downward and slightly backward, using a cotton bud. This gentle pressure will flip the lid inside out, and if you adjust your pull on the eyelashes slightly upward, the eyelid will remain everted. Now wipe the inside of the eyelid gently with a clean tissue or the tip of a cotton bud (moistened so that you do not leave residual fibers) to remove the offending piece of grit, which is often so small that you cannot see it. Finally, pull the eyelashes gently outward and down so that the lid returns to its normal position.

Although it sounds complicated, this maneuver is actually quite simple, provided that both you and the affected person stay relaxed and avoid sudden movements, and that you perform each step without force. A pad to protect the eye for 24 hours will usually heal any scratch on the corneal surface, but if symptoms persist an expert opinion should be sought.

WORKING ABROAD

Safety standards may be different abroad. If you intend to work abroad, or to take part in any activity involving a risk of injury to your eyes, make sure that you take along any protective or other safety equipment that may be needed—and be sure to use it.

PREEXISTING EYE PROBLEMS

It almost goes without saying that persons on regular ophthalmic medication for conditions such as glaucoma and ocular inflammations should make sure that they have an adequate supply of medication for their trip, carried in hand luggage for safekeeping. Many ophthalmic preparations that are readily available at home may be scarce or unobtainable abroad, and drugs may often be dispensed in a different form or dosage. Patients with complicated medical conditions should also therefore carry a note with them explaining their diagnosis and current treatment.

EYEGLASSES

Losing eyeglasses or having them stolen—an increasingly common experience—may also be a great annoyance, and for some people may be a calamity. The most sensible precaution is to have a spare pair available or to carry a recent prescription, since in many parts of the world new glasses can be made up very quickly without a great deal of expense.

CONTACT LENSES

Those who wear contact lenses know that their eyes can tolerate so much and no more. Rigid gas-permeable lens wearers who have overworn their lenses know how intensely painful this mistake can be. Lens wearers can develop irritable eyes with infection or allergy from cleaning, soaking, and rinsing solutions.

Discuss your trip with your contact lens practitioner before you leave. Travelers who normally wear contact lenses should take a spare pair, and also an up-to-date pair of eyeglasses in case of trouble, as well as a pair of sunglasses for protection from dust, wind, and sunlight. At the earliest sign of irritation or discomfort, leave the lenses out for as long as necessary. The commonest problems for rigid lens wearers are overwear and dust particles trapped under the lens. Remind yourself to keep blinking to circulate fresh tears under the lens. In overwear, the cornea, which has high oxygen demands, suffers from edema—corneal swelling. This can be extremely uncomfortable—symptoms are very similar to overexposure to UV light. Treatment involves removing the lens, and resting with your eyes closed—there may be too much discomfort to do anything else! Mild painkilling tablets will help a little.

A scratch on the cornea from a dust particle trapped under the contact lens may feel much the same. A gritty sensation when you blink, a feeling that the particle is still in there, and excessive watering will usually make you keep your eyes closed. After removing the lens, a soft pad fixed by adhesive tape will rest the eye; but keep the eye closed under the pad. If you keep both eyes closed they move less, allowing the scratch on the cornea to heal more quickly.

An additional problem on long flights is that contact lenses tend to dry out. Humidity aboard an aircraft can be as low as 2 percent, because the air supply is drawn from the rarefied outside air by compressors in the engine, and it circulates continuously. Always keep a lens case and lens solutions with you in your hand luggage when you fly; on most long-haul flights, it is more comfortable to wear eyeglasses.

Aerosol insecticide sprays are sometimes used on board aircraft, in accordance with international regulations, to clear the cabin of unwelcome stray insects. In a confined space, these aerosols may be absorbed by soft contact lenses and irritate the eyes, so it is sensible to keep your eyes closed during spraying and for a minute or so afterward.

Recent reports have highlighted the painful condition of keratitis, which is an inflammation of the cornea. Keratitis caused by bacteria (usually staphylococci) and viruses (either *Herpes simplex*, which also causes herpes blisters, or Adenovirus, responsible for the common cold) is not uncommon, whether you wear contact lenses or not. This sort of keratitis is treated either with antibiotic drops (such as gentamicin or neomycin) or antiviral ointment (acyclovir).

Particular interest has centered on a rare but serious cause of keratitis called *Acanthamoeba*, which most frequently occurs in contact lens wearers, though it has also been found in corneal ulcers following minor trauma. *Acanthamoeba* is a protozoal organism that lives freely in the soil and in water, and does not normally cause infections in man. Because contact lenses cause the cornea to become more vulnerable, the organism is able to gain access to the corneal substance and establish a colony. All contact lens wearers should therefore be particularly careful to remove their lenses before bathing in swimming pools, hot tubs, and even in fresh water, and they should never moisten their contact lenses by licking them, since *Acanthamoeba* has even been isolated from normal saliva. It has also been found in contact lens solutions that have been left open for a while, but not in unopened bottles of sterile distilled water.

If you should develop an intensely painful red eye, with blurred vision and acute sensitivity to light, the chances are that you may well have a form of keratitis. If the degree of pain is out of all proportion to the apparent inflammation, particularly if you are a contact lens wearer, it is just possible that you may have this rather unusual corneal ulcer caused by *Acanthamoeba*. Whatever the cause, you should stop wearing your contact lenses and you should seek professional help without delay.

Do not rely on being able to obtain supplies of your usual cleaning, rinsing, and soaking solutions at your destination, and take along an ample supply. Do not attempt to concoct your own solutions under any circumstances.

Do not depend on heat sterilization of lenses when you travel, since adequate facilities may not always be available; there are now

CONTACT LENSES: SOME TRAVEL TIPS

- In general, daily-wear lenses are preferable to extended-wear (sleeping-in lenses) as they are less likely to cause long-term physiological changes to the eye. Daily wear reduces the potential for serious complications like bacterial infections and ulcers.

- If you wear contact lenses and will be traveling under extreme conditions of poor hygiene, you may be better off adopting extended-wear lenses: this can mean anything from keeping contact lenses in for an occasional night, to a regime of six nights' wear followed by one night's rest, or wearing lenses for longer than a week at a time. Not all types of lens are suitable for this wearing pattern, and you should consult your contact lens specialist before you travel. Alternatively, you may have to consider reverting to eyeglasses.

- Disposable lenses are very useful for travel: they allow a large number of spare lenses to be carried in case of loss, damage, and poor cleaning facilities, and are rapidly becoming the first choice of all contact lens wearers for whom they are suitable.

Gillian Whitby, Optometrist
London

several chemical regimes to choose from that are better suited to travel (including solutions based on macromolecular preservatives that do not penetrate the contact lens matrix, and therefore have a very low potential for causing allergy) and you should discuss the best choice with your practitioner.

Many problems when traveling under conditions of poor hygiene can be avoided by using disposable contact lenses that do not require daily removal and cleaning.

EYE-CARE ITEMS TO PACK

Depending on where you are going, and how long you will be away, it is wise to take certain simple medications and equipment as part of an eye kit:

- sunglasses that screen blue and ultraviolet light (UVA and UVB)
- spare eyeglasses or contact lenses, a copy of your current prescription, and your optometrist's telephone number
- eye bath

- eye pads
- lubricant eyedrops (artificial tears)
- antibiotic eyedrops and ointment
- an adequate supply of any regular medication and supplies (such as contact lens solutions) as well as written details of existing eye problems and any treatment.

Note that in countries with no restrictions on the sale of medicines to the public you may be offered eyedrops and ointment containing steroids; these may be dangerous and should be used only on specialist advice.

GYNECOLOGICAL PROBLEMS

Gynecological problems are common in women travelers. Most problems are not serious, but even a supposedly minor problem can ruin a trip.

Dr. John Naponick is a public health physician with specialist training in gynecology, obstetrics, and tropical medicine. He has worked in the USA, Canada, Cameroon, Malaysia, Bangladesh, Thailand, Burma, and El Salvador. He currently works in Bangladesh.

Ellen Poage is a registered nurse and a health educator. She has traveled and worked in Central America, Africa, and Asia, and now lives in Fort Myers, Florida.

Women travelers who plan a long trip abroad, or who plan to live in a country where good medical facilities may not be easily accessible, are well advised to have a gynecological checkup before they leave home—preferably six weeks or so before departure; it is always a good idea to begin a trip with a clean bill of health. Those with previous gynecological problems should have a clear understanding of their medical history, or should carry a written note of any problems.

MENSTRUAL PROBLEMS

PERSONAL SUPPLIES

Women should make a careful estimate of their likely requirements for personal hygiene. Although women throughout the world menstruate, not all of them take the same approach to feminine hygiene. So if the traveler to a remote area is not sufficiently adventurous as to be willing to experiment with the only facilities that may be available locally—such as balls of cotton wool, cloths and towels tied on with strings, or even handfuls of leaves—she should be certain to ensure an uninterrupted supply of her own preferred variety of tampon, sanitary napkin, or pad.

In developing countries locally made menstrual supplies are usually available in most major cities, although the standard varies. In relatively more advanced countries such as Thailand and Malaysia they may be of high quality. In poorer countries such as Bangladesh, napkins are beginning to replace the more traditional towel-and-string methods in the wealthier section of the community; those made locally, however, tend to look (and feel) more like a mattress than the kind of slim-line product with which most women living in developed countries are familiar.

MENSTRUATION

Some women travelers prefer not to have periods at all while traveling; this can be accomplished by taking the Pill continuously, without a break between packets (p. 433); unless you are already on the Pill, however, this is generally worthwhile only if you will be away for three months or longer.

Women who travel to game parks should consider this option or should avoid close proximity to predatory animals (bears, lions, tigers, etc.) while menstruating. There have been a number of reported attacks on menstruating women. Likewise, if they swim or dive in shark-infested waters, they are at increased risk of attack by sharks.

In some parts of Southeast Asia, such as Indonesia, women may be asked not to enter local temples if they are menstruating.

IRREGULAR BLEEDING

Periods may stop completely in travelers. Often, the cause of this proves to be pregnancy. However, an irregular cycle is usually the result of the hormonal changes that follow any disruption of normal routines, and may even be partly psychological in origin. One example of this phenomenon has been studied extensively: nursing students who leave home and move into shared accommodation almost always experience some disturbance of menstruation: after a while, a normal cycle returns, with the women menstruating in unison.

HEAVY BLEEDING

A detailed discussion of causes of heavy vaginal bleeding is outside the scope of this book. Suffice it to say that certain types of frequent bleeding may be due to a serious underlying condition requiring surgical treatment, and expert medical advice should always be obtained.

In many cases, this kind of irregular bleeding may be due to a hormonal disturbance, and will respond to hormonal treatment. If you are bleeding heavily, and are in a remote area where no skilled medical advice can be obtained, it is worth trying the following treatment *provided that* you have had a recent checkup, you are otherwise healthy, and you *are certain that you are not pregnant.*

Take one combined oral contraceptive pill, for example Norinyl 1, four times a day for five days. These pills contain standard doses of progesterone and estrogen hormones, and are readily available worldwide.

I call this a medical or hormonal curettage. Bleeding should stop during treatment, and you should have a period by the seventh day after the last day of treatment. If bleeding does not stop during treatment, the problem will require a skilled assessment, and probably surgery or curettage. If you do not have a period within five to seven days of stopping treatment, you may be pregnant.

Remember that even if this treatment is successful, there may still be an underlying problem, so specialist advice should be obtained at the earliest opportunity.

UNINTENDED PREGNANCY

Some women become pregnant while traveling, and others begin their trip in the earliest stages of pregnancy. Those who choose not to allow the pregnancy to continue are advised to be very careful. A termination of pregnancy in a developed country, where technical facilities and specialist skills are widely available, is generally a safe procedure; a termination of pregnancy performed without these facilities, and under unhygienic conditions, can cause life-threatening complications and may have serious implications for the mother's future health and fertility. Remember that it is your responsibility to ensure that the facilities you choose are clean and safe—even if this means traveling on to a country where better facilities are available, or returning home.

Also remember that, in most cases, time is on your side. Up to six weeks from the last menstrual period, a simple menstrual regulation procedure can be performed. In countries where it is available, RU486 can be used up to nine weeks from the last period (see p. 439). Up to 12 weeks from the last period the termination procedure is safe, although you should definitely avoid delaying any further than this (see p. 439). In exceptional circumstances, action can be taken at up to 20 or 24 weeks, depending upon local laws (see Map 10.2, p. 438).

Those who are happy to continue with their pregnancy should make sure that they have access to adequate medical care (p. 440).

GENITAL AND URINARY TRACT INFECTION

YEAST

Yeast infection or vaginal candidiasis is one of the most common gynecological problems encountered by travelers in hot, humid, tropical conditions. It is caused by overgrowth of a yeast normally found in the female genital area. Several factors promote growth of this organism: heat, humidity, the oral contraceptive pill, certain antibiotics, and diabetes. The best way to prevent the problem is to keep the genital area dry and cool; cotton underwear which absorbs perspiration is strongly recommended, and synthetic fabrics should be avoided.

A yeast infection is characterized by a red rash, itching, and a thick, white "cottage cheese" vaginal discharge.

Treatment Daily vinegar douches (1 tablespoon vinegar per quart of water—or roughly 30 ml. per liter) may be sufficient to relieve the itching, and return the vagina to its correct pH (acidity). If nothing else is available, yogurt may also provide relief. When stronger treatment is required, clotrimazole (Mycelex-G) 100 mg. intravaginally, daily for seven days, or nystatin 100,000 units intravaginally for 14 days may be used. Despite treatment, the condition may recur if the predisposing factors mentioned above have not been rectified.

CYSTITIS

Cystitis, also called urinary tract infection or the "urethral syndrome," is a common condition in women and may be particularly distressing and inconvenient in travelers. It often follows an unaccustomed increase in sexual activity. Symptoms usually consist of frequent urination. The infection is usually due to contamination of the urinary passage with bacteria from the patient's own anal area, but may occasionally be the result of a sexually transmitted disease. If possible, cultures should be performed.

Pain on urination without frequency may be due to vaginal infection, or to genital herpes. Seek a thorough examination.

Treatment Drink plenty of fluids. Cranberry juice is sometimes helpful because it alters the acidity of the urine and may provide some symptomatic relief; cranberry juice is not always available outside the USA, and citrus fruit juices are an acceptable substitute.

Self-treatment with antibiotics is usually inadvisable. If there is no prospect of skilled medical care, and if symptoms persist, tetracycline 500 mg. by mouth four times a day for seven days (total dose 14 g.) or doxycyline 100 mg. by mouth twice daily for seven days may be taken; these drugs will cover the important possible causes of urinary symptoms, including gonorrhea, which has always to be considered. It is essential to complete the full course, and this treatment should not be used in pregnancy; milk products interfere with absorption of these drugs.

Only if there is no possibility of a sexually transmitted disease would I advise using more conventional antibiotic treatment for a urinary infection—such as trimethoprim/sulfamethoxazole (Septra, Bactrim, etc.), two tablets every 12 hours for five days—without a laboratory diagnosis.

Self-treatment should be resorted to only in an emergency, and advice from a qualified medical practitioner should be obtained at the earliest opportunity.

SCHISTOSOMIASIS (BILHARZIA)

Schistosomiasis (pp. 94–99) can sometimes produce itchy or ulcerated swellings in the skin, particularly the labia and genital region, where they are often mistaken for warts. They may appear long after exposure, and several travelers have recently been affected.

CHOOSING A DOCTOR ABROAD

Unfortunately, it is not safe to assume that the high standard of medical ethics and professional behavior you may be accustomed to in your home country will automatically apply to all doctors in every country you visit. For obvious reasons, when dealing with gynecological problems in a strange country it is important to choose your doctor with care. Your embassy or consulate (or staff who speak your language from another embassy or consulate), expatriates, and local residents may be able to recommend a suitable physician; often, the most reliable recommendations are those from satisfied patients. If you can find a female doctor so much the better.

Always insist on a chaperon when being examined; use your common sense, but be prepared to refuse if you are asked to submit to what seems to you to be an unreasonable procedure.

OTHER HAZARDS

Female travelers appear to be at slightly *less* risk of malaria infection than male travelers; one possible explanation is that they take greater care to observe the necessary precautions!

LIVING ABROAD

Screening procedures normally taken for granted at home may not be offered as a routine to long-term residents abroad. All women should request screening for cervical cancer, and be familiar with the technique of breast self-examination. Periodic mammography is advisable—certainly for women over 50. In developing countries, good-quality tests of this type, and appropriate safety standards for equipment and quality control, are not always readily available. A gynecological examination on return home is a sensible precaution; be sure to tell your physician where you have been.

FEVER

Although fever can be harmless, it may be an early feature of serious illnesses, especially malaria, where a delay in treatment can result in death. Fever in anyone who has visited the tropics should always be taken seriously.

Dr. Martin S. Wolfe *has been the tropical medicine specialist for the Department* *of State and the World Bank for 23 years. Prior to this, he worked in Ghana and Pakistan. He is the Director of the Travelers' Medical Service in Washington, D.C., and has a consulting practice in tropical medicine.*

Febrile illness is a common problem in travelers, either during the trip or following return home, and is usually caused by infection. Fever in a traveler is often caused by diseases that are not specifically related to travel and that might just as likely occur at home (see below). Some "tropical fevers" are simply due to viral or bacterial infections that lead to a brief, mild, self-limited illness, and the specific cause is never determined. However, certain more serious causes of fever must always be considered. Heat illnesses causing fever are discussed on pp. 306–8.

THE MOST IMPORTANT FEBRILE ILLNESSES TO CONSIDER

MALARIA
Malaria is potentially the most significant and life-threatening febrile illness in travelers (see pp. 121–32). The minimal incubation period, from the time that one is bitten by a malaria-carrying mosquito until the onset of typical malaria symptoms (fever, chills, sweats, headache, etc.), is seven days. Anyone with no exposure to malaria from a previous trip, who develops a fever during the first week of arrival in a malarious area, therefore can only be suffering from some other kind of infection.

Malaria drug prophylaxis is essential for travelers to malarious areas, but increasing resistance means that complete protection cannot be assured; malaria may still occur, and the possibility should not be removed from consideration simply because medication was taken. Measures against mosquito bites are extremely important in prevention, but malaria may still be a possibility even with the most careful precautions.

Emergency self-treatment If symptoms of malaria develop while traveling (and after at least seven days following arrival in a malarial region) medical care should be sought immediately so that appropriate diagnosis and treatment can be received. There is no simple, safe, and universally available drug for emergency self-treatment, should medical care not be available in a remote area. Some of the options are listed on pp. 126–27, but the choice is difficult. A new drug, halofantrine (Halfan), may well be the most suitable, though it is not yet widely available. Fansidar has been recommended in the past, but cannot be taken by those allergic to sulfa, and malaria parasite resistance to it is increasingly widespread. Mefloquine (Lariam), perhaps the most effective prophylactic drug for most (but not all) malarial areas, is not recommended for emergency self-treatment because of its potential for causing convulsions or hallucinations as side effects. Oral quinine could be used, but requires a three-day course of treatment and frequently causes troublesome side effects.

Other Considerations After leaving a malarial area, drug prophylaxis must be continued for four weeks to prevent the life-threatening form of malaria caused by *Plasmodium falciparum*. Two other forms of malaria, caused by *P. vivax* and *P. ovale*, have a latent phase in the liver that is not eliminated by the drugs taken for prophylaxis. The only available drug to destroy these liver-stage parasites is primaquine. The longer the period of travel, and the greater the exposure to malaria, the higher the possibility of contracting *P. vivax* or *P. ovale* malaria. Infection with these forms is unlikely, though still possible, in short-term travelers with no intense exposure. Since these forms can lead to infection of the blood and symptomatic malaria up to three years after exposure, malaria must be considered in any febrile illness during this period if primaquine has not been taken after return.

Any traveler who develops a fever or other symptoms after leaving a malarial area should report this promptly to a physician. Malaria is known to be a great mimic, and can produce misleading symptoms like cough or diarrhea; people with malaria are frequently thought to have "the flu" or some other common and less serious infection. In some tragic cases, delayed consideration and inadequate diagnosis or treatment have resulted in death from falciparum malaria.

TYPHOID AND PARATYPHOID
Enteric fever caused by *Salmonella typhi* (typhoid fever) and *Salmonella paratyphi* (paratyphoid fever) is usually contracted from contaminated food or water in developing countries. The incubation period ranges from 10 to 21 days. Enteric fever symptoms can be

similar to those of malaria, including fever, chills, headache, abdominal pain, and cough; diarrhea may or may not be a prominent feature, and may contain blood.

VIRAL HEPATITIS

Viral hepatitis, with or without jaundice, has a more prolonged incubation period—about 28 days or more. Travelers who visit rural areas of developing countries or who eat poorly cooked shellfish or drink contaminated water even in major cities are most likely to contract hepatitis A, or the much less common hepatitis E (see p. 58). In the early symptomatic period, high fever and chills can occur, with nausea, and vomiting—these often improve when jaundice develops, and the diagnosis becomes more easily apparent. The urine becomes dark. Serologic tests are required to define the specific type of hepatitis (hepatitis A being by far the most common).

Hepatitis A is eminently preventable with the pre-travel immune globulin injection (see pp. 506–7)—perhaps the most important preventive immunization measure a traveler can take. The newly developed hepatitis A vaccine is not yet available in the U.S.

Hepatitis B is usually transmitted in a similar way to HIV infection, by sexual contact, contaminated needles, or by blood transfusion. A vaccine is available (see p. 509) and its pre-travel use should be considered by those who might have sexual contact or other intimate contact with the local population in the developing world.

DYSENTERY

Entamoeba histolytica is a leading parasitic cause of diarrhea in travelers (see pp. 39–40) and can also infect the liver, causing an amebic liver abscess. The incubation period is over 21 days. This infection should be considered in the presence of fever associated with a tender liver (pain or tenderness in the upper abdomen, on the right); unlike viral hepatitis, jaundice is very uncommon.

Bacterial dysentery caused by *Shigella, Campylobacter,* or *Salmonella* can have an initial onset with fever and chills, followed by diarrhea and other gastrointestinal symptoms.

With both kinds of dysentery, the diarrhea often contains blood.

INSECT-BORNE VIRAL INFECTIONS

Fever may be the initial symptom of a large number of viral infections, usually after an incubation period of 10 days or less.

WARNING SIGNS OF A SERIOUS INFECTION REQUIRING IMMEDIATE EVACUATION TO A SATISFACTORY SOURCE OF MEDICAL CARE INCLUDE:

• Fever which does not subside with the above specific treatment or remains elevated above 103°F. for 12 hours or more

• Jaundice

• Persistent diarrhea or vomiting

• Severe continuous headache

• Continued abdominal pain

• Cough with pus or blood in the sputum

Many kinds of insect-borne viruses (arboviruses) are present worldwide in the tropics and are a leading cause of febrile illness in travelers (see pp. 132–34). Confirmation of a specific viral agent as the cause requires specialized blood tests that are not usually readily available. Most of these viruses cause a rather short, self-limited illness with no serious complications or consequences, and for which no specific antiviral drugs are available.

Dengue is the arbovirus that travelers are most likely to come across, and is a significant risk in many parts of the world: it has been increasing in the Caribbean and Latin America in recent years. Dengue is sometimes known as break-bone fever, because of the severe aching body pains it can cause, along with fever, chills, headache, and frequently a rash. There is no vaccine yet available to prevent dengue, nor is specific treatment available.

Japanese B encephalitis is much less common, but can occur particularly in longer-term residents of the Far East, and can lead to severe neurological problems. A vaccine is available, but is not usually indicated for short-term travelers (see pp. 510–11).

MENINGITIS
Meningococcal (spinal) meningitis is a rare risk to travelers. Symptoms include headache, neck stiffness, increased sensitivity to light (photophobia) and sometimes a rash. Sudden deterioration may occur, and prompt treatment is essential (see pp. 102–4).

Those going to areas where meningitis epidemics occur should take meningococcal meningitis vaccine.

LESS COMMON FEBRILE ILLNESSES

Tuberculosis is an uncommon cause of fever, particularly for short-term travelers. Fever with cough, night sweats, and weight loss would raise the possibility of this infection, and a chest X-ray would then be necessary.

Tick typhus is a particular hazard to those on safari in eastern and southern Africa. The incubation period is five to seven days. There is often a black crusted sore at the site of the vector tick bite, associated with high fever, chills, headache, body aches, and a typical rash. There is no vaccine for this infection, but if considered or diagnosed, there is a very rapid improvement with tetracycline drugs.

African trypanosomiasis (sleeping sickness) was diagnosed in only 15 American travelers between 1967 and 1987. All acquired their infection from tsetse fly bites in East Africa and 11 of the 15 were participants in safaris. The estimated incubation period is 6–28 days. Fever occurs initially, along with a rash, headache, and fatigue. If unrecognized, infection can spread to the brain, leading to confusion and personality changes (see pp. 156–59).

Brucellosis is a febrile bacterial infection contracted by ingestion of unpasteurized cows' or goats' milk or soft cheese made from such milk. Symptoms include fever, chills, sweats, body aches, headache, weight loss, and fatigue, and can be recurrent (see p. 20).

Schistosomiasis (bilharzia) is contracted from swimming in fresh water, particularly in tropical Africa, and can have initial onset about four weeks after infection (see pp. 94–99). Symptoms can include high fever, headache, hives on the skin, wheezing, and joint pain.

COSMOPOLITAN FEVERS

A number of febrile infectious diseases that are common in the United States should also be considered in travelers returning from

COSMOPOLITAN CAUSES OF FEVER

Sinusitis
Otitis media (ear infection)
Strep throat
Upper respiratory infection,
    bronchitis, pneumonia
Infectious mononucleosis
Cytomegalovirus infection
Meningitis
Endocarditis
Appendicitis, diverticulitis
Inflammatory bowel disease
Gallbladder disease
Pancreatitis

Alcoholic hepatitis
Urinary tract infection
Pelvic inflammatory disease
Acute HIV infection
Secondary syphilis
Other sexually transmitted diseases
Skin infections
Lyme disease
Legionnaires' disease
Histoplasmosis
Collagen vascular diseases
Drug fever (drug reaction)

abroad with fever. These "cosmopolitan" causes of fever are just as likely to occur in the U.S. in nontravelers, and the most important examples are listed below.

WHAT TO DO IN AN EMERGENCY

It can be difficult enough for a well-trained physician, let alone a nonmedical traveler, to make a rapid, accurate diagnosis and initiate specific, appropriate treatment for an acute febrile illness. Any traveler with suspected malaria or any acute illness with a high fever (greater than 102°F., 38.9°C.) while traveling should seek immediate medical attention. American, European, and other English-speaking embassies can usually recommend a physician who is speaks English and is Western-trained.

Self-treatment can cause many problems. In particular, it can interfere with laboratory tests, making specific diagnosis impossible; it may also result in side effects, and may cause a false sense of security when symptoms subside, if the illness has not been adequately treated. Self-treatment should be attempted only in those remote situations where adequate skilled care cannot be obtained.

Malaria self-treatment (and its difficulties) have been referred to above. If antimalarial drugs do not improve the fever or other symptoms within two or three days, it is very likely that some other infection is present. Perhaps the single best antibiotic to cover a wide spectrum of infective organisms is ciprofloxacin. A dose of 500 mg. twice daily could be helpful as initial emergency self-treatment for enteric fever, bacillary dysentery with fever, certain pulmonary infections, urinary tract infections, and mild to moderate skin infections. Ciprofloxacin may be associated with hypersensitivity allergic reactions, even following a single dose, and it should be discontinued at the first sign of a skin rash or other allergic reaction (see also pp. 520–21).

Other supportive treatment should include aspirin (not for children) or Tylenol every four hours, and for persistent high fever, measures to reduce temperature such as a sponge bath with tepid water, air-conditioning, or a fan. Fluid intake should be increased. A thermometer should be used to monitor the fever pattern.

10 SEX AND CONTRACEPTION ABROAD

SEXUALLY TRANSMITTED DISEASES

Travelers are at increased risk of acquiring sexually transmitted diseases. All travelers should know how to reduce the risks if they do not intend to avoid them.

Dr. John Naponick is a public health physician with specialist training in gynecology, obstetrics, and tropical medicine. He has worked in the USA, Canada, Cameroon, Bangladesh, Thailand, Burma, and El Salvador. He currently works in Bangladesh.

When Christopher Columbus returned from his voyage of discovery to the New World, an epidemic of syphilis swept Europe. Ever since, historians have debated whether or not Columbus and his sailors were to blame. One thing that *is* certain, however, is that today's traveler is at as great a risk as ever of acquiring a sexually transmitted disease.

Sexually transmitted disease (STD), still popularly known as VD (venereal disease), has reached epidemic proportions in many countries and is a major problem worldwide, encompassing a wide range of infections. Everyone has heard of gonorrhea and syphilis, but more recently recognized diseases such as chlamydia infection—often harder to document—may be twice as common. Herpes, until recently the focus of much public concern, has almost totally been eclipsed by the specter of AIDS. Although HIV may be transmitted by contaminated needles, blood products, and from mother to fetus, and is discussed in greater detail on pp. 419–30, it is still above all else a sexually transmitted disease. Changing attitudes to sexual behavior, as well as promiscuity, prostitution, and homosexual practices, have each contributed to the present pattern of sexually transmitted disease.

As far as the individual traveler is concerned, however, the public health aspects of sexually transmitted infections are less important than their immediate implications.

RISK FACTORS

All STD risk factors depend on individual behavior. If you do not intend to place yourself at risk, you do not need to read this chapter. The only absolute ways of avoiding STD are abstinence, or sexual intercourse with a partner who is known to be disease-free and is completely faithful. Any other type of behavior will place you at risk of infection. Risk factors include:

Travel People behave differently when they travel. Tourists travel to seek adventure and new experiences, and to make new friends. Sex is certainly part of the attraction. Sex is sometimes even the sole purpose of travel, as evidenced by the continuing growth of the "sex tourism" industry to certain parts of Asia. The usual norms of the home environment no longer control behavior. Travelers separated from their families—for example, business travelers, the military, seafarers, and immigrants—are all at particular risk.

Number of sexual partners The more sexual partners a person has, the greater the risk of acquiring—and passing on—an STD. Rates of infection are very high in promiscuous homosexuals. Prostitutes in some Asian cities have infection rates reaching 100 percent. Even in 1987, 90 percent of Kenyan prostitutes were found to be HIV-positive. Even if you have only one contact with a prostitute you are at high risk of contracting an STD.

Frequency of sexual contact The greater the frequency of sexual contact, the greater the risk of acquiring an STD. For example, men have a 20 to 35 percent chance of acquiring gonorrhea from each contact with an infected partner. Two exposures would obviously increase the risk.

TABLE 10.1. SEXUALLY TRANSMITTED DISEASES

Disease	Causal agent	Occurrence
Gonorrhea	*Neïsseria gonorrhoeae*	worldwide (250 million people affected at any one time)
Chlamydia	*Chlamydia trachomatis*	worldwide
Syphilis	*Treponema pallidum*	worldwide (50 million cases each year)
Chancroid	*Haemophilus ducreyi*	subtropical and tropical
Lymphogranuloma venereum	*Chlamydia trachomatis*	subtropical and tropical
Herpes	*Herpes simplex* virus	worldwide
Trichomoniasis	*Trichomonas vaginalis* (a protozoan)	worldwide
Nonspecific vaginitis	*Gardnerella vaginalis*	worldwide
Anogenital warts	human wart virus	worldwide
Scabies	*Sarcoptes scabiei* (a mite)	worldwide
Pubic lice	*Phthirus pubis,* (the crab louse)	worldwide
Intestinal infections	*Campylobacter jejuni* *Shigella species* *non-typhoidal salmonella* *Entamoeba histolytica* (amebic dysentery) *Giardia lamblia* (giardiasis)	worldwide in those who practice anal-oral sex as well as by nonvenereal transmission
Others: AIDS	HIV	worldwide
Hepatitis B	Hepatitis B virus	worldwide

Age The highest incidence of STD is found in the 15-to-30-year-old age group. The incidence declines as age increases. Theoretically one could reduce the risk by choosing a more mature partner.

Choice of partner Certain groups of people are known to be at high risk. They include intravenous drug users, homosexuals, prostitutes, young people with multiple sex partners, and bisexual men; special categories of high-risk groups for HIV include people who have

Incubation	Likely symptoms	Complications
2–7 days	buring on urination, penile and vaginal discharge	infertility; arthritis; pelvic abscess
5–7 days	same as gonorrhea but may be milder	infertility
10 days–10 weeks	painless ulcer, rash	occur late; cardiovascular problems or mental changes
3–14 days	painful necrotizing ulcers, painful swelling of lymph nodes	localized
3–30 days	small painless ulcer	stricture of rectum; genital elephantiasis
2–12 days	painful multiple ulcers	recurrence; cancer of cervix (possible)
4–20 days	vaginal discharge and irritation	local only
7 days	odoriferous vaginal discharge	local only
1–20 months	cauliflower-like growths	localized
2–6 weeks	itching, skin eruptions	local infection
1–2 weeks	itching	local infection
varies	diarrhea, jaundice, etc.	depend on disease
2 weeks–5 years (or more)	fever, weight loss, etc.	opportunistic infection, death
2–6 months	jaundice	carrier state; chronic liver disease

received multiple blood transfusions, hemophiliacs, or anyone who has had regular sexual intercourse with individuals in the above categories.

In addition to an increased risk of acquiring an STD, travelers face many other difficulties. They may be going from an area of modern medical care to an area with less sophisticated medical facilities. The medical professionals may or may not be as well trained, and the laboratory backup services may be nonexistent. Language barriers may pose an obstacle to communication.

DISEASES

A wide variety of diseases can be transmitted sexually, and some are considered in Table 10.1. It is beyond the scope of this book to give exhaustive information about each disease; medical texts and lay publications are available for that purpose.

Bacteria, viruses, protozoa, and arthropods may all be transmitted by sexual contact. Sexual intercourse is the usual mode of transmission, but any close contact that allows transfer of infected materials or secretions can transmit disease. The disease can establish itself wherever it finds a suitable environment—usually those areas of the body that are warm, moist, dark, and lined with a mucous membrane, such as the genital area, the mouth, the rectum, etc.

The spectrum of diseases that can be contracted is immense and there is no limit to the number with which one may be afflicted at any one time. Furthermore there is no such thing as immunity toward most of these diseases, so reinfection is likely unless precautions are taken.

Some sexually transmitted infections, such as crab lice, are merely a nuisance. Herpes may recur, may be particularly troublesome, and is possibly linked to cancer of the cervix. Gonorrhea and chlamydia can cause infertility and painful, incapacitating pelvic infection. Lymphogranuloma venereum can result in genital deformity. Syphilis can lead to insanity and damage to the nervous system, the heart, and major blood vessels. HIV infection is not a "gay plague," it is a hazard that every sexually active male or female traveler must take seriously; AIDS kills. These complications are presented not to scare you, but merely to make you aware of the far-reaching consequences that these diseases have.

GEOGRAPHICAL DISTRIBUTION
It is unfortunately not possible to construct a world map showing global distribution of risk. While some places certainly have a higher incidence of STD than others, it is important to bear in mind that risk depends on behavior, not geography.

HIV has been reported from almost all countries. The highest incidence is in the USA (New York and California), the Central African countries of Zaire, Rwanda, Burundi, Central African Republic, Congo, Zambia, Tanzania, and Uganda, and Haiti. In the USA, it is mainly a disease of homosexual and bisexual men, but introduction into the heterosexual population has begun. In Africa, HIV is transmitted by contaminated needles, blood products, and from mother to fetus. Heterosexual transmission of HIV appears to be most common in Central Africa, but is growing worldwide.

Hepatitis B is spread by the same route, occurs all over the world, and is probably more easily transmitted.

Lymphogranuloma venereum (LGV) and granuloma inguinale (GI) are diseases of the tropics and subtropics. LGV is found in West Africa, Asia, the southern USA, South America, Singapore, and major seaports; GI is found in India, the Pacific Islands, Papua New Guinea, West Africa, the West Indies, South America, and the southern USA; chancroid also occurs mainly in the tropics and subtropics, but small outbreaks do occur elsewhere.

Most other STDs occur worldwide; gonorrhea and syphilis in particular are found more often in urban settings, seaports, and trading centers; the young (15 to 35 years) are most often infected; males outnumber females; male homosexuals are at great risk.

While it would be nice to give a "top ten" country-by-country guide to STD, I think it safer to look warily upon easy sex as the greatest risk: sexually transmitted diseases are a worldwide problem.

PREVENTION

PUBLIC HEALTH MEASURES
China is the only country in the world that claims to have eradicated syphilis and possibly also gonorrhea. Its campaign involved eliminating prostitution, providing health education and treatment on a large scale, exerting pressure on health workers and the general public to identify cases, and actively discouraging premarital and

extramarital sex; this situation is changing, however, and prostitution is again on the rise. In any case, the success of such measures has few immediately obvious benefits for the traveler: finding a consort may be difficult in countries where the risk of contracting an STD is low!

PERSONAL PROTECTION

The only sure way to avoid STD is to avoid sexual contact altogether, or to keep to a mutually faithful relationship with one partner known to be disease-free. Anyone not willing or able to do either should know how to minimize the risks and maximize protection.

Marsha Blachman of the University of California, San Francisco, says that dealing with HIV by deciding to be celibate is like trying to deal with being overweight by fasting, it may work for a while, but eventually you get so hungry you eat anything you can find.

It is important to acknowledge the risk factors already described, and to avoid sexual contact with individuals who are at highest risk. In the USA the usual advice on avoiding HIV includes limiting the number of partners, using condoms, and avoiding anal intercourse; choice of partner is the most important factor and this applies to all STDs.

In attempting to choose a partner belonging to a low-risk category, bear in mind that surveys have shown many people are prepared to lie in order to have sex; one survey of young, sexually active Californians showed that 47 percent of the men, and 60 percent of the women, claimed that they had been lied to for the purposes of sex; 34 percent of the men and 10 percent of the women admitted that they themselves would also be prepared to lie; 20 percent of the men said that they would lie about having a negative HIV-antibody test, and nearly half of both men and women said that they would understate their number of previous partners. Of those who had been sexually involved with more than one person at a time, more than half said their partners did not know.

Clearly prostitutes constitute a high-risk category, and in many Asian countries up to 90 percent of all sexually transmitted infections result from contact with prostitutes. Brothels, massage parlors, and singles bars offer a high probability of infection.

While it is worth trying to examine a prospective partner for sores, ulcers, pus, or other signs of disease, remember that patients with a wide variety of infectious conditions, including HIV, often look and feel healthy. It is more important to try to find out about their sexual history.

Safe sex STDs (including HIV) are transmitted by body fluids such as blood, semen, vaginal secretions, urine, and saliva. The term "safe sex" is used to describe sexual acts that do not allow exchange of body fluids. Examples of safe sex are mutual or simultaneous masturbation, and consistent and correct condom use from start to finish of sexual contact (vaginal, anal, or oral). This approach should be the rule in all casual encounters; in a recent study of returning Swedish travelers, however, 74 percent of those who had sex with a new partner abroad had not used a condom.

CONTRACEPTIVE MEASURES

The condom is particularly valuable in helping to prevent infection and is also safe, cheap, effective, and widely available. HIV will not pass through an intact condom. If used correctly—throughout sexual contact—a condom appears to reduce the risk to men of acquiring syphilis or gonorrhea by a factor of 10. Risks to women are also reduced; so when necessary, women should insist that their male partner wear a condom.

Even with a condom, anal intercourse between an infected individual and an uninfected partner poses a risk of transmitting HIV and other infections because condoms may break.

The following recommendations for proper use of condoms to reduce the transmission of STD are based on current advice provided by the CDC, Atlanta:

- Latex condoms should be used because they offer greater protection against viral STD than natural-membrane condoms.
- Condoms should be stored in a cool, dry place out of direct sunlight.
- Condoms in damaged packages or those that show obvious signs of age (e.g., those that are brittle, sticky, or discolored) should not be used. They cannot be relied upon to prevent infection.
- Condoms should be handled with care to prevent puncture.
- The condom should be put on before any genital contact to prevent exposure to fluids that may contain infectious agents. Hold the tip of the condom and unroll it onto the erect penis, leaving space at the tip to collect semen, yet ensuring that no air is trapped in the tip of the condom.

- Adequate lubrication should be used. If additional lubrication is needed, only water-based lubricants should be used. Petroleum- or oil-based lubricants (such as petroleum jelly, cooking oils, shortening, and lotions) should not be used, since they weaken the latex.
- Suppositories and vaginal or rectal preparations that are oil- based are likely to damage condoms and contraceptive dia- phragms made from latex rubber, reducing their contraceptive efficacy as well as reducing protection from STDs.
- Use of condoms containing spermicides may provide some addi- tional protection against STD. However, vaginal use of spermi- cides along with condoms is likely to provide greater protection.
- If a condom breaks, it should be replaced immediately. If ejacu- lation occurs after condom breakage, the immediate use of sper- micide has been suggested. However, the protective value of post-ejaculation application of spermicide in reducing the risk of STD transmission is unknown.
- After ejaculation, care should be taken so that the condom does not slip off the penis before withdrawal; the base of the condom should be held while withdrawing. The penis should be with- drawn while still erect.
- Condoms should never be reused.

A diaphragm (cap) can also provide a mechanical barrier to infection, as well as a chemical barrier if used, as recommended, in conjunc- tion with a spermicide. Women who use a diaphragm or whose partners use a condom contract gonorrhea only one fifth as often as users of oral contraceptives or IUDs. Spermicides will kill most organisms that can cause STD, including HIV.

Oral contraceptives (the Pill or progestogen-only Pill) do not protect women from STD. However, oral contraceptives do have one pro- tective effect in that they cause thickened cervical mucus. This thick mucus may protect against pelvic inflammatory disease (PID) as it inhibits the spread of STD infections up the cervical passage to the uterus. PID is the consequence of an STD infection spreading up to the fallopian tubes and ovaries and producing fever, abdominal pain, and eventual fibrosis, adhesions, and scarring. Scar formation may be the cause of later infertility.

One survey showed that women who use an oral contraceptive for 12 months or longer can halve their risk of PID.

Long-acting progestogens (p. 436) in the form of implants may also help to prevent PID. The lack of menstruation and thickened cervical mucus may be factors.

IUDs, on the other hand, increase the risk of PID by a factor of almost four, especially if there is exposure to STD.

Other, time-honored methods of STD prevention include washing the genital area and urinating immediately after the sex act. These are sensible measures, although keeping a full bladder during the sex act is a prerequisite for the latter, and is not always comfortable or possible; but avoiding transfer of body fluids is much more reliable.

When consulting your physician prior to travel for advice on the most suitable contraceptive method (pp. 430–39), it is worth taking into account the possible need for protection against STD.

IN CASE OF INFECTION

If you think you have caught an STD, or even if you just suspect you have been exposed, you should seek examination by a fully qualified medical practitioner. Early, prompt treatment is essential if the disease process is to be arrested and permanent complications are to be avoided. Incorrect, inadequate, or inappropriate treatment may mask the symptoms and allow the disease process to advance. Some diseases, such as syphilis, disappear for long periods of time after the initial symptoms, as if cured, only to reappear again in a more serious form at a later date. There is no effective treatment following exposure to HIV.

Travelers sometimes face a problem in obtaining correct diagnosis and treatment. Some sexually transmitted infections take weeks to appear, and by then the traveler may have moved on to a different country, where the disease may be unfamiliar: several infections favor hot climates, but unfortunately many physicians know only about locally occurring diseases. It is always advisable to tell the physician exactly when and where exposure took place.

You should try to locate the best possible medical facilities: expatriates, diplomats, medical associations, and local businesses may be helpful in directing you to qualified practitioners. In areas where STDs are common, STD clinics can be found more easily. You should not be reluctant to attend a clinic if you think you have a disease: we all think it will never happen to us, but it can.

DIAGNOSIS

Some diagnoses can be made on simple inspection, some require microscopes and cultures, and some a blood test. The more reliably a diagnosis can be documented, the greater the likelihood that treatment will be effective. I would recommend keeping detailed records of any symptoms you have had, any diagnoses that have been made, any laboratory examinations done, and all treatment. This information may be valuable to your physician upon your return home should you fail to get better.

DANGERS OF SELF-DIAGNOSIS AND TREATMENT

I would discourage you from attempting either self-diagnosis or self-treatment. If you found yourself alone on a desert island you would have to decide for yourself what to do in those circumstances, but such situations are rare, and you should usually be able to obtain some sort of medical advice. Drugs are available in some countries without prescription, but you may do yourself much harm by making the wrong diagnosis and giving yourself the wrong treatment.

There are several reasons for this. First, there is no one drug that will treat all sexually transmitted infections, and use of the wrong drug may not cure the infection or may not completely cure it.

Second, no drug is free from side effects, and if you use the wrong drug you may expose yourself to undesirable effects without obtaining any benefits.

Third, there is the problem of *resistance* to certain antibiotics and other drugs. Diseases unfortunately appear capable of keeping one step ahead of medical science. When penicillin first became available in the 1940s, small doses of the drug were capable of killing a wide range of microbes. Since then, certain strains of organism have become resistant to penicillin—i.e., they are able to escape the lethal effects of the antibiotics. This has happened to some strains of gonorrhea, and *especially those found in many parts of Asia.*

Indiscriminate, inappropriate, or incorrect use of a drug against bacteria that have developed resistance to that drug may mean that (1) the infection is not cured (at least using normal doses) and (2) drug resistance is further encouraged, thus increasing the public health problem. Few people have butts large enough to receive injections of penicillin in the doses that would now be required to treat infection with penicillin-resistant gonorrhea.

Once a drug becomes useless, doctors have to switch to using another drug, but unfortunately bacteria that have developed resistance to one antibiotic have a tendency to develop resistance to others as well—for example, some strains of gonorrhea have become resistant not only to penicillin, but possibly also to tetracycline and to spectinomycin. Ultimately, more expensive, more potent drugs—with more side effects—have to be used.

A fourth reason for avoiding self-diagnosis and -treatment is that you may give yourself a false sense of security that your disease has been cured when in fact it has subsided only to reappear at a future time in a more dangerous form.

Prophylactic treatment For similar reasons, you should also avoid the prophylactic use of antibiotics or other drugs in an attempt to prevent infection: the drug you choose may well not be effective against any infection you pick up; it will give you a false sense of security, probably increasing the risk of infection, and its indiscriminate use will encourage the development of drug resistance.

CORRECT TREATMENT

When prescribed a treatment, the most important thing is to take it in the correct amount for the correct time. Taking a drug for a shorter time than advised may not effect a cure and may encourage drug resistance.

It is usual during treatment to have the symptoms subside after 24 to 48 hours, so it is often tempting to stop the treatment then rather than complete the full course—especially if the medicine you are taking is one that makes you feel lousy.

The standard treatment schedules of the Centers for Disease Control and Prevention and the World Health Organization are listed in Table 10.2 on pp. 416–17. I have provided these *not* so that you can treat yourself, but rather to enable you to compare them with any treatment you are offered abroad. If you are diagnosed as having an STD and are offered treatment which appears to be substantially different, request an explanation.

Anyone given treatment for an STD should always return to a clinic for a follow-up examination—to confirm that treatment has been successful.

Sexual activity should be avoided during treatment, both to prevent further spread of disease and to avoid confusion: it is rather easier to distinguish recurrence from reinfection if one remains celibate during treatment.

TABLE 10.2. RECOMMENDED TREATMENT SCHEDULES FOR VARIOUS SEXUALLY TRANSMITTED DISEASES

Disease	Recommended treatment
Chlamydia	tetracycline hydrochloride: 500 mg. by mouth, four times a day for at least seven days or doxycycline: 100 mg., by mouth, twice a day for at least seven days or erythromycin: 500 mg., by mouth, four times a day, for at least seven days
Gonococcal infections	ceftriaxone: 250 mg. by im injection, plus doxycycline: 100 mg. orally twice daily for seven days or tetracycline hydrochloride: 500 mg. by mouth four times a day for seven days
Nongonococcal urethritis	tetracycline hydrochloride: 500 mg. by mouth, four times a day for at least seven days or doxycycline: 100 mg., by mouth, twice daily, for at least seven days or erythromycin: 500 mg., by mouth, four times a day, for at least seven days
Gardnerella vaginalis infection	metronidazole: 500 mg., by mouth, twice daily for seven days or clindamycin 300 mg. by mouth, 2 times a day for 7 days
Trichomoniasis	metronidazole: 2 g., by mouth in a single dose
Syphilis	benzathine penicillin G: 2.4 million units total, injected intramuscularly in a single dose or tetracycline hydrochloride: 500 mg., by mouth, four times a day for 15 days
Vulvovaginal candidiasis (not considered a STD)	miconazole nitrate (200 mg. vaginal suppository) intravaginally at bedtime for 3 days or clotrimazole (200 mg. vaginal tablets) intravaginally at bedtime for 3 days or butaconazole (2% cream 5 grams) intravaginally at bedtime for 3 days

Table 10.2— *continued*

Disease	Recommended treatment
Chancroid	erythromycin: 500 mg., by mouth, four times a day or ceftriaxone 250 mg. by im injection in a single dose or trimethoprim sulfamethoxazole (cotrimoxazole) (Septra, Bactrim, etc.): one double strength tablet (160/800 mg.) by mouth, twice daily for at least 10 days and until ulcers and/or lymph nodes have healed
Lymphogranuloma venereum	tetracycline hydrochloride: 500 mg., by mouth, four times a day for at least seven days or doxycycline: 100 mg., by mouth, twice daily for at least two weeks or erythromycin: 500 mg., by mouth, four times a day for at least two weeks or sulfamethoxazole: 500 mg., by mouth, four times daily for three weeks
Scabies (see also p. 178)	lindane (one percent) lotion or cream: one ounce (30 g) applied thinly for eight hours; wash off thoroughly or crotamiton (10 percent): apply thinly overnight for two nights, wash off thoroughly 24 hours after second application or sulfur (6 percent) petrolatum: apply paringly for three consecutive nights, washing thoroughly 24 hours after the third application
Pubic lice (crab lice) (see also p. 178)	lindane (one percent) lotion or cream: as for scabies above or lindane (one percent) shampoo: apply for four minutes and wash off or pyrethrins and piperonyl butoxide: apply to infected area and wash off after 10 minutes

Note: Tetracycline and doxycycline should not be used in pregnancy.

TRAVEL, SEX, AND CANCER

A study has shown that wives of frequent travelers are at higher risk of contracting cervical cancer than other women. For example, wives of airline pilots were four times more likely to develop the disease than wives of civil servants or schoolteachers. A sexually transmitted virus is believed to be partly responsible, so that having multiple partners is a major risk factor. The study did not show, however, if the high rate was caused by husbands who passed the virus to their wives on return home, or by the wives themselves taking advantage of their husbands' absence to find other partners.

CONTACT TRACING

In some countries, it is the law that all sexual contacts of individuals who have contracted an STD be named, traced, and treated. This is good practice, as it is the only way to stop the spread of the diseases. Even where it is not the law, mere concern for others should prompt anyone who is being treated for an STD to tell contacts so that they can seek medical advice in turn. Although this may be embarrassing, it is to be highly recommended.

END OF JOURNEY

I strongly advise travelers with any possibility of exposure to STD to take the precaution of seeking a physical and laboratory examination on their return home—to protect subsequent, unsuspecting sexual partners from unwelcome gifts from abroad.

CONCLUSION

The best protection against sexually transmitted diseases is education, and a commonsense approach to prevention combined with prompt treatment of both partners if treatable disease occurs.

Risk for STD and HIV is determined by what you do, not by who you are or where you go. If you are not monogamous or abstinent, you must use condoms regardless of your sexual orientation. Both male and female travelers who consider sexual contact a possibility on their travels should carry condoms with them and use them every time they have sex.

If you have difficulty resisting temptation abroad, you should consider traveling with your usual partner whenever possible.

WHAT TO DO IN AN EMERGENCY

In the unusual situation of a traveler developing symptoms of a sexually transmitted disease in a remote place, where no medical advice can be obtained and no laboratory facilities are available, but there is access to a supply of medicines, I advise the following approach—bearing in mind the warnings given in the text regarding self-treatment:

- **Penile discharge in males** The most likely causes of this are gonorrhea and chlamydia. One antibiotic treatment that could cure both is tetracycline hydrochloride, 500 mg. by mouth, four times a day for at least seven days. This treatment would give you a period of seven days to seek medical advice. Even if treatment succeeds, I strongly recommend a checkup after your travels. You might have contracted syphilis at the same time, and this treatment would not have eradicated it. Some strains of gonorrhea are resistant to tetracycline.
- **Vaginal discharge in females** I would advise the same treatment as given above for males, for the same reason. If this treatment fails I would then give 2 g. metronidazole (Flagyl) by mouth, in a single dose to treat Trichomonas. If that failed, I would then give treatment for vaginal yeast infection. If this also fails, then medical advice *must* be sought, even if this means changing your travel plans.
- **Genital ulcers** In addition to penile and vaginal discharge, the other major manifestation of STD is genital ulceration. There are several diseases that can produce genital ulcers. A good treatment to start with would be tetracycline hydrochloride, 500 mg. by mouth, four times a day for 15 days. This would treat syphilis and lymphogranuloma venereum. If this treatment failed you could take a treatment for chancroid: erythromycin 500 mg. by mouth, four times a day until the ulcer has healed. These treatment schedules should give you enough time to find medical assistance.

Finally, I would caution you once again to seek medical assistance if at all possible, and not to attempt to diagnose and treat yourself unless there is no alternative. There are side effects to all medicines. These treatments may not be suitable in your particular case, and tetracycline is unsuitable for use in pregnant women.

ACQUIRED IMMUNODEFICIENCY SYNDROME (AIDS) AND ITS CAUSE: HUMAN IMMUNODEFICIENCY VIRUS (HIV)

AIDS has attracted much publicity since its recognition in 1981 because it is still relatively new, it is serious, and it mainly affects young adults. The number of cases reported from countries the world over is rising rapidly. HIV infection is a worldwide problem and the risks to travelers depend more upon their own behavior than upon their choice of destination.

Dr. D. Peter Drotman has been a medical epidemiologist with the Centers for Disease Control and Prevention, Atlanta, since 1979. He has worked exclusively with AIDS since 1982.

Acquired immunodeficiency syndrome (AIDS) is the name given to a group of health problems first recognized in the United States in 1981. By mid-1993, more than 280,000 cases had been reported to the Centers for Disease Control and Prevention (CDC) from all over the United States. In 1981, the World Health Organization (WHO) received reports of AIDS cases from eight nations. By mid-1993, that figure had risen to 209 countries, 44 of which had reported more than 1,000 cases (Table 10.3).

Persons with AIDS have developed a specific defect in their natural immune (defense) system that has left them vulnerable to illnesses that would not otherwise be a threat. These illnesses are referred to as "opportunistic" diseases. The cause of the defect is an infection with a virus called human immunodeficiency virus (HIV). HIV preferentially infects certain cells of the immune system (T-helper lymphocytes, often referred to as CD4 cells) and destroys them. When a sufficient number has been destroyed, the characteristic immunodeficiency results.

WHO IS AT RISK?

Nearly all reported cases of AIDS occur in people who:

1. have had heterosexual intercourse with an infected man or woman;
2. have had sexual intercourse with gay or bisexual men;
3. have used intravenous (IV) drugs and have shared needles;
4. have been treated for hemophilia (or certain other severe bleeding disorders) with clotting factor concentrates;
5. have received transfusions of whole blood or its components (in countries where donations are not adequately screened);
6. were children born to mothers infected with HIV.

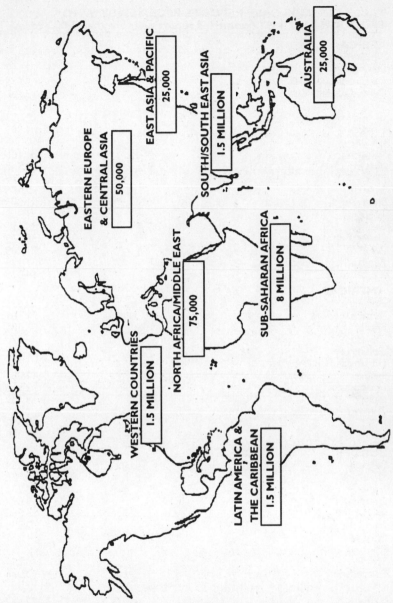

Map 10.1 Cumulative HIV infections, mid-1993, based on estimates by the WHO Global Program on AIDS.

**TABLE 10.3. AIDS CASE REPORTS RECEIVED BY WHO
THROUGH JULY 1993 (countries reporting more than 1,000 cases)**

AFRICA:

Burkina Faso	1,307
Burundi	7,131
Cameroon	2,174
Central African Republic	3,730
Congo	5,267
Côte d'Ivoire	14,655
Ethiopia	4,861
Ghana	10,285
Kenya	31,185
Malawi	26,955
Mali	1,479
Rwanda	9,486
South Africa	1,803
Togo	1,953
Uganda	34,611
United Rep. Tanzania	38,719
Zaire	21,008
Zambia	7,124
Zimbabwe	14,023

AMERICAS

Argentina	2,456
Bahamas	1,161
Brazil	36,481
Canada	7,770
Colombia	2,957
Dominican Republic	1,839
Haiti	3,086
Honduras	2,510
Mexico	13,259
Trinidad and Tobago	1,228
U.S.	289,320
Venezuela	2,342

EUROPE

Belgium	1,364
Denmark	1,182
France	24,226
Germany	9,697
Italy	16,860
Netherlands	2,575
Portugal	1,255
Romania	2,353
Spain	18,347
Switzerland	3,028
UK	7,341
Australia	3,697
Thailand	1,569

Worldwide, the largest portion of HIV infections is attributable to heterosexual intercourse. The age of those diagnosed with AIDS ranges primarily from 25 to 44 years. All races and ethnic groups have been affected.

In industrialized nations, HIV infections are more common among gay men and IV drug users. In nonindustrialized nations, infection also occurs in these populations, but tends to be more prevalent in heterosexuals with multiple sex partners, especially prostitutes employed in the sex industry.

In Africa, men and women are affected in about equal numbers, and transmission via heterosexual contact and unscreened blood transfusion seems most common, along with transmission to newborn babies from infected women during pregnancy. The precise magnitude of the AIDS problem in Africa is poorly documented, but accumulating evidence indicates it is substantial. WHO estimates that the cases that are officially reported represent only about 10 percent of the true number.

Although the number of AIDS cases reported from Asia has so far been small, sexual and needle-sharing transmission have both been documented. In Thailand in 1985, 2–3 percent of IV drug abusers were infected with HIV. By 1988, that figure had risen to 30 percent. A mainstay of the economy in several Southeast Asian countries is sexual tourism. Many prostitutes including the majority in some brothels are HIV infected. HIV appears to be increasing on the Indian subcontinent.

The problem in South America is growing rapidly. Brazil is second only to the United States in the number of reported cases in the Americas.

AIDS has been reported from Eastern Europe. One particularly striking outbreak has been investigated in Romania, where about 1,000 AIDS cases in children have been diagnosed. The children were infected with HIV through reuse of needles and syringes used to administer large numbers of injections of antibiotics and vitamins in state-run orphanages.

In summary, AIDS and HIV infection are global problems and are increasing. The World Health Organization estimated that more than 13 million adults worldwide were infected with HIV by mid-1993, of whom approximately 1 million were in North America. Sexual and drug-using behavior, rather than geography, determines the risk that most travelers face.

HOW IS HIV TRANSMITTED?

Epidemiologic and laboratory evidence clearly shows that HIV is transmitted from one person to another sexually (between gay men, heterosexually both from women to men and from men to women, and less commonly between lesbian women). It is also transmitted through exposure to blood or blood components; and before, during, and shortly after childbirth, when infected women may transmit the virus across the placenta to the fetus or to the infant at the time of birth and through breast-feeding. The most important behavioral risk factors for contracting HIV infection include having multiple sexual partners and sharing needles among drug users. In countries where disposable medical equipment is not available, reuse of needles, syringes, or other blood-contaminated items presents a potential route of transmission. Moreover, in many of these same countries, safe alternatives to breast-feeding may not be available, and this contributes further to the local problem.

HIV is not transmitted via casual contact. Several studies of the families and communities of AIDS patients, and of medical personnel involved in AIDS patient care, show no virus transmission via casual contact, household contact (including sharing kitchens, utensils, toilets, and baths), or other means such as mosquito bites. Animals, food, water, air, the environment, schools, the workplace, public areas, public transportation, coughing and sneezing, and swimming pools have not been associated with HIV transmission.

WHAT ILLNESSES MOST OFTEN AFFECT AIDS PATIENTS?

Various "opportunistic" diseases may affect patients with AIDS. Nearly two thirds of patients studied in North America have had at least one of two opportunistic diseases: a type of cancer known as Kaposi's sarcoma, and *Pneumocystis carinii* pneumonia, a parasitic infection of the lungs.

Other opportunistic infections in AIDS patients include unusually severe infections with mycobacteria (such as tuberculosis), candida (yeast), cytomegalovirus, herpes simplex virus, and toxoplasma. Milder infections with these organisms do not suggest immunodeficiency and are not considered opportunistic.

Kaposi's sarcoma The opportunistic diseases that characterize AIDS are not new. Kaposi's sarcoma was first described over 100 years ago. Before 1980 in Europe and North America, it primarily affected elderly men and was seldom fatal, even five or ten years after diagnosis. A more severe form was also seen in children and young adults in some parts of equatorial Africa and in a few other locations.

Kaposi's sarcoma usually occurs anywhere on the surface of the skin or in the mouth. In the early stages, it may look like a bruise or a blue-violet or brownish spot. The lesions grow larger and may ulcerate. It may arise in other organs, including lymph nodes, causing them to enlarge. Some AIDS patients with Kaposi's sarcoma have responded to treatment with interferon, an immune modulating drug.

Pneumocystis carinii pneumonia (PCP) affected a few hundred adults and children in the developed nations each year before its increase was noted in the United States in 1978–79. Until this time it usually occurred only in patients with a severe underlying illness (such as leukemia) or in patients receiving therapy with drugs known to suppress the immune system (such as those used to prevent rejection of kidney transplants). In fact, an increase in cases of PCP without such underlying predisposing factors was one of the earliest clues that the AIDS epidemic was beginning.

Pneumocystis carinii pneumonia has symptoms similar to those of other forms of severe pneumonia, especially fever, cough, and difficulty in breathing. Specific antibiotic treatments for this pneumonia include trimethoprim/sulfamethoxazole, pentamidine, and several experimental drugs, but the case-fatality rate is still high, and *Pneumocystis carinii* pneumonia remains the leading cause of death in AIDS patients in many countries. Patients whose T-helper lymphocyte count falls below 200 cells per microliter of blood should receive chemoprophylaxis with a regimen of trimethoprim 160 mg./sulfamethoxazole 800 mg. tablets twice daily or respiratory treatments with aerosolized pentamidine every four weeks. In the United States, additional information on treatments is available from the U.S. Public Health Service, National Institutes of Health ([800] 874-2572), or from the American Foundation for AIDS Research, which publishes the AIDS/HIV Treatment Directory. (Copies may be ordered from AmFAR, 733 Third Ave., 12th floor, New York, NY 10017-3204.)

HOW SERIOUS IS AIDS?

AIDS has a very high fatality rate, and no credible reports have been published of any patient with AIDS who has regained lost immunity. There is no cure for AIDS or HIV infection as yet, but experimental trials are under way with drugs that interrupt the replication of HIV. One such drug is zidovudine (often called AZT), which both prolongs the lives of AIDS patients and forestalls the onset of AIDS in HIV-infected persons with T-helper lymphocyte counts below 500 cells/microliter. It is now licensed in many countries. However, it is expensive, has toxic side effects, and must be taken indefinitely. One regimen recommended as of 1993 is 100 mg. five times a day (every four hours while awake). Other antiviral treatments are available with didanosine (DDI) being used as a backup for persons who no longer respond to or tolerate AZT. Eventually, more such drugs and zalcitabine (DDC) in various combinations and sequences will be used to extend therapeutic benefits, and to minimize toxicity and development of viral drug resistance.

SYMPTOMS AND DIAGNOSIS

Infection with HIV typically begins with a flu-like illness that resolves spontaneously. The infected person is then symptomless for up to 10 years or more. However, an infected person can transmit HIV to sex partners and needle-sharers during this long asymptomatic period. There are no clear-cut symptoms that indicate the loss of immunity, but many patients who have AIDS have experienced fever, loss of appetite and weight, extreme fatigue, and enlargement of lymph nodes. These symptoms, which often occur over a period of months, may be severe enough to result in hospitalization or disability. In parts of Africa (mainly East Africa), this condition is sometimes called "slim disease" because of the characteristic weight loss. When patients develop a severe wasting syndrome or any of the opportunistic diseases—such as Kaposi's sarcoma, *Pneumocystis carinii* pneumonia, or cryptococcal meningitis—or have T-helper cell counts that fall below 200 cells/microliter, they are then classified as having AIDS.

HIV can infect the central nervous system directly and produce various disorders including dementia, encephalopathy, sensory-motor deficits, and other problems. This central nervous system involvement also prompts an AIDS diagnosis.

TESTS FOR HIV INFECTION AND AIDS

Tests to detect antibodies to the virus that causes AIDS became available in 1985. This test does not indicate the presence of the virus directly, but a repeatedly reactive and confirmed antibody test provides evidence of infection. This test is used to screen donors of organs, blood, plasma, and other tissues for transfusion, transplantation, or manufacture of clotting-factor concentrates for people with hemophilia and of other blood products. It is used to diagnose HIV infection and to assist in prevention-oriented counseling of sexually active men and women at risk of HIV infection, women contemplating pregnancy, intravenous drug abusers, and others.

Some countries require HIV-antibody testing before granting certain classes of visas (usually longer-term immigrant, resident, work, or student visas). However, the World Health Organization does not endorse or approve of this practice. Travelers should check with appropriate consular authorities to determine testing requirements of nations on their itinerary.

No single specific test is available for diagnosing AIDS. The basic pathology of AIDS is that the number and function of certain white blood cells decrease. Although this decrease can be measured (e.g., by T-helper lymphocyte count), these tests are not generally available outside industrialized nations, nor are they perfectly sensitive and specific. They can be expensive, and are usually done in central laboratories or major research centers. However, the technology and expertise to provide accurate T-helper cell counts are diffusing more widely. Other tests may also help the physician to establish the diagnosis of AIDS and its opportunistic diseases.

SPECIAL ADVICE FOR HIV-INFECTED TRAVELERS

HIV-infected persons, as well as other immunodeficient persons and those taking immunosuppressive medicines or radiation treatments, should consult a physician well in advance of undertaking any long, distant, or arduous journey. Because they may develop opportunistic diseases or more severe manifestations of many other illnesses, such persons should adhere strictly to the advice in this book as well as the advice of their personal physician. In general, such persons should not receive live viral (e.g., oral polio) or bacterial (e.g., BCG) vaccines (see Table 13.3, p. 513). An important exception to this axiom is that HIV-infected children should receive live measles vaccine, alone or in combination with mumps and rubella vaccines, because measles is common, especially in developing countries, and it is particularly severe or even fatal in HIV-infected children or adults.

Before traveling, HIV-infected children should have received the "usual" childhood vaccines against diphtheria, pertussis (whooping cough), and tetanus on schedule, but they and their household should receive the injectable inactivated polio vaccine instead of the live oral vaccine.

Pneumococcal vaccine is recommended for any HIV-infected person over the age of two years (one injection only). Annual influenza vaccinations are recommended for symptomatic HIV-infected children and all HIV-infected adults.

Yellow fever vaccination poses a dilemma for HIV-infected or otherwise immunosuppressed persons. In theory, the live yellow fever vaccine virus presents a risk of encephalitis. However, no data or cases support this theory. The decision to immunize should be weighed against several factors, including the necessity for such persons to travel to yellow fever–infected zones, their likelihood of being exposed to the virus, and degree of adherence to mosquito-avoidance measures. Asymptomatic HIV-infected persons who are unable to avoid exposure to yellow fever virus should be offered immunization and monitored for adverse effects. The physician should consider measuring the neutralizing antibody to the vaccine because it may be less than sufficient to provide protection.

HIV-infected persons should not receive the BCG vaccine but should take precautions to avoid exposure to tuberculosis because they are at special risk for infection and serious complications, including death. Such precautions should include being monitored for TB infection with skin tests and chest X-rays and strictly following infection-control measures in health-care settings (e.g., hand-washing and wearing masks, gloves, and gowns when indicated). No one should consume milk that is not pasteurized, boiled, or cooked, including milk used to make ice cream, cheese, yogurt, or other products. In many developing countries, milk remains a vehicle for transmission of TB as well as many other microorganisms.

SUMMARY OF ADVICE FOR TRAVELERS

- Travelers are normally at no special risk for HIV infection or AIDS unless they engage in sexual or drug-taking behavior that puts them in contact with people who might be infected with HIV.

- Gay men and sexually active heterosexual men and women should take particular note of the recommendations listed above. Engaging only in safer sexual practices, in particular using condoms for all sexual intercourse (vaginal, anal, or oral), can reduce the risk of infection with HIV and other sexually transmitted organisms.

- Intravenous drug abusers risk multiple health problems outside the scope of this chapter. Suffice it to note that needle-sharing is very dangerous.

- When living or traveling in countries where reuse of medical equipment is common, it is important to make sure that medical staff who look after you are trained in and practice good infection-control techniques, such as sterilizing needles, syringes, and surgical equipment before reuse. Blood transfusion abroad is discussed further on pp. 534–36.

- Unless you are certain that new or sterile equipment is being used, skin piercing, such as tattooing, ear piercing, acupuncture, or electrolysis should always be avoided.

- An epidemic of HIV infection precedes an epidemic of AIDS by several years. HIV infection is usually not clinically obvious; travelers should not assume that AIDS is an insignificant risk in countries that may have reported only a small number of cases, and should always take appropriate precautions.

PREVENTION

Many public health services have adopted the following recommendations for prevention of HIV infection:

- For maximum safety, establish a mutually monogamous sexual relationship with a noninfected person.

- Use condoms for all other sexual relationships. Condoms reduce, but do not eliminate, risk of HIV transmission.

- Do not have sexual intercourse with people who have or might be suspected of having AIDS or HIV infection.

- Do not use needles to inject drugs, or have sexual intercourse with people who use them.

- Be aware that having multiple sexual partners increases the chance of contracting AIDS or HIV infection.

- Do not donate blood or plasma or organs for transplantation if your behavior puts you at risk of HIV infection.

- Blood transfusions (see p. 534–36) should be given only when medically essential and should be screened.

- Use extreme care when handling hypodermic needles. Do not recap, bend, or clip needles. Dispose of them into impervious containers.

- Advice for travelers is summarized on p. 429.

CONTRACEPTION AND TRAVEL

Contraception is a neglected aspect of health care for travelers, but can make all the difference between an enjoyable trip and a miserable one. Not all methods of contraception are equally problem-free in travelers, and an appropriate method should be chosen carefully before departure.

Dr. Elphis Christopher *has been involved with contraception for over 25 years. She lectures to medical students and has made numerous radio and TV appearances to discuss sex education, birth control, and related topics.*

Glossy brochures use covert promises of sexual adventure to sell travel. Away from everyday stresses and routines, and far from the influence of anyone who might disapprove, vacations and travel bring relaxation of inhibitions, a sense of freedom, and are undoubtedly a time of increased sexual activity both for couples and for men and women traveling on their own.

Too many travelers leave home unprepared. Single people—particularly women, who are most at risk from the consequences—may be unwilling to anticipate a sexual adventure on vacation, on the grounds that "I am not that kind of girl"; they may find it difficult to believe that pregnancy might begin on a vacation, or that contraceptive precautions may be necessary in advance of a romantic attachment. Others, men and women, simply don't bother.

Avoiding an unwanted pregnancy, an unintended souvenir of an otherwise enjoyable vacation, is not merely a question of chance;

traveling prepared must not be confused with promiscuity, and it is always better to be safe than sorry.

If you are sexually active and settled on a particular contraceptive method, all you may need to do is visit your own physician or family planning clinic for a checkup and obtain any contraceptive supplies you will need while away—and also confirm that the method you are using is appropriate for the length and nature of your trip. For prolonged stays abroad it is worth finding out what is available in the country or countries you intend to visit before you leave: the International Planned Parenthood Federation (IPPF) can provide information on this.*

Traveling may reduce the effectiveness of contraceptive precautions which are otherwise perfectly adequate at home, and the specific problems that arise for each method are discussed below. Normally these problems are not serious enough to warrant changing from your established method, but you should be aware of them, and perhaps travel prepared to switch to an alternative method in an emergency.

Once you have decided upon a method, or if you plan to switch to a new method, it is worth getting used to it well in advance of your trip, to enable any side effects or problems to reveal themselves in time to be sorted out. This is a particularly important consideration with the Pill—nausea and tiredness and slight spotting (breakthrough bleeding) are common when taking it for the first time, but usually settle by the third packet—and with the intrauterine device (IUD).

The various methods available are discussed below along with their advantages and disadvantages, although travelers may well need to consult their physician or clinic in order to make the most suitable choice for their own circumstances.

It may be advisable to travel with *two* methods to ensure against failure of one of these methods.

THE COMBINED ORAL CONTRACEPTIVE: "THE PILL"

The Pill is a popular method of contraception, familiar and convenient to use; with correct use its reliability is 99–100 percent. If you

---

* IPPF, 105 Madison Avenue, New York, NY 10016. Tel. (212) 679-2230.

are on the Pill be sure to travel with an adequate supply, because further supplies of your particular brand may not necessarily be easy to obtain—especially in remote areas. Make allowances for delays and any unexpected extension of your trip.

If you run out, keep an empty pack so that a doctor or a pharmacist can identify your brand—brand names of the same variety of the Pill usually differ from country to country. Thus a widely prescribed variety like Levlen occurs under no fewer than 20 other brand names around the world. If exactly the same Pill cannot be obtained and a different one is prescribed, do not leave a seven-day gap between packets, but go straight on to the new Pill regardless of any bleeding. Other contraceptive precautions will not then be necessary.

Stomach problems and diarrhea affect most travelers at some time or another. *Stomach problems and severe diarrhea reduce absorption of the Pill, and may leave the traveler without protection.* All travelers on the Pill should be aware of this, and should be prepared to use an alternative method when necessary.

A barrier method (see below) should be used to protect intercourse over the duration of the stomach problem and for seven days after it has ended. If vomiting occurs within three hours of taking a pill, an additional pill should be taken. If vomiting continues, another method of contraception will have to be used.

Antibiotics such as tetracycline or ampicillin also reduce the absorption and effectiveness of the Pill, and another method of contraception should be used during a course of antibiotics and for seven days afterward. Antifungal medication, such as griseofulvin, and antiepilepsy drugs may also reduce the effectiveness of the Pill. Additional precautions are needed when these are being taken.

In both instances, if the seven days coincide with the seven Pill-free days, do not take a break of seven days but carry straight on with another packet of pills. Do not worry if there is no withdrawal bleeding.

Time zones cause another potential hazard to travelers on the Pill. When time zones are crossed, make sure that you take a pill every 24 hours, and continue to do so every day at the same time. If that means having to wake up in the middle of the night to take a pill, take it *earlier* before going to sleep rather than later; no more than 24 hours should elapse between doses—particularly with newer varieties of the low-dose Pill—both for protection against pregnancy and to prevent breakthrough bleeding or spotting.

Flight attendants who are continually traveling may find it useful to have two wristwatches, and to keep one of them on "home time" for this purpose.

Travel can interfere with periods even when a woman is on the Pill; so a missed period does not necessarily mean that she is pregnant (pp. 392–93)—provided of course that the daily doses have been taken regularly. Women who prefer not to have periods at all while traveling can take the Pill continuously, without a seven-day break in between packets; *but remember to take extra packets to allow for this.* This is not advisable with the biphasic or triphasic Pills because the dose in the first seven pills is too low to prevent possible breakthrough bleeding; triphasic brands are probably best avoided for long journeys that cross time zones, since the margin of error is less with this type and the risk of pregnancy increases if they are not taken regularly.

High altitude, dehydration, and extreme cold stress are all associated with changes in blood viscosity. Although as yet there is no clear evidence of an increased thrombosis risk among women taking the Pill at high altitude, it would seem wise not to do so.

THE PROGESTOGEN-ONLY PILL (POP)

The progestogen-only Pill, or POP, is sometimes used by women who cannot take the combined Pill, although the same considerations apply. It is *not* 100 percent effective (about 96–98 percent) and it *must* be taken at a fixed time each day, one every 24 hours in order to remain effective. If a pill is forgotten, take one as soon as it is remembered, but use an additional method for seven days. Antibiotics do not affect the progestogen-only Pill.

THE INTRAUTERINE DEVICE (IUD)

Women who already have an IUD should have it checked before going abroad. If it is a copper-bearing device such as a ParaGard T, make sure that it is not due for a change. All-plastic devices such as the Lippes Loop can remain in the uterus for many years provided that there are no problems.

The IUD is about 97–99 percent effective. It has the advantage that it is not affected by stomach upsets or time zones. It can, however, be expelled by the uterus, so it is a sensible precaution to check after each period that the threads can still be felt. If a "hard bit" (part of the IUD itself) can be felt as well as the threads, the IUD may be coming out and will need to be checked by a physician or nurse. An examination is not necessary once the IUD has come out; obviously protection ceases immediately, and another method must be used.

The IUD is not suitable for women with heavy or prolonged periods—it may make these worse. A newly fitted IUD may also cause irregular and sometimes heavy bleeding in the first couple of months—hardly ideal if you are just off on a beach vacation in a new bikini! Heavy or continuous bleeding may make you feel tired and ruin your vacation. It is therefore a good idea to have the IUD fitted well in advance, so that any problems can be sorted out before you travel. Modern studies show conclusively that where a woman is in a mutually faithful sexual relationship infection is not a problem with IUD use. Although an IUD may exacerbate a sexually transmitted disease (see p. 413) it is not the IUD that increases the risks but the woman or her partner, and their sexual practices. The IUD is most suitable for older women who have had children, since side effects such as heavy, painful periods are less common, and there is less chance of the IUD being expelled.

BARRIER METHODS

THE CONDOM
The condom is about 85–98 percent effective when used correctly. It provides some protection against sexually transmitted disease, including HIV (see pp. 429–30), and is particularly useful for the man or woman traveling alone. It can be put on as part of love play.

It is also valuable for women or couples who want to take along a reliable alternative, in case of problems with the Pill, or in case the IUD is expelled. The condom is a good method for the chance sexual encounter, and travels well.

THE DIAPHRAGM AND CERVICAL CAP
The diaphragm, covering the cervix and front wall of the vagina, and the cervical cap, covering the cervix, are useful methods

with about the same effectiveness as the condom. They need to be fitted by a physician or nurse, and the woman must be taught how to use them correctly. A diaphragm or cap lasts for about six months to one year, so on a long trip it may be advisable to take along a spare.

They must be used with a spermicide. These come in the form of creams, gels, foams, vaginal suppositories, or film. Creams may become more messy in hot climates but do not lose their effectiveness. Foams in aerosol containers can be a useful alternative. In addition, vaginal suppositories should be inserted if a second act of intercourse takes place soon after the first. They are designed to melt at body temperature, and this can be an obvious problem in hot countries; brands wrapped individually with silver foil travel best, and should be kept in a cool place.

Foaming tablets also travel well, although if conditions are humid the lid of their container should always be firmly closed: moisture will make the tablets dissolve. The diaphragm and cap provide some protection from sexually transmitted diseases (see p. 412).

THE CONTRACEPTIVE SPONGE

This is an attractive-sounding method that is convenient and easy to use. Unfortunately it is not very effective, but it is certainly better than using nothing.

The sponge, which is impregnated with spermicide, is inserted into the vagina and fits over the cervix. It provides protection for up to 24 hours, and during this time, intercourse may be repeated without need for further measures. Like the diaphragm and cap, the contraceptive vaginal sponge can be left in place for up to 30 hours. This allows for 24 hours of use and the six hours after intercourse guideline.

It does not require a doctor's prescription, and is sold at most pharmacies (in packets of three). It is relatively expensive. It should be disposed of carefully after use.

It is 20 times *less* effective than the Pill; it is most suitable for women over 45 in whom the risk of pregnancy is in any case small, or for women who do not particularly mind when their next pregnancy occurs. A recent study confirms that use of a spermicide-impregnated sponge provides no measurable protection against HIV.

INJECTABLE CONTRACEPTIVES

Injectable contraceptives (Depo-Provera and Noristerat) are virtually 100 percent effective and work in a similar way to the progestogen-only pill.

Depo-Provera is given by injection into the muscle of the buttock or upper arm and remains effective for three months. It is useful for women going on long trips, and crossing time zones frequently. It is not affected by stomach upsets or antibiotics. Side effects often occur, such as irregular and occasionally heavy bleeding, especially with the first injection. With subsequent injections, the periods may stop altogether. This is how the injection *should* work, which makes it an ideal method for the woman who does not want regular periods. If Depo-Provera is chosen, the woman needs to be settled on it before she travels.

A second injectable contraceptive, Noristerat, has similar properties (and side effects) to Depo-Provera and is equally effective. Noristerat is also available in many countries, including some where Depo-Provera is unavailable.

Norplant is a long-acting (up to five years) hormonal method for women. It works rather like the oral contraceptive Pill, preventing ovulation and thickening cervical mucus. Six flexible silastic capsules, each 1.3 inches long, are inserted under the skin in the upper arm, under local anesthesia. The procedure takes 10–15 minutes. It provides a high level of protection against pregnancy (98–99 percent). Its main side effect is irregular vaginal bleeding, which is occasionally prolonged.

A NEW METHOD

FEMALE CONDOM

This is a condom that is put inside the vagina and the area just outside the vagina. There are two soft plastic rings, an inner one to help retain the condom in the vagina, and an outer one to keep its opening in place outside the vagina. It is used once only, and is sold under the brand name *Reality*. When used correctly, its effectiveness in preventing pregnancy and protecting against sexually transmitted diseases (including HIV) is probably about the same as a male condom; however, some people find it difficult to use.

USING CONTRACEPTION FOR THE FIRST TIME

The Pill is probably the most sensible method for a couple going on honeymoon, who have not had sex before and who do not want a pregnancy straightaway. Although honeymoons are often pictured to be idyllic and carefree, in reality they can be a time of great anxiety and stress, with both partners worrying whether sex will be all right.

Sexual adjustment to each other may take time, and methods that directly interfere with intercourse—such as the condom or diaphragm—may interrupt love play and can make that adjustment more complicated. If you choose the Pill, begin taking it a few months in advance, so that any problems can be dealt with before you leave.

EMERGENCY OR POSTCOITAL CONTRACEPTION: PCC

This method of birth control may be used in an emergency. It works by preventing implantation of the fertilized egg in the uterus. It is preferable to abortion but should not be used on a regular basis. It is useful on those occasions when a contraceptive method fails (e.g., a condom splitting), or for the woman who has had unprotected intercourse.

Two tablets of the combined Pill Lo-Ovral (levonorgestrel 250 μg. ethinyloestradiol 50 μg.) must be taken within 72 hours of an unprotected act of sexual intercourse and then another two tablets 12 hours later. The tablets often cause nausea, and if vomiting occurs within three hours of the tablets another two tablets should be taken. The next period may arrive slightly earlier or later than expected but usually within three weeks of prescribing PCC.

Postcoital contraception can be obtained from contraceptive clinics or your own physician or gynecologist. Ideally a follow-up visit should be arranged after receiving PCC.

ABORTION

Travelers who become pregnant abroad and want an abortion may find this difficult to arrange. At the last count 60 out of 128 countries listed by the IPPF prohibit abortion except in extreme circum-

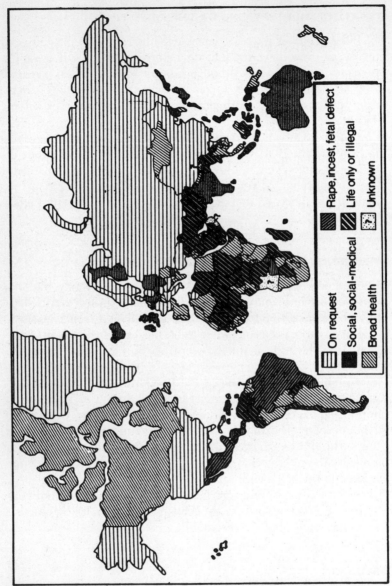

Map 10.2 Abortion: legal status in different countries. (From *Induced abortion, a world review*, C. Tieze and S. K. Hensaw, The Alan Guttmacher Institute, New York, 1986. Reproduced by permission.)

stances—rape, or life-threatening illness. Skilled medical care may be very expensive, or almost impossible to obtain. Map 10.2 (opposite) gives an indication of the legal position in most countries; further information can be obtained from the IPPF, which also publishes a list of family planning offices in different countries.

RU 486 (MIFEPRISTONE, MIFEGYNE): THE ABORTION PILL

RU 486 is a synthetic steroid that counteracts the hormone progesterone. Progesterone is produced naturally in the body and is essential to maintain a pregnancy. By blocking the action of progesterone, RU 486 induces a miscarriage. It is more effective when used with another drug, prostaglandin. RU 486 is given as a single dose (three 200-mg. tablets) by mouth, and a suppository of prostaglandin is inserted into the vagina 48 hours later. The abortion or miscarriage happens spontaneously about six hours later. This treatment can be given to women who are up to nine weeks pregnant and is effective in 95 percent of cases. Side effects include period pains and prolonged bleeding. Less than 10 percent of women have severe pain lasting about an hour. This responds to a strong painkiller. It has no adverse effects on future fertility. It is licensed for use under medical supervision in France and Britain. It has been approved though not as yet introduced for use in China.

‖‖ TRAVELERS WITH
SPECIAL NEEDS

TRAVEL IN PREGNANCY

No woman can be realistically assured in advance that her pregnancy will be trouble-free, and for travel, some extra precautions are necessary.

Professor Herbert A. Brant is Professor of Clinical Obstetrics and Gynecology at University College Hospital, London.

Dr. John Naponick is a public health physician with specialist training in gynecology, obstetrics, and tropical medicine. He has worked in the USA, Canada, Cameroon, Bangladesh, Thailand, Burma, and El Salvador. He currently works in Bangladesh.

Increasingly, we take travel for granted, but its implications for women who are pregnant or may become pregnant while traveling are worth a little thought. Large numbers of women do travel in pregnancy, and they sometimes travel long distances; most have no real problems, but an unlucky few regret having ventured forth. The widely varying standard of medical care and its availability in different countries is more important than the direct effects of travel on pregnancy. But at least being aware of the problems may help you to minimize their effects.

POSSIBLE PROBLEMS

Why should pregnant women be more concerned about travel? The likelihood of a problem needing medical attention arising is greater during pregnancy. On statistical grounds alone, women should hesitate before traveling to any area where medical services will be of doubtful quality or where misunderstandings due to language or cultural problems are going to make communication and therefore diagnosis and treatment more difficult.

No woman can be realistically assured in advance that she will have a trouble-free pregnancy. Although it is not always a popular concept, it is worth remembering that pregnancy is normal only when viewed in retrospect—that is, *after* no problems have occurred.

PRENATAL CARE AND TESTS IN EARLY PREGNANCY

Don't miss out on prenatal care and important tests that should be completed in the first half of pregnancy—postpone your trip if necessary. Serious blood conditions of the fetus such as thalassemia (in those of Mediterranean or Asian origin) or sickle cell anemia (in those of African origin) can be detected early in pregnancy—in time for a pregnancy to be terminated if the fetus is affected. The blood test for spina bifida (AFP) is carried out at 16–18 weeks, and amniocentesis for Down's syndrome in older women at about 16 weeks. Sonography is usually performed during the first 24 weeks (usually at 18 weeks) to confirm the age of the fetus in case of problems later in pregnancy, and also to detect abnormalities that might have arisen during development of fetal organs.

MISCARRIAGE

Spontaneous abortion (miscarriage) is the commonest problem of early pregnancy. It usually occurs during the first three months. If it merely threatens, as evidenced by vaginal bleeding, the eventual outcome will *not* be altered because the woman travels.

Miscarriages in the early months are due to the inevitable errors of a biological system—errors in cell division during the early stages of development of the fetus or the placenta, and errors concerned with the attachment of the placenta to the wall of the uterus. Travel won't cause miscarriage other than *indirectly*, such as through the effect of a high fever associated with infection, or severe dehydration associated with diarrhea.

Of more pressing concern are the immediate complications of miscarriage, which include the occasional life-threatening hemorrhage, the occasional serious infection, or the problems of inept medical treatment employed to cope with them.

Miscarriage, although uncommon at a later stage of pregnancy, can occur at any time, though once the fetus is able to survive, it is termed premature labor; the above complications are more common with later miscarriages. Any pregnant woman who has had a previous late miscarriage, or has any condition predisposing to miscarriage, is ill-advised to travel in mid-pregnancy.

ECTOPIC PREGNANCY

This may be a problem in the first few months of pregnancy, and affects 1 pregnancy in 200. The fetus grows in the fallopian tube instead of in the uterus, and this can lead to life-threatening hemorrhage. If abdominal pain occurs in pregnancy, always consult a physician.

PREMATURE LABOR

If labor starts early but at a time when the resulting baby could live (any time after 24 weeks) then the whole future of the baby can depend on the availability of expert care. Without this, the baby is likely to be seriously mentally or physically handicapped for life— if he or she survives. If expert care is available it can be extremely expensive, especially if prolonged intensive care is necessary. Where good obstetric care is available, treatment can sometimes be given to stop or delay premature labor.

OTHER COMPLICATIONS

In late pregnancy, other possible problems are hemorrhage from a normally situated placenta or from a placenta growing near the cervix (placenta previa); pregnancy-induced hypertension (previously called toxemia of pregnancy); and premature rupture of the membranes. Such complications threaten both mother and fetus, and ready availability of expert care reduces the risks.

Many of the complications that occur in pregnancy may result in hemorrhage and the need for a blood transfusion, and some of the risks associated with this are discussed on pp. 534–36.

BEFORE YOU GO

Women who are pregnant or are contemplating pregnancy should find out as much as possible about medical services at their destination before traveling to foreign parts or deciding to become pregnant during a prolonged stay abroad.

LIVING OVERSEAS

If you are planning to live overseas, you should ensure that you will have access to good-quality prenatal advice and care, and also that your social and emotional environment will provide you with the support you may need.

INSURANCE

Be sure to check that any travel or sickness insurance covers medical care for the consequences of pregnancy; such additional cover will usually need to be arranged separately (p. 495).

IMMUNIZATION

Vaccinations that involve a live virus or are likely to lead to a high temperature should be avoided during pregnancy. A medical certificate can circumvent the vaccination requirements for travel.

Poliomyelitis, measles, rubella, and yellow fever vaccines all involve live viruses. Vaccination against rubella and poliomyelitis should have been carried out *before* pregnancy. Diphtheria and typhoid vaccines may cause fever and should be avoided. BCG (given in some countries against tuberculosis) can affect the fetus, and should therefore also not be given. (See also p. 512.)

ANTIMALARIAL TABLETS

If you are pregnant and are traveling to an area where there is a risk of contracting malaria, it is strongly advisable to take the appropriate medication to prevent infection (p. 128). In some areas malaria is resistant to certain drugs, so seek expert advice on what to take for the area you intend to visit. Chloroquine (Aralen, Avloclor, Nivaquine) and proguanil (Paludrine) are generally agreed to be quite safe in pregnancy. Experience with mefloquine (Lariam) is limited; the balance between benefit and possible risk depends on the exact nature of your trip and circumstances, and expert advice should be obtained, such as from one of the sources listed in Appendix 8.

TRAVEL

AIR

Provided that the cabin is pressurized, reduced pressure on board an airliner (pp. 227–28) should have no adverse effect upon healthy women with a normal pregnancy. If a significant problem with the function of the placenta is suspected, however, air travel should be avoided because the slightly reduced oxygen level may harm the fetus.

Many airlines will not accept you for travel after 32 weeks of pregnancy, but will sometimes stretch this to 36 weeks if you can produce a medical certificate stating that all is well. Policy varies between airlines and also depends on the length of the flight. It is obviously difficult to obtain medical assistance in the air if labor begins unexpectedly.

Pregnant women and those in the first month after delivery have a small but definitely increased risk of developing blood clots in the deep veins of the legs (deep-vein thrombosis). These clots occasionally travel to the lungs via the bloodstream and can prove fatal. When traveling by air, do not sit in a cramped position for a long period, because pressure from the seat and from the fetus slows the circulation in the legs (see pp. 233–35). Tense up the legs and wriggle the toes from time to time; and stand up and walk about at least every hour.

OTHER FORMS OF TRAVEL

Sitting in a cramped position in a car, bus, or train has the same effect of impairing blood circulation in the legs. Stand up and walk about every hour or so; if you are traveling by road, stop the car every hour, get out and take a walk.

Exposure to cosmic radiation at normal flying altitudes (35,000 feet) is more than 100 times greater than at ground level. There has been increasing concern about the effects of low-dose radiation, and it is certainly possible for frequent fliers to build up a significant radiation exposure. Solar flares—bursts of energy on the surface of the sun—account for periodic increases in such exposure, and occur in unpredictable patterns. The radiation exposure for a return trip between London and New York is roughly equivalent to the exposure from a single chest X-ray (0.1 millisievert); a return flight between London and Los Angeles would clock up 0.16 mSv. Because Concorde flies at higher altitudes, radiation exposure might be expected to be higher; this is balanced by the shorter flying time, and overall exposure is generally reduced.

Calculations on the extent of harm associated with radiation exposure are generally based on the effects of much larger doses—such as at Hiroshima. It is difficult to know how such data extrapolate to lower doses, and it is conceivable that low doses may be relatively more harmful. It is also difficult to document the effects, and to know whether subtle changes such as differences in intelligence or minor defects can be attributed to such exposure rather than nature. For this reason it has been suggested that pregnant women should avoid unnecessary long-distance flights during the early, most vulnerable stages of pregnancy.*

R.D.

During pregnancy, women should drive with more care and more slowly, as pregnancy sometimes affects concentration and reaction time in an emergency. Pregnant women should wear seat belts, because in a crash injuries are more serious without them.

NAUSEA AND VOMITING

The tendency to nausea and vomiting in early pregnancy is likely to be aggravated by travel. All travel sickness tablets cause some unwanted effects, such as drowsiness, altered reaction time, dry mouth, and blurred vision, and so should be used only when symptoms warrant (and not at all when driving). Antihistamine preparations such as promethazine (Phenergan) and dimenhydrinate (Dramamine), and drugs based on scopolamine (e.g., Transderm-Scop) are safe for use in pregnancy.

* If you want further information about in-flight radiation, contact High Altitude Radiation Monitoring Service, Inc., P.O. Box 4204, Stamford, CT 06907, Tel. (203) 325-9299.

AT YOUR DESTINATION

FOOD AND DRINK

Dehydration Try to avoid dehydration during air travel or in a hot climate—this aggravates the tendency to thrombosis and also the problem of constipation, which is common in pregnancy. Drink plenty of fluids—preferably in the form of plain water—bottled or boiled if the local supply isn't safe (see pp. 71–77). *Severe* dehydration—such as may follow prolonged diarrhea—increases the risk of miscarriage.

Fiber Take an extra supply of natural bran and increase your intake of fruit and vegetables to counteract the constipation which often goes with changed daily routines and possibly a more refined diet than you are used to at home.

Toxoplasmosis *Don't eat* undercooked meat—the condition toxoplasmosis may result. It causes only mild illness in adults but occasionally has serious effects on the fetus. You could be checked to see whether you are immune, but it is a difficult test, not generally available.

Listeriosis This infection is acquired from contaminated food—particularly poultry which is either fresh or frozen and then *incompletely* cooked. It also occurs in cows' and goats' milk and is not always eliminated by pasteurization. Soft, ripened cheeses often contain the bacteria in high numbers and already prepared salads are not safe, as the bacteria can survive in the refrigerator. All these points should be borne in mind by the pregnant traveler, as the infection has little effect on most healthy adults but can cause serious effects in the fetus. If a flu-like illness develops in pregnancy, then it is probably wise to have antibiotic treatment (such as amoxycillin), just in case.

ALCOHOL, SMOKING, AND DRUGS

Avoid alcohol, not only because of its dehydrating properties but also for its possible harmful effects on the fetus. Smoking, and addictive and recreational drugs also have an extremely detrimental effect during pregnancy. In particular, "crack" cocaine causes serious brain abnormalities in the fetus.

MEDICATION ABROAD

Prescribing habits vary considerably from country to country, and awareness of potential hazards from drug treatment in pregnancy is far from universal; it is safest to avoid medicines altogether if you can, other than iron supplements and vitamins. One group of drugs that may possibly be prescribed for you, but which should be avoided in pregnancy, are the tetracycline group of antibiotics. Other drugs to avoid include bismuth subsalicylate (Pepto-Bismol); metronidazole (Flagyl), which should not be taken during the first trimester unless absolutely necessary; and the fluoroquinolone antibiotics (e.g., ciprofloxacin and norfloxacin). Amoxycillin and ampicillin are safe.

SUMMARY OF ADVICE FOR TRAVELERS

- You will probably have gathered that we are rather against traveling to remote spots at any time in pregnancy, but if a time for a break has to be selected, between 18 and 24 weeks is probably the best. This is after the risk of nausea and miscarriage—and after the necessary tests should have been completed—but before the problems of premature labor loom. You should be back at base for late pregnancy, just in case!

CHILDREN ABROAD

Problems of traveling with children vary according to where you intend to go, how you will be getting there, and how long you will be away. Whether you are moving abroad to live or are merely off on a short trip, careful preparation will be amply rewarded.

Dr. Tony Waterston *is a pediatrician who has worked for several years as a doctor and teacher in Zambia and Zimbabwe and has spent shorter periods in several other parts of Africa. His wife (a physician too) and three children have also contributed to this chapter.*

Dr. Bonita Stanton *is a pediatrician who lived with her family for five years in Bangladesh. She is now Professor of Pediatrics at the University of Maryland in Baltimore.*

Parents traveling abroad appropriately feel many apprehensions regarding their children. Some are concerned with the journey itself, and others with what will happen at the destination. Will the change of environment be good for the children or bad? Will the food be suitable? Will it be safe for them to play outside? What dreadful diseases will they get? How will the baby take the heat?

Fortunately, the reality of traveling with children is usually much better than might be expected and is generally a formative and valuable experience for the whole family. This chapter is designed to answer some of the most common questions about children's health abroad and to help you prepare for your trip, whether you are just going on a short beach vacation or on a long-term posting to some faraway destination in a developing country.

The chapter is divided into three parts. First, what preparations to make, and the journey itself; second, the main health hazards encountered while living abroad; and third, some points about children's diet and baby care.

BEFORE YOU GO

The time spent finding out as much as you can about the country you plan to visit will be amply repaid. The longer you intend to stay away, the more preparation will be needed, and you should try to find out all you can (from friends, employees, or through your embassy) about the following:

THE LOCAL HEALTH SYSTEM

Is insurance necessary (see pp. 492–97)? If it is, will all your family be automatically included and will the cost of return travel home be paid in case of major illness? What are the facilities available for treating sick children? Is emergency medical evacuation covered (i.e., airlift to another country if suitable facilities are not available locally)? Wherever you are, your child may get appendicitis, a fracture, or a severe infection and need specialized care. This care might be available only at a major center and could be a factor in deciding where you are to live.

Can medicines be obtained easily? You will quite likely need antimalarials and antibiotics. A small supply of over-the-counter remedies will come in useful for minor illnesses and should be bought in advance. If you have a baby and are going for more than a few weeks, find out where and how routine immunizations can be carried out (see below for schedule). There should not be any difficulty in obtaining immunization in any country you visit, but you should confirm this in advance. Also, it will be important to find out if you will have access to U.S.-manufactured vaccines. If not, find out from your doctor whether local quality-control standards for vaccines are known to be reasonable. Your doctor can obtain this information from the Centers for Disease Control and Prevention.

In many developing countries, the emphasis in the medical system will be on *primary health care*. This means basic care concentrating on common ailments and on prevention, delivered by workers with a short training. Do not therefore be surprised if you do not see a doctor at a clinic—the health worker you see should be trained to recognize and treat the common childhood complaints.

Be sure to avoid all treatment by injection unless it is absolutely essential, and unless you are certain that the needle has been sterilized (see p. 533). Many people now travel with a small supply of sterile, disposable needles.

DENTAL CARE
Dental care abroad is often expensive or nonexistent. Sanitary conditions are often uncertain. The whole family should have a dental check and receive essential treatment before going (see p. 373).

THE MAIN DISEASES
In Europe and Australia, the diseases are very similar to those encountered in North America, whereas the developing countries of Africa, Asia, and South America share a wide spectrum of infectious diseases that are discussed elsewhere in this book.

Find out what the main problems are in the country you intend to visit and what specific precautions you should take (for example, in many countries throughout Asia and Africa most malaria is now resistant to chloroquine). Do not feel that it would be unsafe to take children to a country where tropical diseases such as malaria and bilharzia are common: simple precautions will protect against these diseases, and it is often more trivial complaints such as cuts, bites, and diarrhea and respiratory infections that become important when you are there. These problems are dealt with below, but you would be wise also to take with you one of the many child-care books which deal with the management of minor illnesses at home.

WATER AND FOOD

Find out whether the local water supply is drinkable—if not, you should pay careful attention to the information in this book about water purification (pp. 71–77). Clean water is essential for young children, as stomach upsets are the commonest disorders encountered. It always pays to be careful about water quality when traveling—even bottled carbonated drinks are not necessarily always safe. It may be wise to stick to tea when in doubt.

What are the major local foods? If they are not of a kind you feel up to preparing (such as maize meal, sweet potato, plantain, yam) you will need to depend on imported foods. Is there always a constant supply of these?

Foreign exchange is scarce in many countries, and infant specialty foods or even wheat may not be at the top of the list of priorities. Can you bake bread? Some basic foods can sometimes be bought in bulk (e.g., sacks of flour or sugar), thus allowing you to live through temporary shortages. You could arrange to have limited stocks of food sent out, but this will prove expensive and it is sensible to try to "live off the land."

Is the milk drinkable, and if not, is powdered milk available? This is something you could quite easily take and may need to if you have a formula-fed baby (see notes below under baby care).

In most cases it is quite easy to provide a balanced diet for children, but it will pay if you learn something about the nutritional content of the foods you will encounter abroad.

IMMUNIZATION

Children should have had the normal schedule of immunization set out in Table 11.1, before traveling abroad—and the same schedule should be used for babies living abroad (but see note on p. 533 about injections abroad).

Tuberculin or "PPD" testing is also normally carried out annually starting at one year of age. BCG is not normally recommended, but can be given at any age from infancy for children going to or born in a country with a high prevalence of tuberculosis. It should always be given intradermally in the left upper arm.

Boosters against tetanus (unless immunized within the last 10 years) and polio should be given before departure.

In addition, yellow fever immunization may be mandatory for the country you are to visit. Protection can optionally be obtained against typhoid, hepatitis A (see below), and rabies. All these additional vaccines may be safely given to children of six months and over, but not earlier. Malaria prevention is dealt with separately below.

THE DOMESTIC SITUATION AND EDUCATION ABROAD

Find out in advance what kind of house you will have and whether you will be put first in a hotel or small apartment. If so, and you have several children, it may be better for them to follow once the house has been obtained. How well equipped will the house be? For a family, a refrigerator is essential, and you may need to take this out yourself.

If you do not intend to employ domestic help, then a washing machine should also be considered and in a developing country it will be much cheaper to take it with you than to buy it there.

If you have school-age children, find out something about the schools, whether there is a choice and whether the teaching is what you are used to. If not, and you intend to return them to their original schools later, seek advice from their teachers on whether books should be taken with you to help bridge the gap. For preschool children, you should take out plenty of books, toys, and playgroup materials, and obtain addresses of mail-order firms that will send things out (for example Sesame Street, Mothercare).

If both parents are to be working, then care arrangements will be needed for preschool children. Domestic help is generally provided by child-minders rather than educators, and you should bear

Table 11.1. IMMUNIZATION SCHEDULE FOR CHILDREN

Birth:	**Hepatitis B vaccine**
2 months:	First dose of diphtheria/pertussis/tetanus (DPT), oral polio (OPV) and *H. influenzae B* (HIB); 2nd dose of Hepatitis B vaccine
4 months:	Second dose of DPT, OPV, and HIB
6 months:	Third dose of DPT, HIB, OPV, and Hepatitis B vaccine
12–15 months:	Measles, mumps, and rubella (MMR)
15–18 months:	DPT, OPV, and HIB booster
4–5 years:	DPT, OPV, and 2nd MMR

this in mind: nursery schools of the quality available at home may not be easy to find. You may find it necessary to organize your own playgroup.

If you have a baby, it may be wise to take several sets of baby clothes to expand into as he or she grows. Cotton clothes are preferable to those made of stretch nylon, and plastic pants should be avoided. A hat or sunshade is a must. Further aspects of baby care are dealt with below.

THE JOURNEY

Traveling long distances with children can be stressful. Some tips are given below on how to reduce the stress:

If you have a baby, breast-feeding on the move is far easier than formula feeding, especially if you are not inhibited about feeding in public. If you are flying, ask for a "sky cot" well in advance (and check again before traveling); otherwise you will be balancing the baby on your knee all the way. Disposable diapers are a must for the journey, and may not always be available from flight attendants on board aircraft. If you bottle-feed, prepacked milk is very useful for the journey.

Suitable books and toys or games should be kept handy, as bored children sitting in an enclosed space for a long period will not stay happy. "Looking at the view" may be fun for parents but not for a two-year-old or even a six-year-old.

A small supply of food and drink should be taken, for example some sandwiches, biscuits, and a bottle of water, as the meals available en route may be neither palatable nor healthful, if you can get them at all.

Travel sickness should be prevented in advance if your children are prone to it. Dramamine chewable (dimenhydrinate) is a suitable medication. Avoid overdosage, which leads to sleepiness, dry mouth, and irritability.

HEALTH HAZARDS AT YOUR DESTINATION

SHORT VISITS (UNDER ONE MONTH)

For short periods abroad, you do not need to be too concerned about exotic diseases—the most likely infections to crop up are the everyday ones. Make sure that you are prepared to deal with problems like diarrhea or respiratory infections (sore throat or ears). The contents of a simple first-aid kit for young children on a beach vacation are shown in the box.

You should *always* be aware of the risk of malaria if you are going to a part of the world where it is endemic: babies and young children must be protected even on a short visit (see below). Check what immunizations are needed, and make sure that children are up to date with tetanus and polio if they will be going to a tropical or subtropical country—boosters are required every 10 years once the primary course has been completed.

FIRST-AID KIT FOR SHORT HOLIDAY TRIPS

- oral rehydration solutions
- acetaminophen tablets or elixir (Tylenol)—for fever
- antiseptic solution (Hibiclens, Phisohex)
- Band-Aids
- sunscreen
- diphenhydramine hydrochloride (Benadryl)
- insect-repellent spray (preferably ozone-friendly)
- antibiotics for ear infections (Ampicillin, Trimethoprim Sulfa)

LONGER VISITS (OVER ONE MONTH)

For longer visits, more careful preparation will be needed, as well as an awareness of the endemic diseases in the country concerned. You will also need to find out about the local health system, and where you will be able to obtain advice after your arrival.

MALARIA

Malaria is fully covered in another chapter (see pp. 121–32), and the manifestations, treatment, and the choice of antimalarial tablets will not be discussed again here, although you should note these points:

- A baby is at risk of malaria from birth, so in a malarial area, protective measures should be taken from then on.

- The main antimalarial drugs are safe for children, in reduced dosages.
- In malarial areas, taking the tablets or medicine should become a routine, like brushing the teeth.
- As with adults, children should commence taking antimalarials one week prior to travel, and for at least four weeks afterward.
- Keep the tablets or syrups in a safe, secure place—even the most trustworthy toddler may swallow a bottleful.

As well as the use of antimalarial tablets or syrups, other control measures should also be used to reduce the likelihood of mosquitoes biting (see pp. 182–92). Netting is valuable (especially chemically impregnated nets). Check for mosquitoes that may have gotten inside the netting each time you place your child to rest. Infants should always be covered with a separate net. It may be wise to take nets with you for use when traveling outside urban areas.

Mosquito control consists of ensuring that there is no standing water near the house to act as a breeding ground, and spraying the bedroom at night.

AIDS AND HIV

The risk to children is mainly from contaminated injections or blood transfusions. Check needle sterility before allowing your child to receive an injection; if necessary take a small supply of needles and syringes with you when traveling to a high-risk country (see p. 533). It is worth knowing your child's blood group, and your own; if they are compatible, you may be able to act as a donor in an emergency.

FEVER

Fever is a much more worrying complaint in children overseas than at home, because of the fear of exotic tropical infections. Although malaria is an ever-present worry (even in the child on antimalarial tablets or syrup), the vast majority of fevers in children have the same causes anywhere, namely viral nose and throat infections (coughs, tonsillitis, and the like). The symptoms of these will usually include cough and a runny nose, with perhaps a sore throat or earache and general malaise with loss of appetite, and sometimes vomiting due to swallowed phlegm. Warning signs of another cause would be these:

SOME SAFETY TIPS

- Children should know how to use child seats and safety belts.
- They should be taught not to go anywhere with a stranger.
- They should know the name of their hotel, and should always know what to do if they get lost. (If necessary, they should carry a written note of their name, address, and other appropriate information.)
- Parents should carry at least one full-face photograph of all children they are traveling with.
- Never leave children alone—to watch luggage, or to keep a place in line.

1. If a child has a very high fever (104°F., 40°C.) with headache (?malaria).
2. If a child suffers from a severe headache and vomiting with neck stiffness (?meningitis).
3. If a child appears jaundiced (with yellow eyes) (?hepatitis or malaria).
4. If a child has blood in stools or severe diarrhea (?dysentery).
5. If a child feels burning on passing urine, or must visit the toilet frequently (?urinary infection).
6. If a baby refuses to feed (?blood infection).
7. If a child has a severe cough with rapid breathing (?pneumonia, ?asthma).
8. If a child suffers persistent abdominal pain (?appendicitis).

If these signs are not present but cold symptoms are, then it is quite reasonable to give the child acetaminophen and extra fluids, keep him or her cool, and carry on as normally as possible (an antibiotic does not help most throat and nose infections, which are usually caused by a virus, but may be needed for severe sore throats or earache). If one of the above features is present, if the fever is in a baby under a year, or if it lasts over two days without improvement and fever is the only symptom, then medical help should be sought. *Any* fever in an infant less than two months old should be regarded as an emergency.

Should a fever in a malarious area be routinely treated with

USING INSECT REPELLENTS WITH CHILDREN

Insect repellents provide valuable protection, but need to be used with care.

It is extremely rare for insect repellents to cause toxic effects, but the majority of cases that have occurred have been in children. The reasons are not entirely clear. It may be that children have a lower threshold for toxicity, or that they metabolize DEET differently. Alternatively, it may be related to the higher ratio of skin area to body weight, especially in cases where DEET is applied to the face (children have disproportionately large heads), resulting in increased absorption. Or it may be more mundane, and result from finger sucking.

Advice on using repellents is given on p. 183.

Dr. Theodore Tsai

chloroquine, just in case it is malaria? This is difficult to answer (see p. 402). Certainly a supply of chloroquine should be kept in the house and you should know how much to give. If medical aid is not readily available, the child has been exposed to mosquitoes, and the features are not typical of a cold, then a chloroquine course should be given *unless* you are in an area of chloroquine resistance, in which case medical assistance must be sought first.

However, a *blood test should, if practicable, always be taken for malaria before giving the chloroquine*—only a few drops of blood on a slide are needed for this. Otherwise it will be hard to decide later whether it was malaria or not. The local hospital or clinic may show you how to take the test yourself.

RESPIRATORY INFECTIONS

These seem to be worse in children living in the tropics, perhaps because of more frequent swimming leading to ear infections, or perhaps because of exposure to a new set of infective agents.

The commonest serious infections are *tonsillitis* (throat infection) and *otitis media* (middle-ear infection), both of which may need antibiotic treatment. Penicillin, ampicillin, and trimethoprim-sulfamethoxazole (Septra, Bactrim) are the most effective antibiotics used for these conditions and they are available worldwide. If your child is allergic to penicillin make sure that this is clear to anyone giving treatment.

DIARRHEA

Diarrhea is extremely common in children when traveling or in another country (see pp. 13–31). "Gastroenteritis" is simply the technical name for a stomach or intestinal infection leading to diarrhea and is not necessarily severe or life-threatening. The seriousness of diarrhea depends on how much fluid is lost from the body: because a child's total fluid volume is greater in proportion to body weight than an adult's, the effect is greater the younger the child. A baby can become dehydrated (dried out) within a few hours of the onset of severe diarrhea.

Diarrheal disease is usually contracted by contact with infected food or fluid, but also from hands that have touched infected material. Feces of an infected person are highly contagious, and careful hand-washing is therefore essential after using the toilet.

Replacement of fluid loss is the most important part of treatment. Drugs are quite ineffective in the vast majority of cases. A suitable fluid-replacement solution may be made with a finger pinch of salt and a teaspoon of sugar added to 250 ml. (about one mugful) of boiled water, with a squeeze of orange juice to provide flavor (and a token amount of potassium). The concentration is very important as the sugar helps aid the absorption of the salt, but too much of either is harmful. Taste the solution before giving to your child, and if it tastes saltier than tears, discard it and start again (see also p. 27 and p. 521).

Special packets of powder (e.g., WHO, Jianas Brothers) for adding to water may be obtained from your doctor or at a pharmacy (with a prescription) before you go and are valuable for journeys. Give one cupful of mixture for each loose stool. Seek medical help

TABLE 11.2. SOME CAUSES OF CHILDREN'S DIARRHEA IN THE TROPICS

Cause	Symptoms
Rotavirus (commonest cause)	mild fever, watery diarrhea, vomiting
Salmonella (food poisoning)	diarrhea and vomiting, abdominal pain, fever, malaise
Shigellosis (bacillary dysentery)	bloody diarrhea, high fever
Cholera	profuse watery diarrhea (leading rapidly to dehydration)
Typhoid	diarrhea or constipation, fever, headache, rash, persistent weakness
Giardiasis	offensive stools, recurrent diarrhea, malaise, abdominal pains (this is a more chronic or lasting condition)

if the child vomits or appears drowsy, has fast breathing, or is dehydrated (eyes become sunken, tongue is dry, skin loses elasticity). Profuse diarrhea in a baby is also a reason for seeking assistance early.

While awaiting assistance or on the way to a doctor, you should give oral rehydration solution in small amounts frequently (even if the child or infant is vomiting, continue to give oral rehydration fluids). A baby may take fluids better by cup and spoon than from a bottle and there is less likelihood of vomiting.

Diet Feeding should be continued during diarrhea if the child feels like eating—especially high-calorie, low-residue foods. Bananas, cereals, bread, chicken, cookies, and eggs are all suitable—concentrate on the foods the child likes most. For infants breast-feeding (or bottle feeding) should be continued. Starving a child suffering from diarrhea is now thought undesirable, although appetite is often reduced.

Drug treatment is necessary only for some of the specific types of diarrhea mentioned in Chapter 2, such as severe dysentery, typhoid, cholera, and giardiasis—all of which are much less likely than a viral cause. Antidiarrheal agents such as kaolin, codeine, diphenoxylate (Lomotil), and over-the-counter mixtures should be avoided in children under five years. Lomotil in particular has toxic side effects (depression of the respiratory system) and should not be used in young children, nor should preventive drugs such as clioquinol (Entero-Vioform).

Prevention The likelihood of diarrhea can be minimized by following these tips:

- Pay close attention to household hygiene—particularly hand-washing before meals and after using the toilet.

- Maintain good hygiene in the kitchen by washing hands before food preparation; keeping stored food in the refrigerator (especially meat); covering all food left out in the open, even for short periods; cooking meat thoroughly; boiling water if there is any doubt about its purity (then keeping it in the refrigerator—it will taste better); washing fresh fruit and vegetables thoroughly before eating; and not permitting flies in the kitchen.

- Avoid precooked foods bought in the streets; milk and milk products (especially ice cream) unless you are quite sure they are manufactured hygienically; salads and other uncooked foods; and cold meat eaten in hotels and restaurants.

VIRAL HEPATITIS

Hepatitis comes in two main forms—named A and B. Of these, hepatitis A or "infectious hepatitis" is more common in children: it is usually spread by the "fecal-oral" route—just like diarrhea. It is not usually a serious disease in children, and indeed may sometimes not be noticed ("subclinical") but is nevertheless best avoided. The features of the illness and how to deal with it are covered in another chapter (pp. 49–60).

Prevention depends mainly on food hygiene and avoiding dubious foods, as discussed under diarrhea. There is as yet only limited experience with the new hepatitis A vaccine in children, which will soon be licensed in the USA, is now available in several other countries (see p. 507). "Passive" immunization with immune globulin provides only short-term protection, and may be given to children aged six months and over. A vaccine is also available against hepatitis B, which is now part of the recommended immunization schedule in the U.S.

SWIMMING HAZARDS

Bilharzia is present in most rivers and lakes in Africa, the Middle East and Asia, and some parts of South and Central America and prohibits swimming with only a few exceptions (see pp. 94–99). Some areas are treated against snails (which infect the water), but be sure you have a reliable local source of information on this. The infective risk of a single brief exposure is not great and may be reduced by showering in clean water immediately afterward, but it is better to be safe than sorry.

Before swimming in pools, check that the chlorine supply has not run out—a common problem in developing countries.

Swimmer's ear occurs quite frequently in hot countries. Children prone to these fungal infections of the ear canal should use an acid solution such as otic Domeboro after each swim, for prevention. Ear plugs are probably not helpful. If your child develops an infection, a one-week course of corticosporin otic solution is necessary.

Your child should avoid submerging his or her head during this period.

Drowning is sadly still a significant cause of accidental death in children, and parents need to be aware of it as an ever-present risk in young children. The first rule is to teach your children to swim at the earliest opportunity. The second is to fence off any swimming pool to which your (or visitors') children might have access. Thirdly, always keep a watchful eye on any young child (below five, or a nonswimmer at any age) when there is water about, whether in baths, in a pool, at a lake, or at the seaside. Toddlers have been known to drown in shallow pools. Babies may be encouraged to swim from a very early age quite safely as long as the water is safe, and you are careful to avoid sunburn.

OTHER HAZARDS

Sunburn is an obvious environmental hazard, particularly in high or mountainous countries where the tropical sun burns very quickly (see p. 323). Also, beware of burning even when it is cloudy. The usual advice of big hats and covering the arms and legs should be followed rigorously until all the children are mahogany-colored. Fair children's hair usually bleaches pale blond, but will darken on returning to cooler climates. Sunscreens, preferably water resistant, are essential when at the swimming pool or seaside. If a child becomes burned, *any* further exposure for a day or two (or more, depending on the extent) must be avoided. Large tense blisters may be popped with a sterile needle; other blisters should be left intact.

Prickly heat is common in hot climates and particularly in humid countries, and can be very troublesome. It is caused by sweating, with blockage of the sweat ducts leading to itching red spots and tiny blisters, usually on the neck, back, and chest.

Treat by washing the area with cool water, and then dry off. If the child is quite uncomfortable due to itching, give Benadryl for symptomatic relief.

Prevent prickly heat by avoiding sweating as much as possible, by frequent bathing, by wearing loose clothing (p. 305), and by drying the skin whenever it becomes wet.

Walking barefoot should be avoided outside your yard or land you know well. Snakes are more afraid of people than we of them, but if stood upon will bite defensively (p. 204).

A more common hazard for the barefoot is *hookworm*, acquired from soil contaminated with human feces (see p. 43). The worm passes through the skin of the feet and circulates through the lymphatics and lungs before eventually settling in the small intestine, where chronic bleeding leads to severe anemia.

Tumbu fly (also known as "Putsi" in some areas) is another infestation commonly picked up from soil in which eggs of the fly have been laid (see p. 172). It does not depend on fecal spread and may occur even where sanitation is perfect (e.g., your yard). Larvae may enter the skin directly from the soil or from eggs laid in clothes left hanging in the shade or laid on the ground to dry. Lesions resembling boils develop under the skin and may be very painful. The main preventive measure is to iron all clothes and sheets which have been left out to dry, so as to kill the eggs.

Cuts, sores, and insect bites are common in hot countries but heal more slowly than at home, probably because of greater sweating. Treat them meticulously in the early stages by cleaning, disinfecting, and covering. Topical antibacterials such as Zephiran or Hibiclens are useful.

For itchy skin lesions and bites, diphenhydramine hydrochloride (Benadryl) is effective.

Bike riding Safety helmets will not be available in most locations and should be brought from the U.S.

Poison prevention Syrup of ipecac is a must for families with young children, and may not be available locally. The dosage is:

• infants 6 months to 1 year: 5 ml.

• children 1–12 years: 15 ml.

• over 12 years: 30 ml.

The syrup should be followed by one to two glasses of water; repeat the dose if vomiting does not occur within 20 to 30 minutes.

Gastric lavage will be necessary if no vomiting occurs within a further 20 minutes.

Pets If you keep a dog, ensure that rabies vaccine is given at the right time and that the dog is dewormed. Also be on the lookout for ticks and remove them immediately (drop into paraffin). They can cause *tickbite* fever in animals and humans.

Cats (as well as undercooked meat) may be a source of toxoplasmosis, which causes a glandular-fever-type illness. An infected pregnant woman may transmit the disease to the fetus, causing congenital deformities, although this condition is rare (p. 446). Cats and dogs may both spread toxocariasis, another parasitic infection, which is a rare cause of blindness in children. Infection may occur through contamination of food by cat and dog feces, so scrupulous hygiene is necessary when handling food if there is a pet around—and be sure to keep animals away from food dishes, and to dispose of their litter effectively.

Stray animals should be avoided and children warned carefully of their risks. Animals in the street should never be petted because of the risk of rabies and other diseases.

CHILDREN'S DIET ABROAD

Children tend to eat less in a hot climate, so it is all the more important to ensure a balanced intake of nutrients. Foods obtainable will generally be healthier (few junk foods and candy) and vegetables and fruit will be abundant and fresh (but always wash them thoroughly if eaten raw). Remember that too many mangoes/guavas/papayas may cause intestinal upsets. Here are some tips:

- *Meat* should be thoroughly cooked, particularly beef, which may carry tapeworms or trichinosis.
- *Eggs* are likely to be readily available.
- *Milk and milk products* (particularly cream and ice cream) should be viewed with caution, and milk boiled unless you are sure it has been hygienically prepared.
- A reasonable *salt* intake is necessary but usually this may be obtained by adding extra to food, without any need for salt tablets.

- *Vitamins* should be readily available from the following sources:

  vitamin A carrots, highly colored or dark green vegetables/ fruit (e.g. mango, guava, papaya, spinach)

  vitamin B nuts, cereals, milk, eggs, meat

  vitamin C oranges, lemons, guavas, potatoes

  vitamin D margarine, eggs, fish, sunlight

  folic acid green leafy vegetables

- *Fluoride* is valuable in preventing dental caries but water supplies overseas are rarely fluoridated. Fluoride supplements are quite safe, but are best obtained before departure: they are recommended from infancy to 12 years of age if the local water supply is deficient. Drops are available for babies. A prescription is necessary (see also p. 380).

BABY CARE ABROAD

In general, the care of babies in hot countries does not differ from anywhere else, but a few tips may be helpful.

BREAST-FEEDING

Breast-feeding should be carried out if possible in preference to bottle, not just because it is better for the baby, but because of the example the expatriate mother sets to the local community. Bottle-feeding is a major cause of death among babies in poor countries because of the difficulty mothers face in boiling water, keeping bottles clean, and just buying milk powder. One reason why the local mother may turn to bottle-feeding is because it carries "prestige"—since expatriate mothers do it.

Extra water is not needed routinely by the breast-fed baby, even in hot climates, unless he or she is feverish or suffering from diarrhea. But the nursing mother must be sure to maintain a high fluid intake herself.

INFANT FOODS

For the same reason, it is preferable to use natural foods rather than commercial cans or jars for weaning the baby—it is also cheaper and probably healthier, as some proprietary foods have a high concentration of salt and other additives. The first food will probably still remain a proprietary cereal but when mixed feeding is commenced, then liquidized vegetables, fruit, meat, cheese, and eggs may all be used quite safely (this will usually be over the age of six months).

DIAPERS AND DIAPER RASH

Disposable diapers may be unobtainable or in short supply, so it is wise to take cotton diapers and diaper liners. Use cotton pants, because plastic pants predispose to diaper rash, and leave the baby without a diaper for some of the time. Most diaper rashes will clear up well if the baby is allowed to play out in the sun without anything on the bottom. For bright red diaper rashes, treatment with an antifungal ointment (mycostatin) may be necessary. Remember to press cotton diapers on both sides with a hot iron, in tropical countries, to kill the eggs of the tumbu fly.

SUNSHINE

Babies have a sensitive skin and burn easily. Always protect them from direct sunlight by using a sunhat or sunshade. Cars left in the sun become very hot inside. *Never* leave your baby alone in a car.

MALARIA PREVENTION IN BABIES

Malaria prophylaxis in babies should be started immediately after birth. Even if you are breast-feeding and taking a drug yourself, an insufficient amount will reach the baby to be effective. Use nets carefully to avoid mosquito bites.

CRIBS

A basket is a better place for a baby to sleep than a crib, as it will be cooler. Often you will find that special baskets can be made locally. If using a straw basket, line the inside with netting to prevent mosquitoes and ticks from getting in. After dark, always put a net over the basket, even in a room with screened windows—mosquitoes are expert hole-finders.

Be sure to take with you items you will need as the baby grows, such as a potty, toilet seat, baby chair, portable crib, car seat, and toddler toys. Clothes should usually be obtainable locally. For the other items, mail order may be possible, but in some countries there may be long delays at customs.

CHILDREN WITH SPECIAL PROBLEMS

If you have a child with diabetes (see below), cystic fibrosis, asthma, or any other chronic disorder, you will need special advice before traveling abroad. Obtain this early from your usual specialist or one of the support organizations, as a lot more advance planning will be required.

CONCLUSION

- Do not let the above list of exotic diseases and problems overwhelm you with horror. Most can be prevented by simple precautions, and on the positive side, there will be the outdoor life, the absence of junk foods and TV, and the exposure to quite different cultures and traditions. You and your children should come back with a much deeper understanding of people of other races and cultures, and of the nature of the problems facing developing countries. It will be worth it.

THE DIABETIC TRAVELER

Provided that a few basic guidelines are followed carefully, travel poses few problems to the majority of diabetics.

Dr. Peter Watkins is a Consultant Physician at King's College Hospital, London, and is an authority on diabetes.

Diabetes mellitus is a very common disorder. In developed countries, 1–2 percent of the population have diabetes, so that in the USA, for example, between 3 and 4 million people are diabetic. Since diabetes is commonest in middle age, there are always a great many diabetic travelers.

TYPES OF DIABETES

There are two main types of diabetes—insulin-dependent diabetes and non-insulin-dependent diabetes. Common to both forms, and the main cause of symptoms in each, is an above-normal level of sugar (glucose) in the blood—a condition called "hyperglycemia."

Glucose arrives in the blood from the intestine after absorption from food and is also made in large amounts by the liver. Normally, the hormone insulin then facilitates use of the glucose as an energy source by various parts of the body: in this way insulin keeps the blood-sugar level under control. Insulin-dependent diabetics are unfortunately unable to make their own insulin, so need daily insulin injections throughout their lives. Without these injections their blood-sugar level would rise uncontrollably, leading to coma and eventually to death.

With non-insulin-dependent diabetes, the cause of the raised blood-sugar level is more complex: insulin deficiency is responsible in some cases, but other factors such as obesity may also play a role. Whatever the cause, the blood-sugar level can be kept in check without resort to insulin injections.

Symptoms are the same with both forms of the disorder: patients describe thirst or dry mouth, pass large amounts of dilute urine, lose weight, and feel tired. Sometimes itching of the genital organs occurs because of yeast infection, and a few people experience blurring of vision.

Treatment is aimed at restoring health by lowering blood sugar to as near normal a level as possible. Dieting is a key part of treatment for both types of diabetes and at the very least, apart from other dietary measures, all simple sugars must be eliminated.

Insulin-dependent diabetics must inject insulin under the skin between one and three times each day. Non-insulin-dependent diabetics may just need a special diet, sometimes supplemented by tablets that help to lower the blood-sugar level. These tablets will not work in diabetics who require insulin injections. Most diabetics monitor their "control" by performing either their own blood-sugar tests after pricking a finger to obtain a small sample of blood, or by testing urine specimens for sugar.

Modern insulins include quick-acting (clear or soluble) insulins and longer-acting (cloudy) insulins. Individual patients will use different combinations of these. When making changes during travel, it is best to confine these to changes of the soluble insulin. Modern insulin "pens" that deliver metered doses from a cartridge make this very simple.

TRAVEL

Traveling generally presents few real problems to diabetics provided that they follow the simple guidelines presented below. It is obviously more difficult for those taking insulin, especially when major time changes occur when traveling long distances by air. No country need be off limits, although places very remote from medical services might not be ideal for those lacking confidence. Those who wish to work abroad can generally do so, but diabetics on insulin ought to remain within reach of medical services, and some remote areas may not be appropriate for long spells. Many of the comments that follow apply only to insulin-dependent diabetics.

BEFORE YOU GO

IMMUNIZATION

Diabetics should be immunized in exactly the same way as non-diabetics (see pp. 498–514). There are only a few reasons for not undertaking immunization and they apply equally to nondiabetics.

SUPPLIES

Ensure that ample supplies of tablets or insulin, syringes, needles, and urine- or blood-testing equipment are carried. It is best to keep some supplies in at least two separate items of luggage in case of loss. Insulin should not be put in baggage that will travel in the hold of an aircraft, where it may freeze.

Storage of insulin is not generally a problem. Refrigeration is not necessary during the journey and in temperate climates insulin will keep for some months at room temperature. Refrigeration (*not* deep freezing) is recommended for long-term storage, especially in the tropics.

INSURANCE

Travel insurance premiums may be quoted at higher rates than normal, but adequate insurance cover is always essential (see p. 492). The American Diabetes Association, 1660 Duke St., Alexandria, VA 22314, Tel. (703) 549-1500, and (800) 232-3472, may be able to advise on suitable travel insurers. Other useful addresses include the Canadian Diabetes Association, 78 Bond St., Toronto, Ontario M5B 2J8, Tel. (416) 362-4440; the British Diabetic Association, 10 Queen Anne St., London W1M OBS, Tel. 071-323-1531; the Australian Diabetes Foundation, P.O. Box 944, Civic Square, Canberra ACT 2608, Tel. 062-475655, 062-475722, Fax 062-573140; and Diabetes New Zealand Inc. (4 Coquet St., P.O.

Box 54, Oamaru, South Island, Tel. 64-3-434 8100, Fax 64-3-434-5821).

MOTION SICKNESS
Diabetics can use the same anti-motion sickness tablets as non-diabetics (see p. 251). These tablets do not affect diabetic control. Don't forget that many preparations cause drowsiness, and it is best not to drive while under their influence. If vomiting should occur, the method of managing the diabetes is described below.

IDENTIFICATION
Some form of identification is most valuable in case of problems. All diabetics should carry with them at all times a clear statement that they are diabetic with details of their treatment, indicating their usual physician or clinic. *Medic-Alert Foundation International* (see address on pp. 219–20) offers a valuable service in this regard, and its bracelet is widely known. Identification will also help if there are any problems with regard to customs officials (syringes and needles may be confused with the paraphernalia of drug addicts). You should not under any circumstances hand over your equipment to any official.

TRAVELING COMPANIONS
Insulin-dependent diabetics traveling to remote parts of the world should ideally be accompanied, so that immediate help is available, especially in the event of a low blood-sugar level (hypoglycemia—see below).

THE JOURNEY

TIME CHANGES DURING LONG-DISTANCE AIR TRAVEL
This will cause minor temporary upset of diabetic control in insulin-treated diabetics.

FLYING WEST
The time between injections can, with little problem, be lengthened by two to three hours twice daily. Regular tests should be performed and if they are very "sugary" a little extra soluble insulin (perhaps 4–8 units) can be given. If the time gap between injections

is lengthened still further, a small supplementary injection of soluble insulin (4–8 units) is given between the usual injections.

FLYING EAST

The time between injections will need to be shortened by two to three hours each time, which could result in rather low blood sugars. Careful testing should be performed, and if required each dose can be reduced by a small amount (4–8 units on average). Regular meals should be taken as normal. Many airlines will make special provision for diabetics if notified in advance.

ABROAD

While on vacation, the chief problems are these:

1. Vomiting, either from motion sickness or stomach upsets;
2. Other illnesses affecting diabetic control, e.g., infections;
3. Hypoglycemia (a low blood sugar);
4. Alterations of diabetic control due to major changes in diet or activity.

VOMITING AND OTHER ILLNESS

The blood-sugar level tends to increase during any illness, even if little food is being taken, and quite often the insulin dose needs to be increased. At the very least, *insulin should never be stopped*, otherwise deterioration of diabetes is inevitable, leading to diabetic ketoacidosis (pre-coma) and hospital admission.

Take the following steps:

- Monitor sugar levels carefully (urine or blood-sugar tests) at least four times daily. If the results are poor (urine sugars persistently 2 percent, or blood sugars greater than 15 mmol./l or 270 mg./ 100 ml.), then extra insulin is needed. This can be done either at the normal times by increasing the soluble insulin by about 10 percent (normally 4–8 units) or as additional doses of soluble insulin at noon or bedtime if tests remain poor then.

- Carbohydrate should be maintained if possible by taking the normal quantity in fluid form. Table 11.3 shows the amounts of various fluids and simple sugar preparations containing 10 grams of sugar (i.e., one carbohydrate "portion").

- If vomiting persists, or if the general condition deteriorates, it is best not to delay seeing a physician or going to a hospital.

HYPOGLYCEMIA

A low blood sugar develops if too much insulin is taken, too little food is eaten, or if there is a marked increase in physical activity. The symptoms fall into three phases: early warning, when the person may shake or tremble, sweat, and note "pins and needles" in the lips and tongue, palpitations or headache; a more advanced phase, with double vision, slurring of speech, difficulty of concentration or even confusion and odd behavior; and eventually, without treatment, the person may become unconscious.

All diabetics taking insulin should be aware of the possibility of hypoglycemia, and all are supposed to carry with them, at all times, some form of sugar, usually as sugar lumps, candy, or dextrose tablets (see Table 11.3). About 10–20 grams of sugar should be taken at the first warning of hypoglycemia; if a diabetic becomes confused, his or her companions should compel the person to take a glucose tablet or sugar lump.

To help people who are seriously prone to troublesome hypoglycemia with unconsciousness, an injection of glucagon (1 mg. intramuscularly) can easily be given by a companion. Glucagon causes a rapid increase of the blood sugar. Glucagon is supplied in a small kit: it must be prescribed by a physician, and those carrying glucagon must learn how to use it before the emergency arises.

ALTERATION OF DIABETIC CONTROL

Lifestyle and routine during traveling are likely to be very different from those at home, and this change may alter diabetic control.

TABLE 11.3. ITEMS CONTAINING 10 GRAMS CARBOHYDRATE

Item	Amount
Milk	one third of a pint
Coca-cola	90 ml. (six tablespoonfuls)
Sugar	two teaspoonfuls
Sugar lumps	three small lumps
Dextrosol	three tablets

If physical activity is much greater than usual (hiking or swim-ming, for example), hypoglycemia is more likely to occur. Food intake needs to be increased, or a small decrease in insulin dose will be required. Most diabetics know that extra carbohydrate is needed *before* considerable physical exertion in order to avoid hypoglyce-mia.

If the level of activity on vacation is much less than usual, then blood sugar tends to increase. This needs to be monitored and, if necessary, a little more insulin given.

Keeping to a diet abroad can be difficult. However, even with foreign foods it should still be possible to keep to the usual amount of carbohydrate. Do your best not to exceed your normal amount.

NON-INSULIN-DEPENDENT DIABETES

There are few problems for those not taking insulin but diabetes should not be neglected, and regular tests should be conducted as if at home. Above all, diabetics should not overeat as this will very probably lead to poor control. If any illness occurs, control must be monitored with special care, and attention from a physician may be necessary. Remember that with this type of diabetes, insulin may occasionally be needed temporarily during an illness, especially if there is an infection.

SUMMARY OF ADVICE FOR DIABETIC TRAVELERS

- If careful preparations are made and proper precautions followed, traveling should not present any problems for diabetics. The major hazard, as at other times, is hypoglycemia—*remember to carry sugar* and make sure someone else knows how to help you if hypoglycemia occurs.

THE HANDICAPPED TRAVELER

Since travel has become a necessity of modern life rather than a luxury, people have begun to realize that physical handicaps are not the insurmountable barriers that they once seemed. As in golf, even with some strokes against you, you're still in the game.

Louise Weiss is a travel writer and author of Access to the World: A Travel Guide for the Handicapped. *She lives in New York.*

Which areas of the world are best equipped to accommodate the needs of travelers with any sort of handicap? This is easy to answer; just imagine a globe: draw a horizontal line under the United States and Canada, over to the British Isles and Northern Europe, curve it down around South Africa, then over to Israel, take in Hong Kong and Singapore, Australia, New Zealand, and the islands that comprise the state of Hawaii. As far as the rest of the world is concerned, leisure travelers would be well advised to consider whether they wish to spend their money attempting to cope with situations completely inimical to their particular handicap. This is in no way to imply that the countries mentioned above are completely barrier-free. They do indeed have fewer barriers, but of no less importance is the fact that they are psychologically more attuned to accepting the handicapped into the mainstream of society.

In the United States alone, government agencies have estimated the handicapped population to be between 35 and 50 million. This may seem mind-boggling until one realizes that handicapping conditions fall into two categories; visible and invisible. Among the most visible, of course, are conditions requiring a wheelchair. Blindness is, too, but deafness less so. Diabetes, heart conditions, kidney disease, and respiratory ailments are not visible to the casual observer, but each presents specific problems for the traveler.

There are differences too, between what has been defined by the Air Traffic Conference of America as "static" and "nonstatic" ambulatory and nonambulatory conditions:

- A static ambulatory condition would be blindness or deafness.
- A nonstatic ambulatory condition describes someone who has recently undergone surgery or had a heart attack but is capable of walking short distances.
- Nonstatic, nonambulatory would describe all stretcher cases as well as seriously ill people who require a wheelchair.
- Static nonambulatory applies to paraplegia, quadriplegia, or any other condition that confines an otherwise healthy person to a wheelchair because of inability to walk.

WHEELCHAIRS

Being confined to a wheelchair is like traveling with a large piece of furniture strapped to one's back. Unless one is simply too tall or heavy, it is best to use a lightweight folding chair, usually called a "junior" model. Battery-operated chairs are heavy and unwieldy and easily damaged in baggage compartments. If such a chair is absolutely necessary, it is imperative to check with the airlines about their rules concerning carriage of batteries. In the United States, wet-cell batteries may now be transported on aircraft if they conform to Federal regulations. A device called a "wheelchair tightener" is invaluable for squeezing out that last half-inch or so that will get the chair through a door. Carrying a few basic tools for making simple repairs is advisable.

BLINDNESS

Logistically, blindness presents fewer difficulties than one might suppose. No furniture problem here. Restaurants are beginning to offer Braille menus, hotels to provide safety instructions in Braille. If flight attendants do not volunteer the information, they should be asked the number of rows to the nearest exit. On United States airlines, blind passengers are allowed to keep their long canes at their seats if they wish. Guide dogs are permitted in passenger cabins on United States domestic flights (except to Hawaii), but whether they can be carried internationally depends upon the destination. The lengthy quarantines imposed by Australia, Hawaii, Hong Kong, Ireland, New Zealand, and the United Kingdom make transporting a guide dog impractical for the vacationer. Bermuda, Denmark, Norway, and Sweden require medical certificates for dogs. It is essential to check with the embassy or consulate of the destination country well in advance of travel. Do not rely on airlines for complete information.

DEAFNESS

The hearing population tends to be unaware of how much information is conveyed through the ear rather than the eye. Announcements of departures and delays, meals and bar service or the lack

DIVING AND THE HANDICAPPED

A growing number of physically handicapped people are discovering that, in the near-weightless conditions of the underwater environment, they are as capable as any able-bodied diver. Also, everybody is deaf under water. HSA International (Handicapped Scuba Association) operates a service, Dive and Travel Fast Facts, which provides information (in English only) about diving opportunities in 25 countries. Call (415) 726-3275 *only* from a fax machine with a key pad. Follow computer voice instructions, then tap "start" and hang up. Printout will emerge. Call from anywhere in the world 24 hours a day. Information is updated every 30 days. The only charge is the cost of the phone call.

R.D.

thereof, fire alarms, "abandon ship" signals, train and bus stops—these are but some of the bits of information that may swirl unheeded around the hearing-impaired traveler. Transportation and hotel staff should be informed about the handicap and asked to make sure that emergency warnings are delivered visually or in person. Many hotels have installed fire and smoke detectors with flashing lights as well as sirens. Hearing guide dogs trained to alert their masters to specific situations, such as a crying child, are becoming more common. The same precautions about traveling with them should be taken as with dogs for the blind, with the caveat that officialdom may need more convincing that these are indeed legitimate guide dogs. In some countries, TTY and TDD telecommunication reservation systems for the hearing- and speech-impaired are available for several hotel chains, railways, and travel agencies.

DIABETES

Major requirements are refrigeration facilities for insulin and 24-hour-a-day access to food. It is best to carry small snacks at all times, since meals in transit may be delayed or even skipped. Daily exercise is also important, a point to be remembered on long bus tours. Foot care should be meticulous, since extended periods of sitting as well as more walking than usual impose added burdens on fragile feet. (See also p. 233.)

HEART CONDITIONS

These should not preclude traveling, unless constant medical supervision is necessary, but it is important to take sensible precautions. Avoid high altitudes and extremely cold weather, keep schedules flexible enough to avoid stress and use luggage with wheels or a collapsible luggage carrier. If you prefer the convenience of an organized tour, but want to avoid the often frenetic pace, consider going with a tour for the handicapped. This can be an excellent choice for heart patients or the elderly who are not mobility-impaired but require a slower pace. Cruises, too, provide an especially low-key mode of travel, but be sure that all decks of the ship are served with elevators.

KIDNEY PATIENTS

With their physician's approval, kidney patients can travel abroad and maintain their dialysis routine at hospitals and renal centers that accept transients. Reservations should be made well in advance. A physician's summary and recommendations for treatment are required, as well as a recent result of a hepatitis B antibody test. If travel plans are delayed or cancelled, the host unit should be notified immediately because a "no show" would disrupt scheduling and inconvenience regular patients. An international directory of dialysis facilities is available for people who wish to travel.*

RESPIRATORY AILMENTS

The medical aspects of flying with respiratory problems are covered on p. 228. This section considers some of the practical aspects. If you use an oxygen-powered respirator, you must make special arrangements with airlines and shipping companies. Most ships, but not all, permit passengers to bring their own oxygen aboard. Airlines require 24 to 48 hours' notice and must abide by strict safety regulations, so it is best to consult as far in advance of travel as possible. Often, only airline-supplied oxygen may be used, for which there may or may not be an additional charge. Dry-cell battery respirators

---

* *The List of Transient Dialysis Centers* is published by Creative Age Publications, 7628 Densmore Ave., Van Nuys, CA 91406-2088; Tel. (818) 782-7328. Price $8.00

are permissible on aircraft. If your respirator needs a domestic electrical supply, you must be able to manage without it for the length of your air journey, plus a couple of hours leeway in case of delay in takeoff or landing. While the United States and Canada use a 110-volt electrical system, most other countries operate on a 220-volt electric current. A converter is necessary to use a respirator on incompatible current, plus adapters for differently shaped plugs even with similar current.

PLANNING AHEAD

Successful travel depends upon careful planning, and planning depends upon correct information. Ask questions that are sufficiently detailed, for instance:

Airplanes Is there a ramp or sleeve for boarding? A wheelchair-accessible lavatory? An aisle chair for moving handicapped passengers to their seats? Does any leg of the journey involve a small aircraft which may not be able to accommodate a collapsible wheelchair? What are the oxygen regulations? Is a companion necessary?

Buses Is there a mechanical wheelchair lift? Are employees permitted to lift passengers manually? On group tours, are buses available in which passengers can remain in their wheelchairs, and can these be safely secured to the floor? Do rest stops have accessible lavatories and restaurants?

Ships How wide are the cabin doors, the bathroom doors, and the elevator doors? Is there turn-around space for a wheelchair to get into the bathroom? Can wheelchairs fit at restaurant tables? Are there ramps over door sills? If not, are portable ramps available? Are wheelchairs allowed on tenders when ships cannot moor at docks? Is there accessible transportation for sightseeing in port?

Trains Are there accessible lavatories? Where are they located? Can food be brought to the passenger? Is there a difference in height between the platform and the train? Do the stations have accessible lavatories? Are porters available?

SUMMARY

The population of industrialized countries is getting older, and medical and technological advances have increased the abilities of people who might once have been totally incapacitated by congenital defect, illness, or accident. Rising expectations increase pressure on society to accommodate the needs of those who are less than physically perfect.

In the USA, the newly enacted *Americans with Disabilities Act*, though not specifically a travel law, affects such travel-related entities as hotels, restaurants, museums, and others in a broad category of "public accommodations" that are required to make their premises and services accessible. Accessibility standards for Amtrak (railroads) and buses have been upgraded, and newly constructed or renovated buildings occupied after January 1993 must be free of architectural barriers. There is an increasing trend toward similar legislation in other countries.

While not everyone can do everything, more and more travel experiences are opening up to people with a wide range of handicaps.

USEFUL ADDRESSES

1. *USA*

   Accent on Information
   P.O. Box 700
   Bloomington, IL 61702
   Tel. (309) 378-2961 (computerized information service for the handicapped)

   Amtrak (National Railroad Passenger Corporation)
   Reservations and information: (202) 906-3000
   Toll-free: (800) 872-7245 (U.S. and Canada)
   Teletypewriter for the deaf: (800) 523-6590 (U.S. only)
   Special assistance for disabled passengers may be arranged by asking for the special services desk.

   Mobility International USA
   P.O. Box 3551
   Eugene, Oregon 97403
   Tel. (503) 343-1284

   Travel Information Service
   Moss Rehabilitation Hospital
   1200 West Tabor Rd.
   Philadelphia, PA 19141
   Tel. (215) 456-9900

   Wheelchair Getaways Inc.
   P.O. Box 819
   Newtown, PA 18940
   Tel. (215) 579-9120
   Toll-free: (800) 642-2042 (U.S. and Canada)
   (Rental vans adapted for disabled drivers and passengers, available nationwide.)

2. *UK*

   RADAR (Royal Association for Disability and Rehabilitation)
   25 Mortimer St.
   London WIN 8AB
   Tel. (071) 637-5400

Holiday Care Service
2 Old Bank Chambers
Station Rd.
Horley, Surrey RH6 9HW
Tel. 0293-774535

3. *Australia*
Australian Council for Rehabilitation of Disabled
P.O. Box 60
Curtin ACT 2605

Further information sources for the handicapped are listed in *Access to the World* (see Further Reading, p. 593).

12

BEING AN EXPATRIATE

BEING AN EXPATRIATE

Expatriates are often better able than other travelers to avoid disease hazards, but psychological and cultural pressures take their toll. A degree of "culture shock" is inevitable, but good preparation, careful briefing, and an understanding of some of the factors involved in adjusting to a new culture can contribute much to the success of an overseas posting.

Barbara Hornby is an editor and writer and a partner in a human resources consultancy and training organization. Her first cross-cultural experience took place when she moved to England as the American wife of a Briton. She has also lived in India, Nepal, Indonesia, and Malawi and traveled extensively throughout the world. She and Nancy Piet-Pelon are the authors of Women's Guide to Overseas Living. *Nancy J. Piet-Pelon is a cross-cultural trainer and a population/family planning consultant. She now lives in Bangladesh. Her first experience of living outside the USA occurred when she accompanied her husband to Indonesia, and she has also lived in Pakistan, Egypt, and Nepal.*

Being an expatriate can be one of life's great experiences if one is prepared for it. Although the strict meaning of "expatriate," as defined both by Webster's and the Oxford English Dictionary, is one who has been banished from his homeland, it has now come to mean a person who lives outside of his own culture. Millions of people from all over the world live in countries or cultures other than their own. Large numbers of them are men and women in business, development assistance, and government who pursue their careers abroad. With them are spouses and children who may or may not share their career dedication. Yet because of the importance of family and personal relationships, the spouses agree to accompany them. And they experience problems.

Those familiar with the challenges of overseas living know that many people return home before completing their contracts, often because the family was not adequately prepared and one or more members cannot adjust. They recommend orientation programs that deal with such things as expectations, culture shock, household management, and daily life overseas. They stress the importance of providing this orientation for the whole family, not just the breadwinner. They increasingly advocate some sort of pre-selection testing to see if the worker and his or her spouse can live and work effectively in another culture.

There is no doubt that pre-selection testing and orientation programs can ease transition, but what are the problems and what can *you* do to lessen them?

It is essential to be prepared. The other chapters in this book have prepared you admirably for the physical problems you may encounter. We want to address the more mental and emotional ones, the ones that can be caused by what is known as *culture shock*.

CULTURE SHOCK

Culture shock is very real and runs far deeper than just being upset by the power failures, germs in the food, and absence of supermarkets. Everyone experiences it in some way in each new culture and country to which he or she goes—and, usually, upon returning home.

Culture can be defined in many ways. For the purpose of this book we define it as *all the ways of living that have been developed by a group of human beings and that are transmitted from one generation to another.* But culture is not taught like the "three Rs." No one sits a child down and says, "Now it is time to learn culture." Rather it is learned through a process of observing, doing, and being told how to behave in specific situations. It indicates the norms of human behavior that prevail in a society. Table manners are a part of culture, as are social graces and greetings. But so are values and value-based behavior and the entire system of relationships among people.

In its simplest form, culture shock occurs when our cultural cues, the signs and symbols that guide social interaction, are stripped away. We embark from our home country surrounded by the warmth of love and emotion that go along with fond and difficult farewells. We know how to say *goodbye* in our own culture. The shock comes in disembarking in the new country and not knowing the acceptable way of saying *hello*. We become children again, not knowing *instinctively* the right thing to do. Enormous amounts of energy must suddenly be spent on small tasks, simple social etiquette, and relationship-building. The stress, and it is real, caused by this effort is called culture shock.

Culture shock is a process that can be analyzed by stages. There are minor points of difference on these stages among the experts, but there is basic agreement on the kinds of emotions and concerns that you will experience as you try to adjust to living overseas.

First comes the *honeymoon* stage, when the world is seen through the rose-colored glasses of excitement and anticipation. It is exhilarating just to arrive, a relief to have that planning, packing, and saying goodbye behind you. You may feel somewhat like a tourist, seeing new and interesting sights, being entertained, anticipating the next interesting event—and ignoring the realities of becoming established in your new life.

Would that it could stay that way! But it does not. The honeymoon stage can last anywhere from a few hours to a few months, or it may not happen at all. Most of us are lucky if it lasts a few weeks. One unpredictable day, the rose-colored glasses shatter and reality confronts us and introduces us to the second stage, the *anxiety* stage. The newcomer begins to feel bewildered and irritable. Things that seemed "quaint" only a week ago now look "dirty." The market that seemed colorful is now "crowded," "smelly," or "inconvenient." Typical symptoms are insecurity, frustration, and impatience.

Anxiety generally arises from problems you cannot define and therefore feel you cannot do anything about. Simply stated, things do not work. The furniture you ordered does not arrive on time; the servants do not understand you; the repairs are done incorrectly; you feel cheated at the market; the children want macaroni and cheese for supper (a manifestation of their own anxiety?) and all you can find at the market is a bag of bug-infested noodles. And where are all those new friends who appeared like bees around a jam jar during the first few weeks? Sad to say, once newcomers are greeted, taken shopping and helped to order a few things, they are often left completely on their own. To the old-timer, the newcomer seems a part of the community long before he or she feels that way.

All of this leads to the next stage, *rejection*. A rebellion occurs. Unable to determine what is really wrong, the newcomer projects the problems onto the handiest scapegoat—the local culture—and develops what is often an intense dislike and even hostility. The same woman who was happily poking around the market and taking her children to nearby parks during the honeymoon stage now shops only in duty-free shops, buys Western-style food in cans and packages, and allows her children to play only in expatriate facilities.

Everything negative that happens is personal. The electrician who arrives late is deliberately trying to make your life miserable. The taxi driver who cannot find the street you want is part of a diabolical scheme designed to infuriate you. Things are judged in "black and white" or "we and they" terms. Everything at home is good, everything about this new country is bad. You may not be able to resist acting out your resentment in juvenile ways, perhaps because in trying to cope with a new culture you have really become a child again.

The fourth stage of culture shock is called *regression* and often occurs concurrently with the rejection stage. It is a time of retreat in which one does everything possible to avoid contact with the local culture and people. You spend long hours in a "safe haven" such as the American Club. Contact with servants is cut back severely and many people dismiss them at this time. Language classes begun with zeal during the pre-departure or honeymoon stage are dropped with such excuses as "I'll never use the language anyway" or "I know enough to get by."

What brings on this extreme negativism? Often it is a growing sense of being trapped. It hits you squarely that you are in this new country for some time. It is not a vacation. You cannot pack up and go when things get difficult.

There are people who never move beyond regression, even though they live overseas for years. But hopefully it is at this point that you slowly, often painfully, enter the final stage of the culture shock process, *adjustment*. This starts as you begin to feel comfortable in your new surroundings. How does it happen? For some people it seems to be simply getting to know their way around. It is a good feeling to get into a taxi and know where you want to go, how to get there, and what it should cost.

Language learning can be a major factor in successful adjustment. Lessons tend to begin again at this stage. You learn to speak enough to work your way around the market and engage in light-hearted conversation with the vendors. You begin to feel a degree of acceptance and it becomes easier to learn about the culture, its values and customs, its economic and political realities.

Ultimately, it is learning about the culture that is the major factor in your adjustment. You not only know your way about the town, you are beginning to know your way about the culture.

There appear to us to be two critical steps in dealing with culture shock and adjusting to life overseas. One is a willingness to view the values, attitudes, and behavior of your host culture as *different* from yours, rather than worse or wrong. The second is self-understanding, or, more precisely, cultural self-awareness. As examples of what this means, let us look at two basic cultural orientations that have a strong impact on cross-cultural interactions.

TIME ORIENTATION

For most Westerners, time is a fixed element. We segment and schedule it. We look ahead and are strongly oriented toward the future. Time is handled very much like materials: we earn it, spend it, save it, waste it.

We value promptness very highly. If people are not prompt, it is taken either as an insult or as an indication that they are not quite responsible.

Being kept waiting is usually seen as an insult to a Westerner. Waiting in anterooms is one of the most difficult experiences Westerners, especially Americans, have to deal with in many countries. In business meetings, the seemingly endless socializing their hosts require can tax to the limit the patience of a straightforward, let's-get-down-to-business American.

SPACE ORIENTATION

People's use of space differs from culture to culture. The distance people maintain from each other when riding in an elevator, stand-

ing in line or carrying on a conversation (often called "social distance") is culturally determined.

It is common when abroad to feel that our personal space is
being violated. Japanese trains are a good example of this. When
this occurs, we feel threatened at a very primitive level of awareness.
In some cultures—the Middle East, for example—personal space
begins inside the body, so that touching is not threatening. In most
Western countries, personal space begins some inches away from
the body (sometimes called an "envelope" of personal space), so
that being touched by strangers can be quite disconcerting.

Understanding our own orientation to space is important. We
may never grow to enjoy being jostled but we may come to feel that
we are not being threatened.

BEYOND CULTURE SHOCK: THE OTHER ADJUSTMENTS

Culture shock is a major hurdle to overcome while settling in overseas, but it is not the only one. Here are some of the other adjustments you should be prepared to make.

EVERYTHING IS NEW, LIKE IT OR NOT

There are few things more exhilarating than something new—a
new house, a new location, a new dress. But everything new at once
can be overwhelming. When faced with too many new and unfamiliar things, children can cling to their beloved blanket or teddy.
Adults are not so lucky. We need to plan how to make ourselves
and our families feel as secure as possible from the first day. Some
people take some "security" with them in the suitcase—favorite
pictures, loved pieces of bric-a-brac, even special pillows.

PRIVACY

Many people experience a significant loss of privacy when living
overseas. We tend to need time alone; we carefully cultivate privacy.
In many cultures, particularly in Asia, the idea that there is pleasure
in being alone is almost incomprehensible. In fact, in many lan-
guages there is no word for "private." Joy and contentment are
found in the presence of others and in the extended family.

Our sense of privacy may be violated by household help. Until
you become accustomed to having servants around, you may want
to stay out of the way while they are working.

LIVING WITH IMAGES

Wherever you go overseas you will have to live with the images people have of your country and its people. These images, or stereotypes, have been implanted by others who have gone before you and by the products of our cultures that have been sent abroad in large quantities. Unfortunately, it is often the worst of our cultures that has been exported: movies filled with sex and violence, lurid stories about entertainers and public figures. It is common all over the world to meet people who are certain that every Westerner is rich, lives in a mansion with a garage stocked with a fleet of expensive cars, uses drugs, and believes in "free love."

BARGAINING AND "BAKSHEESH"

In many countries, bargaining or haggling is an essential part of shopping. Many people who go to such countries find this one of the most uncomfortable aspects of their new lives. Others take to it easily and carry the habit back home with them—where it often works just as well! The best preparation for shopping in a bargaining culture is to have some idea of the going rates for things before you set out. You can get these from expatriates who have been in post for some time or from host country people with whom you work.

The giving of "baksheesh," which some call tips and others call bribes, is common in many, often poorer, countries. Here again one needs to ask long-term residents what is acceptable and when.

LOOKING DIFFERENT

In countries where your physical characteristics mark you clearly as different, you may feel a discomfort you have never experienced before. It takes time to get used to being different, to knowing that you will be stared at no matter how conservative your dress or unassuming your manner. Something as unexpected as the hair on a man's arms can cause a stir in a country where the men's skin is hairless. Once you understand why people react to you in the way they do, you will probably feel more comfortable and be able to learn from the experience of being in the minority.

STATUS OF WOMEN

In one country, the structure of the society was described to us by a national in this way:

"The most respected men are those who are doctors, then teachers, then other professional men. Farmers are next and finally laborers. People who have the least respect are those who have no employment to occupy them and thus are parasites on the rest of society."

"Where do the women come in?" was our innocent question. "Somewhere below the parasites" was the answer. Whether we like it or not, the status of women in the countries we go to will have an impact on us. To be comfortable, we need to find out what the rules are and adhere to them as much as possible.

LONELINESS

In an overseas post, surrounded or even overwhelmed by people, we can still be lonely because the old network of people to whom we once turned is not there. We are strangers in a strange land. A secretary with the U.S. Foreign Service expressed it this way: "If I were to give one piece of advice to women, especially single women, it would be to be prepared to be alone and face yourself."

BAD NEWS FROM HOME

When we learn that something is wrong at home, the normal stress and anxiety is magnified by distance. We can rarely fly off and take care of the situation. Even though international communications are improving daily, it can still be unsatisfactory and frustrating when we are trying to get critical information or comfort a loved one. The best and perhaps only way to deal with bad news from home is to be as fully prepared as possible. Steel yourself to think the unthinkable and decide ahead of time what you will do if it becomes reality.

MEETING THE CULTURE

Workers and spouses make contact with the local culture in different ways. The worker meets nationals in the office or other work contexts. Those they meet tend to be experienced with Westerners and able to accept or at least forgive cultural gaffes because, if nothing else, they value the worker's technical expertise or management skills. A spouse interacts with a different set of people, in trying to manage the home with a limited language ability and the willing but slow assistance of a new household staff and his or her own wits. There is little appreciation and understanding and no admiration for any managerial skills! The spouse thinks the culture is difficult while the worker thinks the spouse is not adjusting well. It is imperative that they stop and examine their lives from each other's perspective and try to understand how each perceives and interprets the experiences overseas.

FEELING OUT OF TOUCH

Hourly news reports, daily papers, and weekly periodicals keep you up-to-date at home. No matter how simple or esoteric your interests, sources of new and useful information are readily available. Not so overseas. If you do not have an official or "safe" mail service, news is old by the time you hear it, if it ever reaches you at all. You begin to feel out of step with your own country and the changes taking place there. Fads come and go and you have missed them completely! You may want to make arrangements to minimize this feeling by subscribing to a local newspaper from your home town, which although late will still let you know what has been happening, and by keeping in touch with friends and family with frequent letters.

CRIME AND VIOLENCE

The expatriate is vulnerable to three broad categories of crime and violence: household intruders, street incidents, and political terrorism. The chances of any of these happening to you can be minimized by being prepared and taking the advice of long-term residents as to precautions to be taken. Common sense is just as useful overseas as it is at home in avoiding the places and situations in which crime and violence are likely to occur (see also p. 274).

MANAGING STRESS

Living overseas is a stressful experience even for individuals and families who make careful decisions and prepare for the transition. Stress is a "fact of life," something built in, that must be dealt with in the normal course of living overseas.

Some of the most common warning signs are:

• anger that is difficult to control
• excesses in eating, drinking, and/or smoking

- nervous tensions
- physical illness
- withdrawal or denial
- marital problems
- depression

What can you do when you find yourself experiencing any of these signs? How can you cope and turn stress energy into positive action? Here are some suggestions that have been helpful for others.

STOCKTAKING
It may be time to sit down and take stock. Identify the good and bad, the positive and negative in your situation. List what makes you feel good about yourself and what is difficult. These lists can lead on to positive actions to improve things.

LEARN YOUR WAY AROUND, AND LEARN THE LANGUAGE
The cardinal rule for every newcomer is to learn your way around and to learn the language as soon as possible. But there is so much to learn at once that it may seem overwhelming. The only antidote to that feeling is to take control of the learning process and do it systematically.

MOVE WITH THE RHYTHMS OF THE COUNTRY, AND RELAX
Do not try to maintain the culturally based time orientation with which you grew up. Do not expect all deadlines to be met. When they are, consider it a bonus! Take time to relax, particularly during the busy settling-in period. The desire to get settled and start living is natural, but you need to take time out.

MAKE TIME FOR YOUR FAMILY
The social whirl that overtakes one in the expatriate community can be breathtaking. It is possible to go out every night of the week. One price you pay for succumbing to this pace is the loss of time with the family. You and they suffer. You have to make an effort to ensure that family time is sufficient for the children to adjust as well as you.

SEEK A SUPPORT GROUP
The family is a major support group. But if you are on your own or find that there are needs that cannot be met within the family,

you need to develop relationships with people with whom you feel comfortable. Avoid like the plague people whose major purpose seems to be complaining and gossiping.

ASK FOR HELP

If you cannot deal with the problems that are causing stress, seek help as soon as possible. You may only need a skilled listener such as a doctor, a pastor, or a friend. In some expatriate communities there are counselors and psychologists. Pack your favorite book on stress management techniques. And be assured that seeking help is not an admission of failure.

A SENSE OF HUMOR

Finally, you need a well-developed sense of humor, particularly the ability to laugh at yourself. From the day you arrive, funny things will happen, though they may not seem so at the time. You may have to work at getting the laughter going, but persist because it is truly the best medicine.

We hope we have not overemphasized the problems at the expense of the rewards of living overseas. Implicit in almost everything we have said is this message: living overseas is an exciting and enriching experience for the person who approaches it with a clear head and a flexible attitude. There is a quality of dynamism about living in another culture that can have a powerful and long-lasting effect on your life.

RETURNING HOME

The process of returning home is really an additional step in cross-cultural adjustment, occasionally referred to as *reverse culture shock*. Most people find that returning home has as many, if not more, pitfalls than the move overseas. This is usually because they have not prepared for the return with the same care they used in preparing for entry into a new culture. When they find that life at home is not as they imagined it, the ensuing depression and discouragement are harder to live with because they are unexpected.

Returning home is much easier if you have made the effort while away to keep in touch. If this has not been done, returning can be overwhelming, particularly for children who may be complete strangers.

Do not fall into the group known as the "when we's." These people are constantly talking about their travels and adventures, oblivious to the raised eyebrows, sighs, and shrugs of indifference. Strive to live in the present and not dream of the place you just left. As you complete the cycle of your overseas sojourn with your return home, you will need the same open-minded, interested attitude you had when you went overseas for the first time.

SUMMARY OF ADVICE FOR EXPATRIATES

- Be prepared to experience culture shock and know the stages you may go through on the way to adjustment.
- Look out for the signs warning that you may be unduly stressed. Take stock and seek help if necessary.
- Prepare for the return to your home country with the same care you took when going overseas.

13 PREPARATIONS FOR TRAVEL

HEALTH INSURANCE FOR INTERNATIONAL TRAVEL

Costs of health care abroad can be very high. Make sure that all your requirements are adequately covered *before* you travel.

Aaron Sugarman is a Senior News Writer for Condé Nast Traveler magazine, New York.

Dr. Richard Fairhurst is the Chief Medical Officer of the Travelers' Medical Service, and was formerly the Chief Medical Officer of Europ Assistance, London.

The modern traveler typically has a corporate or private health insurance policy, a wallet full of credit cards, and a sense of security that these will protect him in case of an accident or illness while on the road. This assumption is risky at best. There are gaps and loopholes in such coverage that can leave a traveler stranded, refused care by foreign hospitals, or stuck with a staggering bill for emergency care. To make matters worse, even policies marketed specifically for travelers may have crucial shortcomings.

Putting together proper insurance coverage need not be a maddening or time-consuming task. There are two basic steps: evaluating your needs, which includes a review of the coverage you already have, and evaluating policies available on the market.

THE RISKS

Why bother? Insurance company records suggest that 1 in 500 travelers will call his insurance or assistance service while abroad with a medical problem, 1 in 10,000 will require repatriation by air ambulance for medical reasons, and 8 in 100,000 will die abroad. In other words, while most travelers get by without mishap, the odds of an accident's happening are not impossibly long. And the price of being unprepared is too high to ignore: if you are incapacitated and need to be evacuated by an air ambulance, the cost can easily reach $30,000; and in many countries with modern medical facilities, hospitals often require payment in full, in local currency, either before they will treat a patient or before they will discharge one.

EVALUATING YOUR NEEDS

The first order of business is to review the coverage you already have. When polled, 55 percent of Condé Nast *Traveler* readers did not know if their health insurance plan covered travel outside the United States; call your insurance company or agent to find out. Corporate and private health insurance policies often cover foreign hospitalization and other medical expenses, but do not cover the cost of emergency evacuation. Medicare generally does not pay for hospital or medical services outside the USA.

If you are covered abroad, find out if your insurer will guarantee payment direct to a foreign hospital, and whether or not it will provide a cash advance: some policies only reimburse expenses after the traveler has paid the bill, which won't do you any good if the hospital insists on payment *before* treatment. Also check whether or not your insurer provides an emergency assistance hotline, or assistance with referral to English-speaking doctors abroad.

You should also check what coverage your credit cards provide. A standard American Express card, for example, gives you $100,000 in death and dismemberment coverage when you purchase a ticket with the card, but no hospitalization. Travelers carrying an American Express Platinum card, or a Gold MasterCard, generally receive free emergency evacuation coverage (check with the card provider for specifics, as there may be restrictions and coverage limits).

The next step is to consider your needs. These will be determined by your destination, the nature of your trip, and the extent of your existing coverage. If traveling to a country where medical care of a good standard is difficult to find, you should make certain that you are covered for emergency evacuation. For a trip to a European capital, such coverage is less crucial, though even in countries with socialized medical care, you may still have to pay for all treatment. Even if you do not require evacuation, you will still have to pay costs such as rearrangement of your travel plans. If you are traveling with members of your family, are they covered by existing policies, or will they need additional insurance? Does your policy have any gaps—that is, are there specific destinations (Libya, say, or Vietnam) or activities (skiing, scuba diving) that are not covered?

FILLING THE GAPS

Travelers uncomfortable with their existing level of coverage should shop for a supplemental policy. There are several reputable companies offering plans that combine travel insurance with foreign assistance programs. In general, they offer 24-hour emergency hotlines and help with referral to hospitals or English-speaking physicians, they arrange for payment of medical expenses, and if necessary, they organize and pay for repatriation by air ambulance. Some also tack on fringe benefits like legal assistance and lost-baggage insurance.

Costs vary depending on coverage and length of trip. A basic policy with Access America (a subsidiary of Blue Cross–Blue Shield; Tel. 800-284-8300) starts at about $50 for $10,000 coverage for a trip of 9–14 days. A family plan with $20,000 in coverage, plus full evacuation costs, starts at around $100. USAssist (Tel. 800-225-5911), International SOS Assistance (Tel. 800-523-8930), AMEX Assurance (a subsidiary of American Express, Tel. 800-234-0375), and Mutual of Omaha/Tele-Trip (Tel. 800-228-9792) all offer variations on the theme, with varying amounts of coverage and extras. Call several—or all—of them to compare the details.

Though you will obviously save money if you can manage to

avoid paying a second time for coverage you already have, this is sometimes not possible. You may find that you only need an emergency-evacuation policy, for instance, but that you can only get it as part of an entire package of insurance benefits. Still, it is undoubtedly better to be overprotected than undercovered.

RESTRICTIONS AND EXCLUSIONS

Before buying supplemental insurance, check the fine print for policy exclusions. Preexisting conditions are rarely covered. If you are in any doubt about whether a specific problem will be covered, it is better to find out in advance, and to know exactly where you stand. Get written confirmation that your insurer will cover the expenses relating to it. The general rule is this: if coverage for a condition or situation is not specifically spelled out somewhere in the policy, you should assume it is *not* covered. In special circumstances, you may need to have a policy customized to your exact needs, though you can expect to pay a substantial premium for it.

PREGNANCY

Pregnancy is a particularly tricky area. Some insurance companies consider it a "preexisting condition" and don't cover it, while others will cover only some types of care. In the event of a traveler giving birth while abroad, the odds are her insurance will not cover any costs incurred directly by the child even if it does pay for care of the mother. If this is a concern, you must have a policy specifically written to cover both mother and child.

You should bear in mind that a baby born prematurely may require several weeks of intensive care or hospitalization, during which repatriation may not be feasible: the costs may be extremely high.

THE YOUNG, THE ELDERLY, AND THE DISABLED

In general, children and young people are accepted on the same terms as adults, though there is sometimes a discount for children. The elderly obviously have an increased chance of making a claim under a health insurance policy and are more likely to have preexisting medical conditions (see following page). Disabled people in general are no more likely to become ill than anyone else, though disabilities can sometimes cause problems with repatriation, and it is therefore advisable for disabled people to notify insurance companies of their disability in advance.

PREEXISTING ILLNESSES AND MEDICAL CONDITIONS

Policies almost always exclude cover for "risks that could be reasonably foreseen by the client," or "travel against the advice of a physician." If you have any kind of preexisting medical condition, it is vital to notify the insurance company in advance, and to obtain written confirmation the problem *will* be covered. A letter from your physician stating that you are not likely to need medical treatment during the trip (rather than one that simply says you are fit to fly) is likely to be helpful in satisfying the insurance company.

There is also a moral issue here. Is it reasonable for insurance companies or physicians to encourage people with preexisting illnesses to travel abroad on vacation? Often a person who is ill perceives the vacation as being a valuable part of convalescence, and looks forward to the benefits it will bring.

No less often, however, neither the patient nor the physician gives adequate consideration to what will happen if the patient becomes ill again outside his own home environment. Even in countries with good medical facilities, being ill in a hospital where the doctors do not speak your language and cannot refer to your previous records can be a dangerous and unpleasant experience. In countries where medical facilities are poor, what was conceived as a period of convalescence and relaxation can be transformed all too readily into a nightmare.

People with a preexisting illness—and their physicians—should therefore satisfy themselves that adequate facilities for treatment really will be available if the condition recurs or deteriorates, and should think carefully about whether or not the risks are justified.

RISKY DESTINATIONS

Few policies cover acts of war or terrorism, and there are some places deemed too high-risk for coverage. At press time, Access America policies were not good for travel to Afghanistan, Cambodia, El Salvador, Iran, Iraq, Laos, Lebanon, Libya, Myanmar (formerly Burma), Nicaragua, Nigeria, North Korea, Yemen, and Vietnam.

SPORTS AND HIGH-RISK ACTIVITIES

Motorcycle riding, skiing, scuba diving, para-sailing, climbing, and the like are often excluded from travel-insurance policies. Some may also exclude driving, or driving rented cars, and many exclude manual labor and work. Of course, people participating in these activities are exactly the ones who most need insurance against accidents. To protect yourself, either find a policy that does not carry these exclusions, or have a policy specially written for you.

LIVING OR WORKING OVERSEAS

If you will be living or working overseas, you will need a form of permanent health insurance that will provide for all of your normal health-care requirements wherever you may be living. This usually includes some form of repatriation coverage, though this may be limited to repatriation to the nearest city where good medical care is available, rather than all the way home. These policies are usually taken out by employers rather than on an individual basis, but if you are going overseas to work, you should certainly demand such coverage as a condition of accepting the post.

YEAR-ROUND INSURANCE

Traditionally, travel insurance has been bought on a trip basis, in other words you purchase fixed-term insurance to cover the duration of a single trip. More recently there has been a trend toward providing year-round policies, albeit with a limit to the duration of any one trip. These annual policies are particularly attractive to frequent travelers, especially because they do not require prior notification of trips, and are always in force.

SUMMARY OF ADVICE FOR TRAVELERS

Accidents, as is their nature, will happen—and even the most cautious traveler may find himself in need of medical care while abroad. Insurance will not prevent accidents or illnesses, but it can help you deal with them when they occur. The best policies offer a support network to help you find proper care and cut through red tape, and can protect you from potentially ruinous financial liability.

IMMUNIZATION

All travelers visiting developing countries are exposed to an increased risk of infectious diseases. Although there are now few formal vaccination requirements for travel, immunization is an effective measure against some important diseases, and there have been many improvements in the vaccines available. All travelers should make sure they receive the recommended immunizations. On the other hand, it is not necessary to be immunized against diseases that are only an extremely small risk, particularly if they can be treated effectively.

Dr. Gil Lea *joined the airline medical service 20 years ago, developing the main British Airways immunization unit to provide the widest range of vaccines and other travel health advice, at what became two of the busiest clinics anywhere (Regent Street and Victoria, London). She is now Consultant Medical Advisor to Trailfinders Immunization Center, London, and to the Communicable Diseases Surveillance Centre of the Public Health Laboratory Service, London.*

Professor Robert Steffen *is President of the International Society of Travel Medicine, and runs the travel clinic at the University of Zurich, Switzerland, where he also conducts research.*

International travel is increasing, and people are choosing more exotic destinations for vacation. Relaxation of international vaccine regulations has made it easier—but not less hazardous—for travelers to visit risk areas without having first to seek specialist advice.

MANDATORY AND NONMANDATORY IMMUNIZATION

There is only one *mandatory* immunization requirement for travel—yellow fever—that countries are permitted to demand under the International Health Regulations of the WHO, and even this vaccine is required only for travel to or through certain parts of Africa and South America. Most of the immunizations available are nonmandatory, but for most overseas destinations outside Canada, Northern Europe, Australia, and New Zealand, one or more of them will probably still be *strongly advised*. In terms of health protection, these nonmandatory vaccinations are often far more important.

Unfortunately travel agents, embassy officials, and staff at national tourist offices tend to mention only the mandatory immunization requirements for a particular country (i.e., those for which a certificate is required), and may not tell you about other advisable precautions. It can therefore be quite easy for travelers to be left with the impression that no vaccinations are necessary for destinations like India or Thailand, simply because there are no mandatory requirements. In fact, several immunizations should be considered, and at the same time, the opportunity should also be taken to seek medical advice about malaria prevention (see p. 121) and other health precautions.

Travel agents and tour companies cannot reasonably be expected to provide detailed information about optional vaccinations and the choice of antimalarial tablets; they should certainly tell travelers about any mandatory requirements, however, and they should also remind them to consult a physician, an immunization center, or a travel clinic. A general outline of the current position is given below and in Appendix 1.

ABOUT VACCINES

Strictly, the word "vaccination" applies only to smallpox; however, the WHO's International Health Regulations refer to other immunizations by the same term, and the words "vaccination" and "immunization" have come to be used interchangeably (other than with immune globulins—see following page).

Vaccination stimulates the body's defense systems by introducing a small amount of the bacteria or viruses concerned (or their components or products) into the tissues. Some vaccines contain organisms that have been killed; others contain live organisms from strains that have been attenuated and are safe for inoculation. The vaccine stimulates antibody production, ready for when the real infection is encountered.

The number of doses required and the spacing between them depend on a variety of factors, like whether the vaccine is "live" or "killed," and whether protection has been received previously. Some vaccines provide long-lasting protection: once the initial courses of polio and tetanus vaccines have been completed, single "booster" doses every 10 years are all that is required to maintain protection. Yellow fever vaccine also protects for 10 years, whereas the injected cholera vaccine provides protection for less than six months.

It is important to realize that not all vaccines provide 100 percent protection, and other precautions, such as care with food, drink, and personal hygiene, are still necessary even when you have been vaccinated.

The only travel shot that is not a vaccine is immune globulin (previously called gamma globulin), which is used for protection against hepatitis A. Instead of stimulating the body's defenses, immune globulin is ready-made antibody. It does not last long in the body after injection, so it has to be given close to departure, and after the other shots.

Not every vaccine is suitable for every person, for reasons such as allergy, pregnancy, age, or because of certain medical conditions; these problems are considered below.

OBTAINING IMMUNIZATION

WHERE?

Yellow fever vaccine needs to be given in specially licensed centers (that can guarantee correct storage of the vaccine). Other vaccines can be given by your own physician, though most family physicians do not generally carry a stock of travel vaccines, and some of these may be difficult for you to track down if you are just given a prescription for them.

Yellow fever vaccine, and many of the other travel vaccines, are usually available at immunization clinics run by city, county, and state departments of health; if not, clinic staff should at the very least be able to tell you where you can get them.

There are now increasing numbers of more specialized travel clinics, mostly in cities with a large population of potential travelers, and some of these are listed in Appendix 8. These range from small clinics run by individual private physicians, to hospital- or university-based centers providing a comprehensive service. Most of the larger clinics carry a complete stock of vaccines, and provide information and advice on both mandatory immunization requirements and nonmandatory recommendations. Telephone numbers of vaccine manufacturers are also listed in Appendix 8, in case of difficulty obtaining supplies.

The major source of vaccine recommendations is the CDC in Atlanta (see Appendix 8), which provides recorded advice for travelers through its telephone and fax hotline, and also offers the option of speaking to a specialist in difficult cases.

WHEN?

All travelers should check their individual needs ideally four to six weeks before departure. A full immunization schedule may take one month or more to complete, but even if less time is available valuable protection can still be gained.

Common reasons for vaccination requests being delayed to the last minute are unexpected business trips, or news of sudden outbreaks of disease. Another reason may be the discovery that "no vaccinations are necessary for your trip" actually means that there may still be optional immunizations that are advised, at which point there may be little time left. Persons who may need to travel at short notice can avoid most problems by keeping their protection up to date by means of booster doses, particularly for the vaccines they are most likely to need: tetanus, polio, (and the new hepatitis A vaccine, where available) only need boosters every 10 years, once the initial courses have been completed; typhoid may also be worth keeping up to date, though its boosters are needed more frequently. Persons who may have to travel at short notice to tropical Africa or South America should also ensure that they have an up-to-date yellow fever vaccination certificate—the certificate is not valid until 10 days after injection but then remains valid for 10 years.

The dates for booster injections are not critical to the exact week and can be taken at any convenient time. If there is only time for a single dose of vaccine before your trip, it is worth completing the course afterward, to avoid the likelihood of the same problem occurring again, and so that only booster doses will be needed in the future.

IMMUNIZATION SCHEDULES

For many destinations, a single visit may be all that is necessary. Two visits spaced four to six weeks apart will allow administration of most commonly needed vaccinations—but a third visit six weeks to one year later will be needed for a traveler taking a first-ever course of polio, and a third visit is also necessary for rabies and

Japanese encephalitis vaccination. Yellow fever can be fitted into a two-visit schedule if required, but an extra visit to allow fewer injections at the same time would be preferable.

Where many vaccines are required, it is probably easier to go to an immunization center if there is one in a convenient location.

Don't forget to bring your previous vaccination certificates and details with you, for every visit.

TABLE 13.1. EXAMPLES OF IMMUNIZATION SCHEDULES (these should be planned individually for each traveler)

A. Overland trip through Africa, with about four weeks before departure:

First attendance:	yellow fever typhoid tetanus (booster) hepatitis A [hepatitis B first dose] [rabies (first dose)]
Second attendance: (one week later)	meningitis [rabies (second dose)]
Third attendance: (four weeks after first visit)	polio (booster) typhoid (second dose if required) [rabies (third dose)] [immune globulin] [hepatitis B second dose]

B. Rushed schedule, with only one attendance possible:

For Africa:	meningitis typhoid tetanus* polio* immune globulin yellow fever
For Asia: (Indian subcontinent or Southeast Asia)	meningitis (some areas) typhoid tetanus* polio* immune globulin
For South America:	typhoid tetanus* polio* immune globulin yellow fever

* These tetanus and polio immunizations should be booster doses, if not, courses should be completed *en route*, but only if hygienic medical facilities can be found (see note on p. 533 regarding injections abroad).

THE INJECTIONS

A surprising number of people are frightened by the thought of an injection. Young adults may not have had a shot since childhood, and the memory may still loom large. However, modern disposable needles are very small and sharp, and anyone who is well practiced can give these shots almost painlessly. Smaller doses of purer vaccines are often used, and adverse reactions are now less common.

Most travel vaccines are given into different layers of the skin, and the outer part of the upper arm is a convenient site. (Preferences vary: the French often give travel injections into the back, just below the shoulder blade.) The only injection given into the buttock is immune globulin, which contains more fluid and is more comfortably given into a large muscle.

Those attending for injections (and especially anyone who is prone to feeling faint) should eat normally beforehand. In general, there are no special rules regarding alcohol before or after an injection. However, if several injections are given in one day it may be advisable to avoid strenuous exercise or alcohol for several hours, but each individual should be guided by how he or she feels. Anyone who feels faint after the injections should immediately lie down with his or her legs raised. Anyone with a tendency to faint should ask to have the shots lying down, and should lie down for at least 15 minutes afterward.

The doctor or nurse who gives the injections should advise about malaria protection without being asked, but it is sensible for travelers to check on this if it is not mentioned; similarly this is a good time to ask about other travel medical problems like travelers' diarrhea, or what medication to include in a medical kit.

INDIVIDUAL VACCINES

YELLOW FEVER (see pp. 134–136)

The only remaining international vaccination certificate requirements relate to yellow fever vaccination. The vaccine provides virtually 100 percent protection for at least the 10 years that the certificate lasts, so it is understandable that many countries maintain their yellow fever regulations, although a traveler visiting only the capital city of a country reporting the disease may not be at risk.

Yellow fever exists only in two endemic zones, one across tropical Africa and the other in the northern part of South America (see

Map 5.2, p. 136). Not all these countries report disease all the time, but when planning to travel through these areas, it is wise to be immunized since epidemics may flare up after decades without a single case. Some countries require a certificate from all travelers; the rest may not require a certificate from those on direct flights from North America or Europe, but may do so for travel from one country to another within the zone; in addition it may be worth taking the vaccine for personal protection even if a certificate is not required (Appendix 1). There are many misconceptions about the

TABLE 13.2. DOSE INTERVALS FOR TRAVEL VACCINES

Vaccine or immune globulin	No. of doses	Primary course — Interval between 1st and 2nd dose	Primary course — Interval between 2nd and 3rd dose	Booster Intervals
Yellow fever	1			10 years
Typhoid (Injected, Vi)	2			3 years
Typhoid (Oral)	4	on alternate days	on alternate days	3–5 years
Tetanus	3	4 weeks	4 weeks	5–10 years
Polio	3	At least 6 weeks	At least 6 weeks	5–10 years
Rabies (pre-exposure)	3	7 days	21 days	2 years
Meningitis (meningococcal)	1			3 years
Japanese encephalitis	3	1–2 weeks	2–4 weeks	1–4 years
Tick encephalitis (East European)	3	1–3 months	9–12 months	3 years
Plague	3	1–3 months	3–6 months	6 months
Hepatitis A	2	6–12 months		5–10 years
Immune globulin (hepatitis A)	1			2–6 months according to size of dose
Hepatitis B	3	1 month	5 months	2–5 years

Note: 1. Recommended regimens vary slightly between vaccine manufacturers and countries. Intervals can in some cases be shortened or lengthened to suit travel arrangements.

yellow fever regulations, and travelers often ask for yellow fever vaccination when they do not need it.

As yellow fever does not exist in Asia, yellow fever vaccination is unnecessary for travel to Asian countries, *provided* travel is by the usual direct routes. However, for travel via Kenya to India, for example, a certificate *would* be required, as India wishes to avoid the introduction of the disease from Africa. There are many "yellow fever receptive" areas outside the zones in which yellow fever infections occur. These are countries that have similar climates (and mosquitoes) to the countries where yellow fever is endemic, and naturally they wish to prevent introduction of the disease.

Staff at embassies have on many occasions appeared to know the regulations only for direct travel to their countries; it is therefore important to find out about yellow fever vaccination from a reliable source, and to be sure to mention all the countries you will visit, in the correct sequence. Travel agents should have reference sources— such as the CDC publication *Health Information for International Travel,* and the *Travel Information Manual (TIM)*—that give up-to-date information; reference sources produced from within the travel industry are less likely to be reliable and up to date.

All of the vaccines mentioned below are optional, except that meningitis vaccination is required for the pilgrimage to Mecca.

TETANUS AND DIPHTHERIA

As tetanus can follow an injury (p. 91) everyone should be protected whether traveling or not. Certain kinds of travel—hiking, outdoor activities, and camping trips, for example—carry an increased risk of injury and good medical facilities may not always be readily available nearby.

Diphtheria vaccine is often combined with tetanus vaccine. It is particularly useful for adults who will be in close contact with children in developing areas, for example nurses and teachers (p. 99). They should take a booster if they have not done so in the last 10 years.

POLIO (see pp. 47–49)

Oral (Sabin) polio vaccine, taken on a sugar lump or as drops on the tongue or in water, is also included with the childhood vaccines, usually starting at two months of age. Any child who has not completed the course should do so prior to travel, and unpro-tected adults of any age should take the vaccine for travel to every-where outside North America, Western Europe, Australia, and New Zealand. Persons who have previously had polio should still receive the immunization: they may have immunity to only one of the three types of polio virus.

There are three types of polio virus and three doses in the initial course of vaccine. Each dose contains all three viruses and one of them has an opportunity to "take" each time. This provides a high level of protection, although sometimes not all types have taken, so booster doses may be recommended after 10 years for travel.

An injected (killed) polio vaccine is also available: this is an up-to-date version of the Salk vaccine used before the oral (live) vaccine was developed. The modern injected vaccine is used by choice in a few countries, and is given especially to those for whom the live vaccine is unsuitable; in the USA, this is the preferred vaccine for adults who have not been immunized previously. The disadvantage is that it may take longer to confer protection.

MEASLES
All children going overseas who have not completed their routine childhood immunization course, including measles vaccine, should do so (see p. 451).

Americans born after 1957 who have not previously been im-munized or had the disease are susceptible to measles and are at significant risk when they travel overseas; they should consult their physician for immunization (this should not be given at the same time as immune globulin).

HEPATITIS A (see pp. 50–53)
Hepatitis A is the most frequent vaccine-preventable infection in travelers: for every month spent abroad, 1 in 300 unprotected trav-elers will be infected. Protection against hepatitis A is particularly important for people traveling overland in developing countries (risk 1 in 50!) and for travelers to rural areas in developing coun-tries; increasing numbers of travelers are now choosing to be im-munized even for short trips, rather than risk a long and unpleasant illness on their return. The risk of dying from hepatitis A is less

than 0.1 percent for children and young adults, but this rate exceeds 2 percent in people aged over 40 years.

Immune globulin is an injection of antibodies that could be expected to provide protection against a number of diseases, but for the purposes of travel it is useful only against hepatitis A. It provides 85 percent protection for up to five months. Its main disadvantages are that protection is short-lived, that repeated doses are necessary, and that injection is often painful.

For frequent travelers, a blood test is available to check immune status and to determine whether or not further immunization is necessary. Unless they have a previous history of the disease, or have lived in the tropics for at least one year, young adults are not very likely to have a positive result, though the incidence increases with age. A positive result means that no further immunization is necessary.

As an alternative to the immune globulin, there is now an almost 100 percent effective new vaccine against hepatitis A that is becoming more widely available. A course of two doses is necessary for long-term protection. The second dose is given 6–12 months later. Protection lasts probably 10 years—much longer than with the immune globulin injection. In addition, the vaccine gives better protection and is less painful, and will be welcomed by long-suffering frequent travelers, who have had to endure repeated injections of immune globulin over the years. It is, however, considerably more expensive. It will shortly be licensed in the USA.

Although both injections protect against hepatitis A, caution with food and water hygiene is still necessary, since other forms of hepatitis are also spread by this route (see p. 51).

TYPHOID
Typhoid immunization is used rather too often as a travel vaccine, in view of the limited risk of infection encountered by travelers (risk 1 in 3,000 to 1 in 30,000) and the low case-fatality rate (less than 2 percent).

As it is a food- and waterborne disease, the risk is bound to be greater where hygiene conditions are poor, and the vaccine is therefore recommended for travel to high-risk areas, mainly the Indian subcontinent, North and West Africa; it is also certainly justified for rural travel through developing countries, and for prolonged stays there.

There are two routes of administering the vaccine: orally, and by injection. The oral vaccine currently used in the USA (Ty21a) is given in the form of four capsules, to be taken on alternate days. (In many European countries the same vaccine is given in three capsules.) Each capsule should be refrigerated until it is taken, or the vaccine may lose efficacy. This vaccine avoids the need for an injection—an idea that is popular with travelers. Reactions are few and efficacy generally considered to be similar to the injected vaccines (roughly 70 percent). The oral vaccine should not be taken during treatment with antibiotics, or on the same day as a dose of mefloquine (Lariam).

The traditional injected vaccine causes frequent reactions, in the form of discomfort around the site of injection for 24–36 hours, and fever, malaise, and headache. Two doses are necessary, and protection lasts three years. A new injectable vaccine has been developed (Vi), that is effective for three years following a single dose and is considered to cause little reaction. This has now been licensed in the USA.

All typhoid vaccines should be regarded as merely an adjunct to hygiene precautions, which are in any case the only way to avoid the commoner causes of travelers' diarrhea.

CHOLERA (see p. 31)
In June 1991 Pitcairn abandoned its international cholera vaccination certificate requirements for travelers coming from infected areas. It was the last territory in the world to do so; any request for a cholera certificate from now on, anywhere in the world, may be immediately identified as being unofficial and outside the WHO International Regulations. However, there have still been reports that Zanzibar continues to require a certificate from individual travelers. Elsewhere, threats of delays or, even worse, of compulsory injections, have virtually disappeared.

It is well known that the traditional injected cholera vaccine provides only about 50 percent protection and that most travelers are anyway at little risk from disease caused by the El Tor 01 strain (risk 1 in 300,000, case-fatality rate 1-2 percent). Although once the most commonly given travel vaccine, it is now seldom used; the primary method of prevention of cholera is by food and water hygiene precautions.

New cholera vaccines are in development, but the situation has been altered by appearance in Asia of a new strain, able to cause more severe illness, and against which these new vaccines may not be effective (see p. 33).

HEPATITIS B
The hepatitis B vaccine tends to be given mostly to travelers going on longer or repeated trips, and is fairly expensive. Hepatitis B is transmitted by the same routes as HIV—such as sexual contact, blood, serum, nonsterile needles and medical instruments, acupuncture, or tattooing. Ideally, anyone who might need medical or dental treatment in a developing country should be protected, as should health-care professionals going to work in those areas, and anyone who might have sexual contact with new partners while traveling. This is discussed in greater detail on p. 53; such travelers should also take full precautions against HIV.

RABIES (see pp. 197–203)
Until recently the only rabies vaccine available was so unpleasant that it was not used until *after* a bite, when the victim was faced with an imminent threat of rabies. The new vaccines are effective and safe, though fairly expensive; they produce very few reactions (a small percentage of people seem to be allergic and should not continue the course). These vaccines makes immunization *prior* to possible exposure to rabies feasible for the first time.

This does not remove the need for treatment after a bite but will reduce the amount necessary (fewer doses of vaccine and no serum injection) and can be expected to be effective even if there is a short delay before post-exposure booster doses of vaccine can be obtained. CDC recommends the vaccine for travelers to risk areas on visits lasting longer than 30 days: the risk of being bitten exceeds 2 percent per year in many places. Vaccination should also be considered by travelers who will be visiting particularly remote areas, more than a day's journey from medical care. It is important to avoid any delay in starting treatment after a bite, especially in people who have had no pre-exposure vaccination.

The antimalarial drugs chloroquine and mefloquine (Lariam) are thought to reduce the antibody response to the vaccine; if these drugs are being taken, the vaccine should not be given by the low-dose (intradermal) method, and the full intramuscular dose should be used.

MENINGOCOCCAL MENINGITIS
The only vaccine available is against the A and C meningococcal strains (or A/C/Y/W-135). The group A strain has caused outbreaks in countries of the endemic zone that stretches across Africa—especially in the meningitis belt stretching from Senegal to Sudan and Ethiopia (see p. 103); from 1989 onward some disease was also reported from Kenya, Uganda, Tanzania, Rwanda, and Burundi, which are south of the usual belt. Brazil has had outbreaks of several strains in the last few decades, and India and Nepal reported some group A meningitis from 1984 onward. There is no vaccine against the meningococcal B type—the commonest strain in most industrialized countries.

In view of the increase in reports of meningitis in the home countries of Muslim pilgrims traveling to Mecca, and the fact that there had been a number of cases in the Middle East the previous year, the health authorities in Saudi Arabia took the unprecedented step of making vaccination against meningococcal meningitis and a vaccination certificate mandatory for those joining the hajj pilgrimage in 1988. Meningitis is not a disease for which an international certificate of vaccination is provided under World Health Organization regulations, and this example illustrates how countries may, from time to time, impose their own restrictions on visas, making them conditional upon additional health certificates and requirements.

Travelers from the USA rarely contract the disease, and in general the vaccine is advised only for those going to areas with outbreaks in progress, or staying in endemic zones during the dry season, particularly if there is likely to be close contact with the local population. (See note on p. 104 regarding protection of travelers who have had their spleens removed.)

JAPANESE ENCEPHALITIS (see p. 139)
This disease is endemic across Asia, affecting many countries from India to Japan. It is seasonal in the temperate zones affected, but may be all-year-round in the tropics.

The virus is transmitted to humans by mosquitoes that have

bitten farm animals or birds, so that prolonged travel through agricultural regions constitutes the highest risk. The disease can be serious or fatal, but it has fortunately been reported only in a tiny number of Western travelers, and as the vaccine has to be imported from Japan in small amounts, a course tends to be rather expensive.

Travelers intending to reside in rural parts of Asia for at least two weeks should inquire about the likely risk before they travel. The vaccine is not licensed in Europe, but can be ordered specifically by general practitioners or taken at a specialist travel clinic. It is available at some clinics in Canada, Australia, and many Asian countries. It is licensed in the USA.

TUBERCULOSIS (see p. 86)

Vaccination against tuberculosis using BCG is seldom given in the USA, and has been gradually disappearing from immunization schedules in many industrialized countries. The main reason is that the vaccine tends to make it more difficult to diagnose tuberculosis if it does occur. However BCG remains part of public health policy in the UK and is recommended to British travelers on longer stays abroad.

PLAGUE (see p. 163)

Plague is transmitted by rodent fleas and the vaccine may be given to relief workers in disaster areas or for other work in plague endemic areas where avoiding contact with rats might be difficult. Only two travelers have been infected by plague in the past 25 years.

TICK-BORNE ENCEPHALITIS

Tick-borne encephalitis is an arbovirus infection that occurs especially in summer in the forests of Central and Eastern Europe (mainly Austria, Germany, and Switzerland), including parts of the Commonwealth of Independent States (formerly the USSR) and Scandinavia. It is a risk to foresters, campers, and hikers using paths not only in the wooded areas, but also through shrubbery on the fringes, where undergrowth can brush against their legs or arms.

SMALLPOX

Smallpox was eradicated worldwide in 1978. There is now no reason for any traveler to have smallpox vaccination under any circumstances.

WHEN NOT TO BE VACCINATED

Each case should be considered individually, but there are some general guidelines.

Vaccines to which the recipient has a known allergy are not normally given, and vaccines should not be given during acute illness. Otherwise, there are no particular circumstances when killed vaccines (see Table 13.3) should be avoided—with the exception of the injected polio vaccine, which contains trace quantities of penicillin and several rare antibiotics.

Gastrointestinal infections at the time of vaccination may inhibit the oral typhoid and polio vaccines from "taking."

Other specific cautions are allergy to eggs for yellow fever, tick-borne encephalitis, and measles vaccines, and to several rare antibiotics for both vaccines and polio.

IMMUNE DISORDERS

People with an impaired immune system, whether due to serious disease, steroid medication, cancer chemotherapy, or radiotherapy, should not usually take live vaccines (see Table 13.3). HIV-positive people are a special category who should avoid BCG and other live travel vaccines where possible; but those requiring yellow fever or polio protection should discuss with their physician the risk/benefit ratio that applies in their individual situation. HIV-positive children traveling should have measles protection.

PREGNANCY

Live and inactivated vaccines are listed in Table 13.3. During pregnancy (see p. 443) live vaccines are generally avoided, but in some circumstances they may still be advisable. There is no evidence that yellow fever vaccine has ever been harmful, and where there is a real threat from the disease (not just a certificate requirement), it may be given. Oral polio vaccine has been used in pregnancy without a problem, and *where urgent polio protection is vital,* experts prefer this vaccine to the injectable one.

Killed vaccines have been used for many years without any known ill effect, although anything causing a fever is undesirable, so the traditional typhoid vaccine has been given by the small-dose method in those few pregnant women who could be exposed to high risk of disease while traveling. Experience during pregnancy with newer killed vaccines like Japanese encephalitis and rabies is limited, and so the vaccines are usually avoided unless there is a definite risk, such as having already been bitten by a potentially rabid dog.

SMALL CHILDREN

Routine childhood vaccinations are very important (see p. 450). Cholera and traditional typhoid vaccines are not usually given under one year of age, and yellow fever not below nine or, occasionally, six months of age. The lowest age at which the oral typhoid vaccine is effective is uncertain—recommendations range from 18 months to six years; it should be borne in mind that the child must be able to swallow the capsules whole for the vaccine to be effective. The issue of hepatitis A protection is debatable, as children usually have no or very few symptoms of this infection, but they may upon return shed the virus and infect others. Children going to live overseas may be vaccinated against rabies, hepatitis B, and Japanese encephalitis, if the areas to be visited are considered to be sufficiently risky.

EXEMPTION

Where a certificate would normally be required, a letter or medical certificate of exemption signed by a doctor is usually acceptable to the authorities. Those who cannot be vaccinated on medical grounds have to consider the risks of travel without protection.

REACTIONS TO VACCINES—WHAT TO EXPECT

Yellow fever, oral polio, the new hepatitis A, the new typhoid, and modern rabies vaccines usually produce virtually no reaction. Chol-

TABLE 13.3. LIVE AND INACTIVATED VACCINES

Live vaccines	Inactivated vaccines
Yellow fever	injected Typhoid
oral Polio	injected Cholera
BCG (TB)	injected Polio
Measles ⎫	Tetanus ⎫ toxoid
Mumps ⎬ MMR	Diphtheria ⎭
Rubella ⎭	Meningitis
oral Typhoid	Rabies
	Hepatitis A
	Hepatitis B
	Japanese encephalitis
	Plague
	Whooping cough

era, tetanus, immune globulin, and the injected polio and traditional injected typhoid vaccines may do the same, but often produce some local soreness of the arm. Rubbing the arm may increase the irritation and should be avoided. A general off-color feeling, sometimes accompanied by a raised temperature, may follow cholera (unless given at low dose) and typhoid vaccines and lasts for up to 48 hours.

Should treatment be necessary, rest, plenty of fluids, acetaminophen tablets or soluble aspirin for adults (unless there is a past history of stomach ulcers) should be adequate. Red marks often appear at the injection sites and may disappear quickly or fade slowly, but, apart from BCG, virtually never produce permanent scars.

SIDE EFFECTS

Isolated cases of more serious side effects have been recorded *but are extremely rare.* Oral polio vaccine has been known to produce polio-like symptoms in some recipients or their close contacts on very, very few occasions (about three per 5 millon doses). It is recommended that unprotected parents take the vaccine at the same time as their babies.

SUMMARY OF ADVICE FOR TRAVELERS

If you are traveling through Africa or South America, check whether you need an international certificate of vaccination against yellow fever.

All other immunizations are optional. Obtain medical advice on planning a course to provide the best protection for your individual trip: for most travelers, it is wise to be immune against tetanus and diphtheria, polio and hepatitis A.

Immunizations are only *part* of your health protection, so don't forget to find out about the other measures you can take to protect yourself, such as food and water precautions, and precautions against malaria.

MEDICINES AND MEDICAL SUPPLIES FOR TRAVEL; INJECTIONS AND BLOOD TRANSFUSIONS ABROAD

What medical supplies should one travel with? Individual needs vary widely, and will of course depend upon precise travel plans: the destination, nature, and duration of one's trip, and whether or

not skilled medical care, medicines, and medical supplies are likely
to be available locally.

Dr. Richard Dawood *devised this project and is the editor of this book. He has
traveled in more than 70 countries around the world—and has survived.*

John A. Becher *is the Drug Service Chief, National Center for Infectious Diseases,
Centers for Disease Control and Prevention, Atlanta, Georgia.**

In this chapter, a number of common problems are considered
briefly, and so are the kinds of remedies that might be worth taking
along for them. A concise checklist of these items is given in Appendix 6 (p. 576).

SOME GENERAL POINTS

SAFETY

All drugs known to have any useful effect may also be potentially
harmful, especially if taken inappropriately or in excess. No drug is
suitable for everyone: if at all possible, you should seek advice from
your own physician about any medication you intend to use abroad.
Read manufacturers' instructions carefully, and take notice of them;
it is sometimes helpful to ask your pharmacist for a copy of the
manufacturer's package insert or a copy of the patient information
sheet.

Don't forget to keep all drugs and medicines out of reach of
children.

Do check the expiration date of any medicines you purchase
abroad. "Out-of-date" medicines can be harmful or ineffective, especially if they have not been stored correctly.

Counterfeit drugs and medicines are a growing problem in developing countries; some products are ineffective, and others are
actually dangerous. There have been a number of recent reports of
cases involving a variety of well-known brand names, particularly
in Africa and the Far East, where drug counterfeiting is believed to
occur on a large scale. It is better to take along anything you know

---

*   The use of trade names is for identification purposes only and does not imply endorsement by the Public Health Service (PHS) or by the United States Department of Health and Human Services (DHHS).

you might need, rather than to rely on being able to buy supplies locally. Inspect all packaging carefully, although fakes have certainly been concealed in authentic packaging. And bear this problem in mind if locally purchased medication fails to produce the desired effect.

DOSAGE

Keep strictly to recommended doses—twice as much is not necessarily twice as effective!

Always complete a full course of treatment if you are taking antibiotics, **but you should always discontinue any drug you suspect of causing adverse effects.**

DRUG NAMES

Most drugs have two names—a *generic*, or scientific name, that is usually the same or similar in most countries, and a *trade* or *brand* name that may vary from one country to another (some drugs are sold under several different brand names even in the same country). For example, in the UK there is a popular motion sickness remedy called *Kwells*; a British traveler asking for this brand name at a US pharmacy might easily be given a bottle of *Kwell*, lotion for killing lice.

To complicate matters still further, tablets containing combinations of more than one drug are sometimes given new generic names. For instance, the antibiotic trimethoprim/sulfamethoxazole is sometimes called co-trimoxazole. Make sure that you get what you *want* at a pharmacy abroad, not just what you have asked for.

Throughout this book, the *generic* name appears first; any names following in parentheses are *brand* names, but where there are a large number of different brands, these are not listed or only the better-known brand names are given; this does not imply endorsement of any particular brand.

PREEXISTING MEDICAL PROBLEMS

Travelers with any preexisting medical condition requiring drug treatment, besides taking with them an adequate supply of their usual medication, should also carry a prescription or written record of their medication giving its *generic* name in case further supplies are needed in an emergency.

It is also a good idea to inform the pharmacist of any preexisting conditions or any medication you are currently taking, whenever buying medicinal items from a pharmacy. The same advice applies when seeking treatment abroad from any source.

PRESCRIPTIONS

Medicines marked with an asterisk (*) are available in the US only with a doctor's prescription. In many countries, however, they can be purchased at any pharmacy or dispensary without restriction.

When traveling with medicines, the risk of customs difficulties can be reduced by making sure that they are all clearly labeled and in their original container, and that a prescription is carried whenever possible.

PACKAGING FOR TRAVEL

It is often more convenient to carry tablets in blister packs rather than loose in a bottle. After a few months of rattling around in a backpack, loose tablets can be reduced to powder. The strip packs can be kept in small sealable plastic bags, together with the manufacturer's instructions. A sealable plastic container can be used to store medicines and first-aid equipment, although backpackers may find a plastic zip wallet or waterproof pouch less bulky.

Jars of creams readily become contaminated with bacteria that grow rapidly in a warm environment and might introduce infection into open wounds. Tubes of creams are less likely to become contaminated than jars and are easier to carry, though care should still be taken to keep the cap of the tube clean and away from direct contact with the skin surface.

Suppositories need to be protected from extreme heat—they are designed to melt at body temperatures.

ATHLETES ABROAD

Athletes packing a travel kit should know that some of the medicines listed here may be banned from use in competitive sport. A list of banned drugs is available from the United States Olympic Committee, One Olympic Plaza, Colorado Springs, CO 80909 (Tel. 800-233-0393).

DIARRHEA

The advantages and disadvantages of the use of antidiarrheal agents for symptomatic treatment of diarrhea are discussed in detail on p. 27. If necessary, one of the following should suffice:

Bismuth subsalicylate (Pepto-Bismol) can be used to decrease the number of loose stools and shorten the duration of traveler's diarrhea by taking one ounce or two tablets (262.5 mg.) every 30 minutes to one hour as needed, up to eight doses in a 24-hour period. It is important not to ingest more than the recommended dosage or to use the drug for prolonged periods because of the danger of salicylate toxicity. Extra caution should be observed in anyone who is also taking aspirin or another salicylate, since any side effects will be additive. Large doses of bismuth subsalicylate can cause the tongue and the stools to turn temporarily black. Other side effects include nausea, constipation, and ringing in the ears. People with aspirin allergy, gout, or who are taking anticoagulants, methotrexate, or large doses of aspirin or other salicylates should avoid taking bismuth subsalicylate. Children should not be given bismuth subsalicylate because of the salicylate content and danger of Reye's syndrome.

Loperamide (Imodium) is a synthetic opioid, available by prescription or over the counter, that is used for symptomatic relief of diarrhea in adults. The dosage is 4 mg. to start, and then 2 mg. after each loose stool as needed, but not to exceed 16 mg./day. It is not recommended for use in children.

*Codeine phosphate** is used primarily as an analgesic or antitussive, but also has constipating side effects. Other antimotility drugs that are used for control of temporary cramping in diarrhea include *paregoric* (camphorated tincture of opium)*, and *deodorized tincture of opium**. All of these products are narcotic agonists and therefore require a prescription. They are all quite closely related to morphine and the regulations regarding their use can vary in different countries. As well as carrying a copy of the original prescription, it is also advisable to have with you a letter from the prescribing physician explaining why they are necessary.

*Diphenoxylate with atropine** (Lomotil). In the recommended dosage, this often causes a dry mouth and headache; it is unpleasant to take, and is now seldom used.

Of all of these medications, loperamide is generally preferable since it is the fastest-acting and has fewest side effects. It acts locally on the intestine, without entering the blood system. It is suitable for use by athletes, since it does not influence the results of drug tests.

These agents should not be used in the presence of a high fever or bloody stools. If diarrhea persists for longer than 48 hours, these medications should be discontinued and the advice of a physician should be sought. They should *not* be used in children.

See below for antibiotic treatment/prevention, and treatment of dehydration.

INTESTINAL INFECTIONS

TREATMENT

Currently recommended antibiotic regimens for treatment of diarrhea include: *trimethoprim/sulfamethoxazole** (e.g., Septra, Bactrim) 160 mg. TMP/800 mg. SMX, twice a day, or *ciprofloxacin** (e.g., Cipro) 500 mg. taken twice a day, or *norfloxacin** (Noroxin) 400 mg. taken twice daily, or *ofloxacin** (Floxin) 300 mg. twice a day until symptoms resolve, for up to three days. Loperamide (Imodium) may be taken at the same time, in the dosage referred to above. Antimicrobials should not be used in the presence of nausea and vomiting without diarrhea. Those allergic to sulfonamides should avoid trimethoprim/sulfamethoxazole. Treatment of diarrhea with antibiotics is discussed in greater detail on p. 25.

*Metronidazole** (e.g., Flagyl), and *trimethoprim/sulfamethoxazole** (e.g., Septra, Bactrim), or *ciprofloxacin** (e.g., Cipro) are useful drugs, and it is probably worth traveling with a supply of these if you are likely to be staying in a remote area for long. Instructions for use are given on p. 26. You should also discuss the appropriate use of these medicines with the physician who prescribes them.

Metronidazole would be needed to treat a bout of amebic dysentery. Three tablets taken three times a day for 5–10 days would be needed to complete a course of therapy.

*Mebendazole** (Vermox) can be used for the treatment of some of the worm infestations mentioned on p. 41 and p. 43.

PREVENTION

Bismuth subsalicylate (Pepto-Bismol) has been shown in several studies to decrease the incidence of traveler's diarrhea by 60 percent and appears to be an effective agent for the prevention of traveler's diarrhea. The dosage is two tablets (or 2 oz.) taken four times a day, with meals and at bedtime. It should not, however be used for periods longer than three weeks. Side effects and precautions are referred to above.

Antibiotics. Prevention of traveler's diarrhea with antibiotics is a controversial subject, and is discussed on p. 25. CDC does not recommend using antimicrobial agents for prophylaxis of traveler's diarrhea, nor do many physicians; however, some physicians do prescribe antibiotics to be taken upon the first sign of infection, where no medical care is available. The benefits of the prophylactic use of antimicrobials must be weighed against the risk of allergic reaction and side effects.

The following drugs are sometimes advocated, and there is evidence that they may prevent as many as 50 percent of attacks, but they should not be used for longer than two weeks:

*Trimethoprim/sulfamethoxazole** One double-strength tablet (160 mg. TMP/800 mg. SMX) (Bactrim DS, Septra DS) can be used for the prevention of traveler's diarrhea. The traveler must be aware; however, of possible serious side effects that could occur. These include skin reactions (e.g., rashes, urticaria, Stevens-Johnson syndrome), gastrointestinal disturbances, hemolytic anemia, neutropenia, and aplastic anemia, as well as photosensitivity (see p. 362). When taking this medication adequate fluid intake must be maintained. Any traveler who experiences skin rashes, a sore throat, fever, or unusual bruising and bleeding while taking this medication should seek the advice of a physician immediately, and should not take any further doses.

*Doxycycline** (Vibramycin) is an alternative antimicrobial for prophylaxis of diarrhea. The prophylactic dose is 100 mg. of doxycycline daily. Doxycycline should be taken with food or milk. Photosensitivity is a common side effect, so the traveler using this drug would be well advised to take precautions to reduce sun exposure by wearing protective clothing, dark sunglasses, and sunscreens (SPF 15 or greater). Doxycycline should not be used by children.

*Ciprofloxacin** (Cipro) taken at 500 mg. once daily or *norfloxacin** (Noroxin), a related drug, taken at 400 mg. once daily are also alternative antibiotics for the prophylaxis of traveler's diarrhea. Ciprofloxacin may be taken without regard to meals, but norfloxacin should be taken on an empty stomach, one hour before or two hours after a meal. Both of these antibiotics should not be taken concomitantly with antacids, zinc or iron preparations. If a skin rash, sore throat, or unusual bleeding occurs, consult a physician. These drugs should not be used by children.

*Trimethoprim** (Proloprim) can also be taken for prophylaxis at 200 mg. once a day.

DEHYDRATION

Most cases of diarrhea are self-limiting and require only the replacement of fluid and electrolyte loss. These can be replenished by drinking fruit juices and soft drinks (preferably caffeine-free) and eating salted crackers. Avoid ice in drinks or drinking anything made with water from a questionable source. Dairy products may aggravate diarrhea and should be avoided. Severe diarrhea causes rapid loss of fluid and salts, which can be particularly dangerous in small children, but can also cause symptoms in adults. Glucose promotes intestinal absorption of salts and water, and an understanding of this mechanism led to the formulation of special oral rehydration solutions. These solutions are easy to prepare, and instructions for making one's own are given on p. 27.

Oral rehydration salts (ORS) provide all the necessary ingredients, in convenient packets, that can simply be added to water, and should be carried in high-risk zones, especially when traveling with children. These preparations are available from Jianas Brothers Packaging Co., 2533 S.W. Blvd., Kansas City, MO 64108. Oral Rehydration Solution packets, recommended by the WHO, are available in stores and pharmacies of most developed countries. These packets should be reconstituted in a quart or liter of boiled or chemically treated water. The solution may be kept at room temperatures for a period of up to 12 hours, or up to 24 hours when refrigerated; discard any unused portions.

Infants with diarrhea have an increased risk of developing dehydration. Dehydration can often be prevented by feeding the infant with soup or watery porridges. Should the infant show signs of mild dehydration (i.e., increased thirst and restlessness), reconstituted ORS should be given frequently. If vomiting occurs, try giving the ORS in small sips. The infant should continue with breast-feeding, formula, and soup feeding through the duration of the illness.

Should the infant develop signs of moderate to severe dehydration (i.e., rapid and weak pulse, sunken eyes and anterior fontanelle, reduced urine output, absence of tears, fever greater than 102°F.

(38.9°C.) or blood in the stools) skilled medical care should be sought immediately.

Salt losses increase under tropical conditions and salt replacement may be necessary. Depending on the nature of your trip, it may be worth traveling with a small supply of ordinary table salt in a small, waterproof container. Salt tablets should not be used—they may take a long time to dissolve and may cause gastric irritation.

CONSTIPATION

Dehydration, readjustment of bowel habits after crossing time zones, dietary changes (including low-residue airline food), and initial reluctance to use dirty toilets may each contribute to this problem. A high fluid intake and a high-fiber diet are preferable to medication; it may be worth traveling with a small supply of natural bran (also available in tablet form). *Senokot* tablets are a safe and effective laxative if one is required.

HEARTBURN AND INDIGESTION

This is a common complaint at home and while traveling, and can be exacerbated by unfamiliar foods and overindulgence in alcohol. There is little to choose between the various antacid preparations; select one that you like and that is not too bulky to carry (e.g., *Tums, Mylanta, Rolaids*).

Gastric acid has a slight protective effect against several intestinal infections, so antacids should not be used unless symptoms warrant—nor should drugs that prevent acid secretion, like *cimetidine** (Tagamet), *ranitidine** (Zantac), *nizatidine** (Axid), *famotidine** (Pepcid), and *omeprazole** (Prilosec).

VOMITING

Specific treatment of vomiting in food poisoning is not generally advised or considered necessary unless symptoms are sufficiently severe as to require skilled medical treatment.

Once vomiting has begun, treatment with tablets is unlikely to afford relief and *prochloperazine** (Compazine) suppositories 25 mg. (5 mg. or 2.5 mg. for children), or *trimethobenzamide** (Tigan) 200 mg. suppositories (100 mg. for children), or *thiethylperazine**

(Norzine, Torecon) suppositories 10 mg. would be an alternative to injections, although they could melt in very hot climates. These products are not to be used in infants and small children of less than 30 pounds. Thiethylperazine should not be used in children less than 12 years old.

*Metoclopramide** tablets (Maxolon, Primperan, Reglan) 10 mg. are occasionally useful to treat nausea unrelated to motion sickness.

MOTION SICKNESS

Motion sickness is, by definition, almost exclusively a complaint of travelers, although people vary considerably in their susceptibility. It is discussed in greater detail on p. 245.

Since different anti–motion sickness drugs appear to suit different people, susceptible individuals may need to try several different pills on successive occasions until they find an effective remedy or regime—and then keep to it. Both phenothiazine-containing pills such as *promethazine** (Phenergan) and antihistamine-containing remedies such as *cyclizine** (Marezine), *meclizine* (Antivert, Bonine), and *dimenhydrinate** (Dramamine)* can have unwanted side effects; in particular, do not drive after taking them, because they may cause drowsiness (see also p. 250). Cyclizine, meclizine, and dimenhydrinate are available as over-the-counter (OTC) or as prescription preparations. *Buclizine** (Bucladin-S) is also very effective and may be dissolved in the mouth, chewed, or swallowed whole.

*Scopolamine** is available in the form of an adhesive patch (Transderm-Scop*) that allows absorption of the drug through the skin and remains effective for up to three days (see p. 251). These should not be used in children or the elderly, and may also cause dry mouth as well as drowsiness.

Some preparations of *Meclizine* (e.g., Antivert, Bonine) contain instructions to chew the tablets for rapid absorption. Otherwise, remember that anti-motion-sickness pills are of little use once vomiting has started—and make a point of taking the pills or applying the patch some hours before your journey begins.

URINARY TRACT INFECTIONS

Symptoms of cystitis are common in women and troublesome when they occur during a trip. Those prone to cystitis should discuss the problem with their own physician before leaving home.

Trimethoprim/sulfamethoxazole* (Septra, Bactrim) in a dose of two tablets or one double-strength tablet (160 mg. TMP/ 800 mg. SMX) twice daily for five days is likely to be effective for most urinary tract infections, but will not treat gonorrhea, which is a possible cause of urinary symptoms in travelers. Dr. Naponick's comments about this on p. 395 are worth noting.

VAGINAL INFECTIONS (CANDIDIASIS, MONILIASIS, YEAST INFECTION)

Like cystitis, this can be a particularly annoying problem when it occurs abroad. Treatment is discussed on p. 394, and it is well worth traveling with a suitable remedy, especially if you are prone to it.

If a vaginal tablet is to be used, one *clotrimazole** 500 mg. vaginal tablet (Gyne-Lotrimin, Mycelex G₃) will clear up an infection. The longer course of therapy (three or seven days) using 100 mg. *clotrimazole* (Gyne-Lotrimin) or 100 mg. *miconazole* (Monistat-7) can be purchased without a prescription.

OTHER INFECTIONS

Causes of fever in travelers are discussed on p. 396. Do not rely on antibiotics to treat a fever without seeking medical advice unless the cause of the fever is obvious. It is probably worth traveling with a course of a "broad-spectrum" antibiotic in the case of skin, sinus, or throat infections, and *ciprofloxacin** is a suitable choice (p. 403). *Trimethoprim/sulfamethoxazole** is a sensible alternative (dosage as in "urinary tract infections," above). *Amoxycillin/potassium clavulanate** (Augmentin) can be taken in most of the situations where trimethoprim/sulfamethoxazole has been suggested; it is actually superior in treating some types of infection, such as those of the skin (the usual dose is one tablet three times a day for five to seven days); it is best taken with food or milk and a full glass of water to reduce the incidence of an upset stomach, a known side effect. It must not be taken by people allergic to penicillin. Generally the first sign of allergy is a rash, and any antibiotic should be discontinued if this develops.

A rash sometimes develops with trimethoprim/sulfamethoxazole following exposure of the skin to strong sunlight, so it is worth using a high-factor sunscreen when taking this antibiotic.

PAIN

Headache, toothache, sunburn, minor injuries, and other causes of mild to moderate pain respond well to *aspirin, acetaminophen,* or *ibuprofen*, which are probably the only three mild painkillers the traveler need consider taking.

Aspirin Buffered preparations may decrease the chance of gastric symptoms, and are absorbed more rapidly. Aspirin also reduces temperature in a fever. It should be avoided by those with stomach ulceration, and should not be given to children or teenagers in the presence of chicken-pox or flu-like symptoms to avoid the possible complication of Reye's Syndrome.

Acetaminophen (Tylenol) has a comparable pain-relieving effect to that of aspirin, and causes no gastric symptoms. It also reduces temperature in fever and may be given safely to children.

Ibuprofen (Advil, Nuprin, Motrin IB) has anti-inflammatory properties that make it particularly useful for treating muscle and joint aches and pains. Like aspirin, it must be avoided by sufferers from stomach ulcers. Ibuprofen is available over the counter as 200 mg. tablets. Preparations containing higher strengths (e.g., Motrin, Rufen) require a prescription.

Codeine phosphate* can be used by travelers as a constipating agent to relieve diarrhea, in a dose of 30–60 mg. every four hours. It is also a valuable remedy for moderate pain. Codeine in smaller doses can be purchased in many countries without a prescription when combined with *acetaminophen* (e.g., Panadeine) or *aspirin* (e.g., Codis); however, in the U.S., codeine-combination products require a prescription (with the exception of cough syrup preparations).

An alternative would be *Hydrocodone*, available in the U.S. in combination with *acetaminophen (Lorcet, Lortab, Vicodin)** or *aspirin (Lortab ASA, Azdone)**. *Dihydrocodeine*, another codeine analog, is also effective as a combination product with *aspirin* and *caffeine (Synalgos DC)**.

These stronger painkillers (codeine, dihydrocodeine, and hydrocodone) are all quite closely related to morphine and the regulations regarding their use can vary in different countries. As well as carrying a copy of the original prescription it is also advisable to have a letter from the prescribing doctor explaining why they are necessary. This would not normally apply to the small amount of codeine in the compound preparations. However, in 1987 there was a single report regarding a nurse who was arrested and fined for carrying 10 tablets of Panadeine (acetaminophen with codeine) into Greece. The Greek government has since explained that this incident was a result of a misunderstanding and that there is no problem with carrying small quantities of such tablets for personal use.

JET LAG

No specific treatment has ever been conclusively proven to be of value. A short/intermediate-acting sedative/hypnotic such as temazepam, a benzodiazepine derivative (see below), may be helpful for the journey, and during readjustment of sleep patterns. (See also p. 238.) Benzodiazepines can produce dose-dependent impairment of recall along with other adverse effects, so they should be used with caution.

SLEEP

Sleeping tablets can be useful on especially long and tiring journeys—particularly across time zones, or overnight journeys in noisy surroundings. Sleeping tablets may also facilitate readjustment of sleep patterns in a new time zone, when used for the first night or two after arrival.

ADULTS

Temazepam* (e.g., Restoril) in a dose of 15–30 mg. (only the lower dose should be used in elderly people) is effective, short-acting, and rapidly eliminated from the body. It causes little or no hangover effect. It should not be taken with alcohol, which enhances its effects. Do not drive a car until the effects have fully worn off. There have been several case reports of short-term memory loss in travelers who have taken triazolam* (Halcion) with alcohol on long-haul flights.

CHILDREN

Promethazine* (Phenergan) in a dose of 5–10 mg. for children aged six to twelve months, 15–20 mg. for children aged one to five years,

The world's worst urban nightmare, or Africa's most vibrant city? The constant roar of traffic, blare of car horns, and wail of loudspeakers competing to summon the faithful to prayer from several thousand minarets have forced 62 percent of Cairo residents to resort to sleeping pills in order to get to sleep, according to a report in the London *Times*. The favored remedy is Valimil, the local brand of Valium, and earplugs are also at a premium.

and 20–25 mg. for children aged six to ten years may be useful occasionally.

MALARIAL PROPHYLAXIS AND TREATMENT

A detailed discussion of the choice and dosage of antimalarial drugs can be found on p. 127.

No drug regimen currently available will guarantee complete protection against malaria, and precautions against mosquito bites are essential. Contact the Centers for Disease Control and Prevention at (404) 332-4553 to obtain complete and up-to-date information on the risk of malaria in various countries around the world. In areas where choroquine-resistant malaria occurs, *mefloquine** (Lariam) is currently the recommended drug.

INSECT BITES

TREATMENT

Crotamiton* (Eurax) cream or lotion is often sufficient to relieve local irritation, and is more suitable than *calamine lotion*. (The FDA has recently ruled that zinc oxide, calamine lotion's main ingredient, is not active against pain and itching from rashes and insect bites.)

Antihistamines may be required if bites are widespread, with persistent, itchy weals. Avoid antihistamine creams and ointments—sensitivity to them can occur. *Chlorpheniramine maleate* (Chlor-Trimeton) tablets in a dose of 4–16 mg. daily, *diphenhydramine* (Benadryl) 25 mg. every four to six hours, or *hydroxyzine* (Atarax) 25 mg. every six hours is often helpful, but causes drowsiness. *Terfenadine** (Seldane) one 60 mg. tablet twice daily and *astemizole** (Hismanal) one 10 mg. tablet daily are effective new antihistamines that do not cause drowsiness. (Terfenadine should not be used while taking oral ketoconazole or erythromycin.)

Steroid creams *Hydrocortisone cream* (Lanacort, Cortizone-5) is a mild steroid cream that may be purchased without a prescription at 0.5 or 1 percent strength; this may not be sufficient for some people, and a more powerful preparation may be necessary.

Antibiotic treatment is occasionally necessary when bites are scratched and become infected. *Trimethoprim/sulfamethoxazole** would be effective in most circumstances (dosage as in "urinary tract infections" above). Under tropical conditions, infected bites and minor skin wounds, especially on the lower leg, need careful local treatment as well, to prevent formation of a skin ulcer that may take many weeks to heal.

PREVENTION

Insect repellents are a most sensible precaution, and are an essential part of any medical kit for travel to a hot country—see p. 182.

The most effective topical insect repellant known is *N,N diethyl-m-toluamide,* commonly called *"DEET."* DEET repels mosquitoes, chiggers, ticks, and fleas. It is widely available—more than 200 separate DEET-containing products are registered with the EPA (the best-known brands include Off!, Cutter's, and Repel).

Products containing high concentrations of DEET last longest on the skin, and are most compact to travel with, but generally have least cosmetic appeal. High-concentration liquids should be used sparingly—especially in children—and not smeared over the entire body surface, because significant quantities can be absorbed (see p. 183). Lower concentrations don't last as long.

Permethrin (Permanone), a pesticide, is sold as a clothing spray for protection against mosquitoes and ticks (see p. 191).

ALLERGIES

Treatment of bee-sting allergy is discussed on p. 219. Travelers who have had a serious allergic reaction of any kind in the past are strongly advised to travel with all they may need in an emergency.

If necessary, this includes adrenaline in pre-loaded syringes, or an inhaler.

Chlorpheniramine tablets *(Chlor-Trimeton)* in a dosage of 4–16 mg. daily are often useful to treat allergic skin reactions, and steroid creams may also be useful (see "insect bites" above).

If you suffer from hay fever, remember to take along any medication you may need. Hay fever seasons vary considerably between different countries.

SUNBURN

Prevention is the most sensible strategy. Sunscreens (see also p. 328) should be applied liberally. Water-resistant sunscreens are now widely available and are especially recommended for children. Stated protection factors usually refer to protection from UVB; check that any product you propose to use also protects against UVA.

Calamine lotion may be helpful for treatment of mild cases. *Aspirin* or *acetaminophen* is useful for pain relief (see "painkillers" above).

CONJUNCTIVITIS

Eye irritation following excessive exposure to sun and dust, and minor eye infections are common in travelers.

Antibiotic eye ointment and eyedrops are worth taking if medical supplies are not likely to be available en route, especially if you wear contact lenses, and the best choice should be discussed with your practitioner. *Chloramphenicol** drops need to be stored in a refrigerator; *gentamicin** eyedrops (Garamycin, Gentacidin) do not need refrigeration and are more suitable for travel.

COLDS/SINUSITIS

Air travelers liable to colds or sinusitis should travel with a *decongestant spray* (e.g., Sinex, Phenylephrine, Neosynephrine) to avoid discomfort from pressure changes during flight.

COLD SORES, HERPES BLISTERS

Strong sunlight, cold, and wind can trigger cold sores. Anyone who is prone to cold sores should use a high-protection-factor sunscreen on the lips. The duration and severity of attacks can be reduced by applying *acyclovir ointment** (Zovirax) at an early stage; this is not widely available abroad. A *lip salve* (e.g., Chapstick) may also be helpful for chapped and sore lips.

EAR PROBLEMS

External ear infection can be a problem for swimmers and divers. Advice on suitable drops to take is given on p. 339.

FIRST AID—CUTS, ABRASIONS, AND ANIMAL BITES

Prompt cleansing of any wound—with running water, or better still, with an antiseptic solution—is the most important step in treatment. Subsequently, keeping a wound clean and dry under arduous traveling and living conditions in a tropical environment can be difficult, but is extremely important.

TREATMENT

Local people sometimes ask travelers to remote areas to treat minor wounds, and it is worth carrying extra supplies of an antiseptic.

Iodine is a valuable antiseptic agent. A dry powder (povidone) *iodine spray* is now available in a small container (Betadine Aerosol Spray); it does not sting and removes the need to touch damaged skin.

SteriStrips and similar adhesive tapes are useful for holding together the edges of a clean, gaping wound if medical care cannot be obtained.

Wound dressings Band-Aids and similar dressings are essential for minor wounds and cuts. It is also worthwhile carrying nonadherent dressings that may be difficult to obtain abroad, together with tape (e.g., Micropore) to secure them. For those engaged in more hazardous activities, a standard wound dressing would be useful in an emergency. Keep wounds clean and dry; if they are oozing, change dressings frequently.

An Ace bandage may provide relief following a joint injury, but anything less than three inches in width would be of little use on a knee joint, for example. Other bandages, dressings, and slings can usually be improvised, and are probably not worth taking.

Larger expeditions may need to consider more extensive first-aid supplies, including inflatable or malleable aluminum (SAM) splints (Seaberg Inc., South Beach, OK).

Antibiotic treatment may occasionally be necessary if infection is more than trivial (see p. 200 for treatment of animal bites).

FUNGAL SKIN INFECTIONS

Antifungal cream and dusting powder are useful for treatment of athlete's foot and other fungal skin infections. See also p. 364.

SOME OTHER THINGS TO TAKE

1. *Water-purification supplies* are discussed in detail on pp. 75–76. The most reliable way to purify water and render it potable is to boil it vigorously and then allow it to cool to room temperature. Do not use ice. To improve its taste, a pinch of salt may be added to each quart.

   When boiling is not feasible, chemical disinfection may be accomplished using either *iodine tincture* or *tetraglycine hyperiodide* tablets. Five drops of iodine tincture (2 percent) to a quart or liter of clear water will achieve a chemical purification. If the water is cloudy or cold, use 10 drops of iodine tincture per quart or liter. Let the solution stand for 30 minutes. (If the water is cold or cloudy several hours of contact time may be required.) Iodine tincture doubles as a useful antiseptic for minor cuts.

   Tetraglycine hyperiodide tablets (Globaline, Potable-Aqua, Coghlan's) are available over the counter in pharmacies as well as from sporting goods stores. Follow the directions of the manufacturer. If the water is cloudy, the number of tablets used to disinfect the water should be doubled. If the water is very cold, try to warm it as well as increasing the contact time before drinking it. If no source of safe drinking water is available, as a last resort hot tap water that is uncomfortable to the touch is usually safe—allow it to cool before using it.

2. *Contact lens solution* Take ample supplies, and do not rely upon being able to obtain your preferred brand abroad. Bottles of sterile intravenous saline can usually be obtained cheaply from pharmacies in most countries, and are useful if other supplies run out. Keep solutions with you on long flights.

3. *Contraceptive needs* are discussed on pp. 430–439.

4. *Feminine hygiene* Take all your likely needs with you, unless you *know* that acceptable supplies will be available locally (p. 391).

5. *Catheter* Male travelers over the age of 65, or who have a history of prostatic symptoms (such as hesitancy or difficulty passing urine, or a poor urinary stream) should talk to their doctor about the possibility of traveling with a sterile urinary catheter that could be used by a local doctor in an emergency. In remote places, and in many developing countries, such items may not be easily available.

6. *Thermometer* If required, a thermometer should be carried in a protective container, and kept away from excessive heat. An ordinary clinical thermometer is not suitable for detecting or monitoring hypothermia (see p. 311); a special, low-reading thermometer should also be taken if it is likely to be needed.

7. *Toilet paper* Away from the beaten track, seasoned travelers take their own. In many parts of the world, toilet paper is not used, or is not readily available.

8. *Alcohol-soaked wipes* in small sachets are useful for cleaning minor wounds, and in a pinch can be used on suspicious-looking plates and cutlery.

9. *Lancets* These are small sterile needles covered with a twist-off plastic cap. They are normally used for pricking the thumb to obtain a small droplet of blood for testing. They are ideal for use by travelers to remove splinters or burst a blister.

10. *Rubs* If much walking will be done, an ointment for muscle aches or sprains can provide relief. There are many preparations on the market, such as *10 percent triethanolamine salicy-*

late (Aspercreme, Myoflex) or *methylsalicylate* (Banalg, Ben-Gay).

11. **Microscope slide** Travelers to remote malarial areas who develop a fever may have to treat themselves presumptively for malaria. A blood film made prior to treatment can be extremely helpful in confirming the diagnosis. The technique is simple to learn, and travel clinic staff may be willing to show you how to prepare your own film.

12. **Specimen containers** Providing a sample for a stool exam or urinalysis can turn into a test of ingenuity in countries where suitable specimen containers are not obtainable; you may need to bring your own.

INJECTIONS ABROAD

• Hepatitis and HIV are important hazards that have been discussed in detail elsewhere in this book. Hepatitis B has occurred in numerous travelers who have received injections with contaminated needles and syringes, and the HIV risk from this route of infection is also high. Disposable pre-sterilized needles and syringes are not widely available in many poor countries, and even when available, may not be provided unless specifically requested (you may also have to pay extra). If you are going abroad to live in such a country or expect that you will need any other medication by injection (including dental anesthesia) while you are away, you should *either* satisfy yourself that any needle or syringe used has been adequately sterilized (i.e., boiled for at least 10 minutes) *or* you should take your own supply. Remember that if you have an accident when driving abroad, a blood test for alcohol may be compulsory—this is the situation in Turkey, for example.

• In the USA and most other countries, a prescription is necessary to obtain needles and syringes; a prescription should *always* be carried when traveling.

• Regardless, it is better to avoid receiving any medication by injection at all—it can almost always be given effectively by an alternate route. Doctors sometimes do strange things: in one case, a traveler in Africa who requested treatment for sunburn was given injections of local anesthetic; he subsequently developed hepatitis B.

BLOOD TRANSFUSION ABROAD

The HIV risks have received much publicity, but are not the only hazard of blood transfusion abroad. Other risks include hepatitis A, B, C, D, E, cytomegalovirus, syphilis, Chagas' disease, and malaria. Transfusion with badly matched blood causes severe reactions and can be fatal, and in women can lead to serious antibody reactions in a subsequent pregnancy; allergic reactions also occur, and are more likely when storage conditions are poor.

- In most of Western Europe, North America, Japan, and Australasia, all donated blood is now screened for HIV antibodies, and prospective blood donors are questioned carefully about their lifestyle and risk factors for AIDS. The World Health Organization is working to improve blood transfusion services in all developing countries, and now believes that every capital city has at least one source of screened blood for transfusion.

- In developing countries, however, adequate facilities for screening donated blood and selecting donors are the exception rather than the rule, and at least two thirds of blood donations are thought to be unscreened. Building up a pool of blood donors requires a motivated and well-educated local population and a well-organized infrastructure. It also requires skills and resources that poor countries do not have. Most developing countries have only the most rudimentary blood-transfusion services, accessible perhaps only in capital cities.

- A clearer understanding of the risk of contamination of the blood supply is beginning to emerge. In a 1992 study of blood donors in Ivory Coast, West Africa, approximately 12 percent of donors tested positive for HIV, compared with rates of approximately 1 percent in sub-Saharan Africa just five years earlier. As the prevalence rises, the risk of infection from *screened* blood also increases, because current HIV tests all have a false-negative rate: laboratory and technical errors occur, and some people test negative while their infection is still incubating. In the Ivory Coast study, between 1 in every 94 and 1 in every 185 screened donations later proved to have been infected. The true risk is higher, however, because most people who need a transfusion need to receive more than one pint—i.e., from more than one donor. For comparison, in the USA in 1992, the incidence of transfusion-related HIV infection was between 1 in 40,000 and 1 in 153,000.

- Blood transfusion should be given only when medically essential: it is often possible to use plasma expanders or other intravenous fluids instead. The risks from a blood transfusion must, however, be balanced against the more immediate risk of NOT having a transfusion after serious blood loss in a life-threatening situation. People who are seriously ill generally find that they have little say in what happens, even in the unlikely event that they are well enough to protest: in England, a woman involved in a car accident recently received a transfusion on the orders of a court that overturned her refusal to have one.

- Don't travel to countries with poor medical facilities if you are pregnant or have a medical problem that might cause bleeding—stomach ulceration, anticoagulant medication, or any condition requiring surgery.

- Accidents are the commonest reason for travelers to need a blood transfusion, and after an accident, other medical facilities of a good standard may also be lacking. Avoiding accidents is the most effective way to avoid needing a blood transfusion, so take extra precautions, especially on the roads: wear seat belts, don't drive in the dark, don't drive too fast, and don't drink and drive (see also pp. 262–273). Peace Corps volunteers have recently been banned from driving mopeds or motorcycles, and there has been a dramatic reduction in their injury rate.

- It is possible to travel with plasma substitutes and intravenous fluids for use in an emergency, though such products require skill to use, and an adequate supply is bulky and heavy. In an emergency, supplies can sometimes be obtained from embassies. Likewise, sterile equipment to administer transfusions may be scarce; such items are sometimes included in first-aid kits for travel (see above). Large expeditions with trained medical officers may find it valuable to travel with such resources, but these are impractical for the majority of travelers, and this approach is unlikely to help you.

- Knowing your blood type in advance may make it easier to find a blood donor in an emergency—the embassy of your country may keep a record of screened donors who are willing to help. Other precautions include taking out health insurance that provides telephone support as well as evacuation by air ambulance in an emergency.

- HIV, blood transfusion, and contaminated needles have become the focal point of anxiety about medical care abroad, but in reality travelers are more likely to suffer not from medical treatment itself, but from the lack of it, which is why the *preventive* information in this book is so important. In the remote, exotic places that have greatest appeal to the serious traveler, there are no intensive-care units, no MRI scanners, no surgeons, and no ambulances. Fear of HIV should not deter any traveler who is prepared to observe sensible precautions.

FITNESS FOR WORKING ABROAD

Choose an overseas assignment with care, and make sure that you are in peak mental and physical condition before you go.

Dr. Anthony P. Hall is the medical adviser to a large number of companies and corporations; his patients have included included U.S. soldiers in Vietnam, rural Thais, and travelers from all over the world in London.

The success or failure of an overseas assignment often depends on the ability of the individual to remain physically and mentally healthy under difficult circumstances.

Some people cope better than others: think about your fitness and suitability for your assignment well in advance; the wrong decision has far-reaching consequences for your own career and for your employer.

DESIRABLE ATTRIBUTES

The apposite biblical quotation for foreign service is "many are called but few are chosen." Positive attributes for successful overseas service include birth or previous residence in the tropics and a family history of stability and successful accomplishment, especially abroad; a personal record of success in work and play; and a happy marriage.

Your reasons for going are important: a desire for new challenges and interest in your work are better harbingers of success than a desire for money or a need to escape—from a broken marriage or job failure, or after an abortion.

PSYCHOLOGICAL STABILITY

Those who work in the tropics have to adapt to a variety of psychologically adverse stimuli, including heat, humidity, bright light, poor diet, noise, road traffic accidents, boredom, language difficulties, racial tension, and the risk of being assaulted and robbed. Coping with these factors demands a high degree of mental toughness and emotional flexibility. If you are considering working abroad and are not sure whether you possess these attributes, don't go.

Unfortunately, many companies and other organizations regard the Third World as somewhere to send their misfits, so as to get rid of them. Employees may be given inadequate information about a foreign country, the job, and the problems they are likely to face (in fact these may be deliberately concealed), and backup facilities are often poor. Companies who employ such a policy in the selection and treatment of their overseas personnel are likely to meet with disaster—especially in the face of strong competition for the provision of goods and services.

PHYSICAL FITNESS

Everyone is at greater risk of illness in the tropics. In my opinion—based on examining several thousand people before employment abroad—the four most important avoidable risk factors are a high alcohol consumption, obesity, cigarette smoking, and extramarital sex.

ALCOHOL

A high alcohol consumption frequently leads to a deterioration in work performance. Individual responses and tolerance to alcohol are variable but a consumption of more than 20 grams of alcohol daily (contained in about one pint of beer *or* two glasses of wine *or* two single measures of spirits) is often related to an increased incidence of disease.

Psychological stress, less expensive alcohol, and boredom may induce people living in the tropics to increase their consumption of alcohol. Individuals with an existing high alcohol intake (i.e., higher than quoted above) who intend to work abroad are at significant risk of jeopardizing their health and should not go. Companies should avoid appointing heavy drinkers for work in tropical countries.

I advise expatriates to attempt to reduce rather than increase their alcohol intake, and to avoid other recreational drugs such as cannabis, "ecstasy," and magic mushrooms.

OBESITY

Excess fat is a greater hazard in hot than in cold climates. Apart from the higher risk of sudden death due to a heart attack, fat people have a higher incidence of sore rashes in the groin, heat intolerance, and other symptoms that may reduce the capacity for hard sustained work under conditions of heat and humidity.

Measurements of the circumference of the waist and hips are a useful guide to obesity. Most men have excessive body fat if their waist measurements are over 32 inches and women if their hip size is over 36 inches. The body mass index (BMI) is another useful guide.

The BMI is the weight in kilograms divided by the height in meters squared. In my opinion a BMI as near as possible to 20 (around 140 lb. or 64 kg. for a 5 ft. 10 in. (1.78 m.) man or around 126 lb. or 57 kg. for a 5 ft. 6 in. (1.68 m.) woman is desirable for a tropical climate.

A BMI over 25 indicates obesity, except in some very muscular young athletes.

SMOKING

People who use tobacco have a higher incidence of disease including heart trouble, peptic ulcer, lung cancer, and respiratory infections; stopping smoking is likely to improve your health wherever you are living, and going abroad presents a timely opportunity to give up smoking.

In rough terms, an alcoholic has at least twice the chance of becoming ill that a nonalcoholic has, and obesity and smoking carry similar twofold penalties. So an alcoholic obese smoker has eight times the chance of becoming ill that a fit person has. Of course, many companies would not be able to fill all their foreign vacancies if they employed only slim, fit, teetotal nonsmokers. The sort of people who are willing to work on an oil rig or in a remote mining camp are the sort of people who like to drink, smoke, and overeat. Nevertheless, such problems as high blood pressure, irritability, and diarrhea may all lessen if some excess fat is dieted off and if alcohol intake and smoking are halved.

SEX

I now consider that people should work abroad only if they take their spouse, because so many lonely people have unsafe sex and expose themselves to serious risk of infection with HIV and other STDs.

PRE-TROPICAL CHECKUP

A thorough medical checkup is advisable before undertaking any long-term overseas assignment. Spouses and children should also be examined. People with psychological or existing medical problems should not go.

Doctors carrying out pre-tropical examinations should not skimp on giving appropriate, and if necessary strict, advice to intending overseas workers or their employers, nor should such advice be ignored, even if it is not what the individual wants to hear. It is surprising how often the wrong advice is given, and the most unlikely people are passed "fit" for blatantly unsuitable assignments; setting off for the tropics in anything less than optimal physical and mental condition may all too easily result in an enforced early return home, either alive or in a box.

14 DISEASE ERADICATION: WHAT THE FUTURE HOLDS

The fact that travelers no longer have to concern themselves with smallpox or smallpox vaccination is a tribute to the effectiveness of the worldwide campaign that led to the eradication of smallpox, but the campaign's success also depended on many peculiarities of the disease itself. This chapter examines the prospects for eradication of other diseases within the foreseeable future. How soon will the world become a less dangerous place in which to travel, at least as far as disease is concerned?

The authors of this chapter were directly involved in the eradication of smallpox from large areas of the world.

Andrew N. Agle *was the Child Survival Coordinator at CDC in 1980–90, and is now Director of Operations at Global 2000.*

Dr. Donald R. Hopkins *was the Deputy Director of CDC from 1984 to 1987; he is now Director of the International Task Force for Disease Eradication, Senior Health Consultant to Global 2000, and the Guinea Worm Eradication Program Director.*

Dr. William H. Foege *was the Director of the CDC from 1977–83, and is now the Executive Director at the Carter Center and of Global 2000, and Executive Director of the Task Force for Child Survival and Development.*

If an ounce of prevention is worth a pound of cure, the eradication of a disease—the ultimate means of prevention—must be worth tons. Eradication is an absolute, and is defined as the achievement of a status whereby no further cases of a disease occur anywhere, so that continued control measures are unnecessary. For anything less than this, use of the word "eradication" is inappropriate.

BACKGROUND: THE SMALLPOX CAMPAIGN

By now, the story of the eradication of smallpox is well known. This unique achievement means that there is one less disease hazard for travelers to worry about and one less vaccination that is needed. No country now requires smallpox vaccination as a condition of entry.

Smallpox has been responsible for millions of deaths through the ages; it was eliminated as the result of a ten-year international effort coordinated by the WHO. In 1980, more than two years after the last recorded case of smallpox, and following the most careful scrutiny, a Global Commission certified that the disease was indeed no more.

For the first time in human history, a disease had been eradicated. WHO estimates the total cost of the eradication program to have been just over $300 million—considerably less than the *annual* cost to the nations of the world of preventing and controlling the disease.

If this was the first successful eradication effort, it was not the first that had been attempted. In fact, there had been an earlier global program to eradicate smallpox, which had failed. Malaria, yaws, and yellow fever are other diseases that were the subjects of eradication programs that fell short. The smallpox effort will not be the last: several other diseases are now candidates for eradication.

TARGETING OTHER DISEASES

In 1988, the International Task Force for Disease Eradication (ITFDE) was formed to systematically evaluate the potential for global eradicability of candidate diseases, to identify specific barriers to their eradication that might be surmountable, and to promote eradication efforts. The Task Force, based at The Carter Presidential Center in Atlanta, is made up of representatives of leading international agencies involved in health: WHO, UNICEF, the World Bank, the United Nations Development Program, the Rockefeller Foundation, the Institute of Medicine (U.S.), the Centers for Disease Control and Prevention (CDC), the Swedish Academy of Science, the Charles A. Dana Foundation, the Carnegie Corporation, and the Japanese International Cooperation Agency. The Carter Center secretariat consists of representatives of The Carter Center of Emory University and Global 2000, Inc.

Using the success of the smallpox eradication program as a guide, the ITFDE established criteria for evaluating the eradicability of other diseases. These criteria include scientific feasibility, and political, economic, and public support considerations.

WHAT MAKES A DISEASE ERADICABLE?

The following criteria are helpful for assessing the potential eradicability of a disease:

SCIENTIFIC FEASIBILITY

- Epidemiologic vulnerability (e.g., existence of non-human reservoir, ease of spread, natural cyclical decline in prevalence, naturally induced immunity, ease of diagnosis, duration of any relapse potential).
- Effective, practical intervention available (e.g., vaccine or other primary preventive, curative treatment, "vectoricide"). Ideally, intervention should be effective, safe, inexpensive, long-lasting, and easily deployed.
- Demonstrated feasibility of elimination (e.g., documented elimination from island or other geographic unit).

POLITICAL WILL/POPULAR SUPPORT

- Perceived burden of the disease (e.g., extent, deaths, other effects; true burden may not be perceived; the reverse of benefits expected to accrue from eradication; relevance to rich and poor countries).
- Expected cost of eradication (especially in relation to perceived burden of the disease).
- Synergy of attack with other interventions (potential for added benefits or savings, spin-off effects [e.g., polio eradication/Expanded Program on Immunization, Guinea worm/Water and Sanitation Decade, yaws/Primary Health Care]).
- Necessity for eradication rather than control.

Following the examination of 21 candidate diseases against these criteria, the ITFDE judged two of them—Guinea-worm infection and poliomyelitis—to be eradicable; three of them—mumps, rubella, and taeniasis/cysticercosis (tape worms)—to be potentially eradicable; another three—onchocerciasis, yaws and endemic syphilis, and rabies—to be candidates for elimination of transmission or of clinical symptoms; and the remainder not currently eradicable (Table 14.1).

Each of the two diseases deemed eradicable is now the subject of an active global eradication campaign (each benefiting from leadership provided by persons involved in the smallpox program). Guinea worm is still endemic in India, Pakistan, and at least 16 countries in Africa. Poliomyelitis is endemic in most developing countries outside the Western Hemisphere (where it has already been eliminated—no cases of polio have been reported in the Americas since August 1991).

GUINEA WORM ERADICATION

India was the first country to undertake an organized program to eliminate Guinea-worm disease (dracunculiasis), in 1980, as persons at CDC began a campaign for a global eradication effort linked to the International Drinking Water Supply and Sanitation Decade (1981–90). In 1986, WHO officially launched the global eradication program, and in 1991 it adopted an eradication target of 1995. India and Pakistan, the only two endemic countries in Asia, are making great progress with their programs and should eliminate the disease well before 1995. In Africa, Ghana and Nigeria have the longest-established programs, which commenced in 1987 and 1988, respectively. They have reduced their combined total of cases from 850,000 in 1989 to 240,000 in 1992. Most other endemic countries now have active, well-organized programs, except for Chad, Ethiopia, Kenya, and Sudan, where programs are just getting underway. The biggest threat to the program's success is that posed by the continuing internal strife in Sudan, which makes work there particularly difficult.

The program relies on preventive interventions, all of which are aimed at ensuring that no water is consumed that is contaminated with *Dracunculus* larvae. Unsafe drinking water causes immeasurable disease and suffering in the developing world, but none is so preventable as Guinea-worm disease. More than 100 million people are at risk of the disease, and as many as three million are infected each year, contracting the disease through drinking water that is

TABLE 14.1. DISEASE CANDIDATES FOR WORLDWIDE ERADICATION

Disease	Current annual toll worldwide	Chief obstacles to eradication	Conclusion
Guinea worm	10 million persons infected; few deaths	Lack of public and political awareness; inadequate funding	Eradicable
Poliomyelitis	250,000 cases of paralytic polio; 25,000 deaths	No insurmountable technical obstacles; increased national/international commitment needed	Eradicable
Onchocerciasis	18 million cases; 340,000 blind	High cost of vector control; no therapy to kill adult worms; restrictions in mass use of ivermectin	Could eliminate associated blindness
Yaws and endemic syphilis	2.5 million cases	Political and financial inertia	Could interrupt transmission
Rabies	52,000 deaths	No effective way to deliver vaccine to wild-animal disease carriers	Could eliminate urban rabies
Measles	2 million deaths, mostly children	Lack of suitably effective vaccine for young infants; cost; public misconception of seriousness	Not now eradicable
Tuberculosis	8–10 million new cases; 2–3 million deaths	Need for improved diagnostic tests, chemotherapy, and vaccine; wider application of current therapy	Not now eradicable
Hansen's disease (leprosy)	11–12 million cases	Need for improved diagnostic tests and chemotherapy; social stigma; potential reservoir in armadillos	Not now eradicable
Mumps	Unknown	Lack of data on impact in developing countries; difficult diagnosis	Potentially eradicable

TABLE 14.1—*continued*

Disease	Current annual toll worldwide	Chief obstacles to eradication	Conclusion
Rubella	Unknown	Lack of data on impact in developing countries; difficult diagnosis	Potentially eradicable
Hepatitis B	250,000 deaths	Carrier state, in-utero infections not preventable; need routine infant vaccination	Not now eradicable
Neonatal tetanus	770,000 deaths	Inexhaustible environmental reservoir	Not now eradicable
Diphtheria	Unknown	Difficult diagnosis; multiple-dose vaccine; carrier state	Now now eradicable
Pertussis	60 million cases; 700,000 deaths	High infectiousness; early infections; multiple-dose vaccine	Not now eradicable
Yellow fever	≥10,000 deaths	Sylvatic reservoir; heat-labile vaccine	Not now eradicable
Taeniasis/Cysticercosis	50 million cases; 50,000 deaths	Need simpler diagnostics for humans and pigs	Potentially eradicable
Cholera	Unknown	Environmental reservoirs; strain differences	Not now eradicable
Chagas' disease	15–20 million infected	Difficult diagnosis and treatment; animal reservoirs	Not eradicable
Schistosomiasis	200 million infected	Reservoir hosts; increased snail-breeding sites	Not now eradicable
Ascariasis	1 billion infected; 20,000 deaths	Eggs viable in soil for years; laborious diagnosis; widespread	Not now eradicable
Hookworm disease	900 million infected; 60,000 deaths	Laborious diagnosis; adult worms may live 5 years; widespread	Not now eradicable

contaminated by the worm's larvae. The threadlike parasite—which is up to three feet long—rarely kills, but its painful one-to-two-month emergence through an arm, leg, or foot incapacitates its victims, keeping children from school and farmers from their fields. The preferred intervention, provision of safe water sources (usually tube wells) is expensive and slow, and therefore is not sufficient on its own to enable the 1995 target date for eradication to be met. Other interventions include filtering all drinking water through finely meshed cloth, health education to prevent contamination of drinking water sources in the first place, or applying a chemical, temephos (Abate), to water sources at four-week intervals to kill the tiny water fleas (copepods) that carry the larvae.

As a part of the campaign strategy, endemic countries conduct village-by-village searches for cases of the disease nationwide to ascertain the full extent of the problem—i.e., the number and location of all endemic villages, and the number of cases occurring annually. They then train village-based health workers, at least one in each affected village, to conduct health education, to distribute cloth filters, to bandage Guinea-worm wounds, and to report cases every month. In Ghana, where there are more than 2,000 endemic villages, over 85 percent of the villages reported their cases consistently within 30 days of the end of each month, throughout 1992.

Toward the end of each campaign, as the annual number of cases falls below about 1,000 nationally or even within smaller areas, intensive "case containment" activities are undertaken. These are designed to detect each case within 24 hours of emergence of the worm, and to prevent any further contamination of the water supply from each case. A careful history is taken from each affected person, to try to determine the source of the infection (which may have taken place as long as a year previously), and to detect any bodies of water that might have been contaminated by the current infection. Cash rewards are sometimes used to increase the sensitivity of surveillance. Maximal mobilization and education of persons in affected areas is a key aspect of this stage as well as during the main intervention phase of national campaigns.

It is hoped the eventual success of the global campaign to eradicate the Guinea worm by 1995 will encourage and strengthen efforts to eradicate poliomyelitis by the year 2000. The surveillance systems established for monthly reporting of cases in those endemic areas should be a valuable legacy to the polio eradication campaign as well.

POLIO ERADICATION

Approximately 250,000 cases of paralytic poliomyelitis occur throughout the world each year, with an estimated 25,000 deaths (see also page 47). The disease's true extent remains hidden, however, because for every paralytic case there are 100 persons who carry the virus and can infect others, but have no symptoms themselves.

In 1985, the Pan American Health Organization (PAHO) declared a goal of eliminating indigenous paralytic polio from the Americas by 1990. Progress of that effort spurred the World Health Assembly, in May 1988, to declare a goal of global eradication by the year 2000.

The initiative to eradicate the indigenous transmission of wild poliovirus from the Western Hemisphere, using national vaccination days with live, oral poliovirus vaccine (OPV) and intensive surveillance activities, decreased the number of cases of poliomyelitis caused by wild poliovirus from about 1,000 reported cases in 1986 to nine laboratory-confirmed cases in 1991. Eight of the nine cases detected in 1991 occurred in Colombia during January through April; the only other case was in a two-year-old boy in Peru in August. No cases were detected in 1992.

The apparent elimination of wild poliovirus infection in the Americas underscores the feasibility of achieving a similar goal in other regions. The current WHO-recommended strategy for the global eradication effort is based on the experience gained by PAHO and includes maintaining high OPV coverage levels; improving surveillance for acute flaccid paralysis; conducting supplemental vaccination, such as national vaccination campaigns (in addition to the routine program); and establishing a global laboratory network.

Countries in the Western Pacific Region of WHO, including the People's Republic of China, have adopted the goal of poliomyelitis eradication by 1995. Although many countries in the African, eastern Mediterranean, European, and Southeast Asian regions still report endemic poliomyelitis, regional and national elimination plans have been developed and are being implemented. Major challenges facing the global initiative are:

- to generate the necessary political and social will in all countries
- to identify sufficient funds to purchase vaccine and conduct eradication activities
- to seek means of reducing the cost of OPV
- to refine strategies to achieve eradication in the most timely and cost-effective manner.

An improved polio vaccine, especially one that is more stable in tropical heat, would greatly speed the eradication of polio.

THE FUTURE OF DISEASE ERADICATION

Already the pendulum has swung back toward greater receptivity to the idea of disease eradication in international health and development circles, including WHO. The unique ability of an eradication program to marshal resources that would not otherwise be forthcoming is being increasingly demonstrated and understood, thanks to the Guinea-worm and polio eradication efforts. In the case of polio, the obvious self-interest angle for industrialized countries is especially important. This second example (smallpox was the first) of such favorable benefit/cost ratio for an eradication campaign of that type should help mobilize the support of decision makers in North America, Europe, and Japan.

This momentum will increase during the 1990s, with the expected successful eradication of Guinea worm in 1995 and polio in 2000. Major interim benchmarks, the achievement of which will feed that momentum in the meantime, are the elimination of Guinea worm from Asia in 1993; and the dramatic reductions in Guinea worm in Ghana and Nigeria as those two countries move closer to elimination.

In addition to eradication of Guinea worm and polio, by the year 2000 the potential eradicability of measles may have been demonstrated convincingly. Upcoming benchmarks with measles include Cuba's target of eliminating measles by 1990 (not yet achieved); the English-speaking Caribbean's target of eliminating measles by 1995; and the global goal of reducing measles morbidity by 90 percent by 2000. The good success of the Expanded Program on Immunization provides a much stronger base on which to build these immunizable disease eradication targets. Success with Guinea worm and polio will give even greater confidence (and experience) to take on subsequent targets, provided the latter are chosen carefully.

The systematic review of infectious diseases to evaluate their eradicability, carried out by the ITFDE, has already identified other promising candidate diseases "in the wings": mumps, rubella, and *T. solium* (pork tapeworm) cysticercosis (see page 45). Moreover, rapid improvements in technology and use of ivermectin may move onchocerciasis (page 145) to the forefront of the 1990s, especially once the Guinea-worm eradication program achieves the precedent of eradicating a parasitic disease.

One potential source of negative feedback is the ill-advised campaign to "eliminate" neonatal tetanus by 1995. This seems to be making little headway, and its prospects of near-term success are dim in any case. There will be some who will ignore the successes of smallpox, Guinea worm, and polio, and focus on the failures of malaria and tetanus eradication. The announced goal of leprosy elimination by 2000 is another such danger. Care must be taken to reserve declarations of global eradication or elimination campaigns for those that have very good prospects of succeeding. Eventually, the latter will include one or more non-infectious diseases, such as iodine deficiency.

At its first meeting, the International Task Force for Disease Eradication set forth the compelling rationale for eradication campaigns as a public health strategy:

- Control of a disease requires unrelenting effort and investment; eradication is permanent.

- Limited campaign duration, and campaign target dates, make possible concentrated efforts.

- Worldwide eradication targets create a powerful case for cooperation among neighboring countries.

- Eradication campaigns set a standard of success that is unambiguous.

Sequential eradication of diseases would multiply the benefits. Many of the same experienced health workers could be used in successive campaigns, with some of the savings achieved by elimination of one disease devoted to an attack on the next.

CONCLUSION

As far as travelers are concerned, there could hardly be a clearer example of the potential benefits of eradication than the case of smallpox. The eradication of polio will be another welcome development, but the pace of progress is still slow; there are only limited prospects for eradicating the other major travel-related diseases, and for many years to come, responsibility for staying healthy abroad will rest firmly with individual travelers themselves.

APPENDIXES

Appendix I

VACCINATION REQUIREMENTS AND RECOMMENDATIONS

I: Requirements

The only formal requirements relate to yellow fever vaccination.

A. The following countries require a yellow fever vaccination certificate from ALL arriving travelers:

Benin	Liberia
Burkina Faso	Mali
Cameroon	Mauritania*
Central African Republic	Niger
Congo	Rwanda
Côte d'Ivoire	São Tomé and Principe*
French Guiana	Senegal
Gabon	Togo
Ghana	Zaire

B. The following countries require a yellow fever vaccination certificate ONLY for travelers arriving from certain African or South American countries. These requirements do not apply for direct travel from the USA, Europe, or Australasia.

Afghanistan	Antigua and Barbuda
Albania	Australia
Algeria	Bahamas
American Samoa	Bahrain
Angola (R)	Bangladesh

KEY

R = vaccination recommended even if not mandatory

NC, R = no certificate mandatory, only recommended for some areas

* = except for visits shorter than two weeks, with direct travel from UK, USA, or Australasia

T = also required from travelers who have been in transit in infected areas

Infants: in most but not all cases, infants under one year are exempt from producing a certificate; however, the vaccine may sometimes be recommended for their protection.

These guidelines are based on WHO sources but are subject to change. Check the exact regulations that apply at time of travel, and make sure that you have no medical contraindications to the vaccine (see p. 512).

Barbados
Belize
Bhutan
Bolivia (R some areas)
Brazil (R some areas)
Brunei
Burma (see Myanmar)
Burundi (R)
Cambodia
Cape Verde
Chad (R)
China
Colombia (NC, R some areas)
Djibouti
Dominica
Ecuador (R some areas)
Egypt
El Salvador
Equatorial Guinea (R)
Ethiopia (R)
Fiji
French Polynesia
Gambia (R)
Greece
Grenada
Guadeloupe
Guatemala
Guinea (R)
Guinea-Bissau (R)
Guyana (R some areas)
Haiti
Honduras
India
Indonesia
Iran
Iraq
Jamaica
Kenya (R)
Kiribati
Laos
Lebanon
Lesotho
Libya
Madagascar (T)
Malawi
Malaysia
Maldives
Malta
Martinique
Mauritius
Mexico

Montserrat
Mozambique
Myanmar
Namibia
Nauru
Nepal
Netherlands Antilles
New Caledonia
Nicaragua
Nigeria (R)
Niue
Oman
Pakistan
Panama (R)
Papua New Guinea
Peru (R some areas)
Philippines
Pitcairn
Portugal (Azores and
   Madeira only)
Qatar
Réunion
St. Kitts & Nevis
St. Lucia
St. Vincent & the Grenadines
Samoa
Saudi Arabia
Sierra Leone (R)
Seychelles
Singapore
Solomon Islands
Somalia (R)
South Africa
Sri Lanka
Sudan (R some areas)
Suriname (R)
Swaziland
Syria
Tanzania (R)
Thailand
Tonga
Trinidad & Tobago
Tunisia
Tuvalu
Uganda (R)
Venezuela (NC, R some areas)
Vietnam
Yemen
Zambia (NC, R some areas)
Zimbabwe

II: Recommended vaccines

Recommendations vary from source to source; for example, even the WHO and the Centers for Disease Control and Prevention give slightly differing recommendations.

Travelers are strongly advised to seek advice from an up-to-date source at least four weeks prior to departure—an ample choice of suitable sources is listed in Appendix 8. The summary below is intended merely as a general guide.

Region 1: North America, Northern or Western Europe, Australia, New Zealand, Japan

Everyone should be protected against tetanus. No additional travel vaccinations are likely to be recommended except for very rural Japan.

Region 2: Eastern (Asian) Mediterranean and North Africa

Tetanus, polio, hepatitis A, and also typhoid (except Turkey, Tunisia) protection is recommended.

Region 3: Tropical Africa

Tetanus, polio, hepatitis A; in addition, yellow fever is recommended for travel to many parts of Central, West, and East Africa. Travelers to places other than the usual tourist destinations should be immunized against typhoid, and those staying for prolonged visits should be vaccinated against hepatitis B and rabies. In some areas protection against meningococcal disease may be advisable for long-stay travelers, and for short-stay visitors during an outbreak.

Region 4: Middle East

Tetanus, polio, hepatitis A; in addition, travelers to places other than the usual tourist destinations should be immunized against typhoid, and those staying for prolonged visits should be vaccinated against hepatitis B and rabies. Meningitis vaccine is required for the pilgrimage to Mecca and is recommended if there are any current outbreaks in the region.

Region 5: Asia

Tetanus, polio, hepatitis A; in addition, travelers to places other than the usual tourist destinations, and everyone visiting the Indian subcontinent, should be immunized against typhoid; those staying for prolonged visits should be vaccinated against hepatitis B and rabies. In addition, Japanese encephalitis (see p. 139) may be advisable. Meningitis vaccine is recommended for parts of India and Nepal, particularly when trekking.

Region 6: Mexico, Central and South America

Tetanus, hepatitis A; in addition, travelers to places other than the usual tourist destinations should be immunized against typhoid, and those staying for prolonged visits should be vaccinated against hepatitis B and rabies. Yellow fever vaccination is advised for travel to Panama and the Amazon basin area.

Region 7: Caribbean and Pacific Islands

Tetanus; in addition, travelers to places other than the usual tourist destinations should be immunized against typhoid and hepatitis A, and this is especially important for travel to Haiti and the Dominican Republic; those staying for prolonged visits should be vaccinated against hepatitis B, and for certain Caribbean islands, rabies. For the Pacific islands, polio is advisable.

Note: Cholera vaccination is *not* officially required for entry to any country, and the injected vaccine is not recommended by the WHO (see p. 508). There is no longer an "official" cholera vaccination certificate. If you do not want the vaccine, but are worried you might have to show some kind of documentation on your travels, ask your physician to write a letter stating that it is medically inadvisable for you to receive the vaccine.

Appendix 2

MALARIA—RISK AREAS FOR DISEASE AND DRUG RESISTANCE

Countries where malaria occurs

Afghanistan
Algeria
Angola
Argentina
Bangladesh
Belize
Benin
Bhutan
Bolivia
Botswana
Brazil
Burkina Faso
Burma
Burundi
Cambodia
Cameroon
Central African
  Republic
Chad
China
Colombia
Comoros
Congo
Costa Rica
Djibouti
Dominican
  Republic
Morocco
Ecuador
Egypt
El Salvador
Equatorial Guinea
Ethiopia
French Guiana

Gabon
Gambia
Ghana
Guatemala
Guinea
Guinea-Bissau
Guyana
Haiti
Honduras
India
Indonesia
Iran
Iraq
Ivory Coast
Kenya
Laos
Liberia
Libya
Madagascar
Malawi
Malaysia
Mali
Mauritania
Mauritius
Mexico
Mozambique
Namibia
Nepal
Nicaragua
Nigeria
Niger
Oman
Pakistan
Panama

Papua New Guinea
Paraguay
Peru
Philippines
Rwanda
São Tomé and
  Principe
Saudi Arabia
Senegal
Sierra Leone
Solomon Islands
Somalia
South Africa
Sri Lanka
Sudan
Suriname
Swaziland
Syria
Tanzania
Thailand
Togo
Turkey
Uganda
United Arab
  Emirates
Vanuatu (formerly
  New Hebrides
Venezuela
Vietnam
Yemen
Zaire
Zambia
Zimbabwe

Areas where chloroquine-resistant *falciparum* malaria occurs

Central and South America
Bolivia, Brazil, Colombia, Ecuador, French Guiana, Guyana, Panama, Peru, Suriname, Venezuela

Asia
Afghanistan, Bangladesh, Bhutan, Burma, Cambodia, China, India, Indonesia, Iran, Laos, Malaysia, Nepal, Pakistan, Philippines, Sri Lanka, Thailand, Vietnam, Yemen

Oceania
Papua New Guinea, Solomon Islands, Vanuatu

Africa
Chloroquine-resistant *falciparum* malaria may occur in any country in sub-Saharan Africa.

Note: Malaria distribution may vary significantly within countries and from time to time. Use the addresses in Appendix 8 to obtain up-to-date information, and if necessary refer to the CDC or WHO publications listed under "Further Reading" (p. 593). Malaria prophylaxis is much safer than malaria, so if in doubt it is safest to take it.

Further information

Malaria Branch, Centers for Disease Control and Prevention, Atlanta, GA 30333, Tel. (404) 332-4555
Malaria Action Program, World Health Organization, 1121 Geneva, 27-Switzerland, Tel. 791-21-11

Appendix 3

GEOGRAPHICAL DISTRIBUTION OF INFECTIOUS DISEASES

One of the most basic and obvious questions that a book like this could be expected to answer is also the most complex: what diseases occur where?

In one sense, the answer ought not to really matter. Travelers who want to stay healthy should adopt healthy habits wherever they go.

Statistics that filter back to the World Health Organization in Geneva depend upon:

1. An accurate medical diagnosis in the first place, which in turn usually needs doctors and perhaps laboratory facilities for confirmation;
2. A public health bureaucratic infrastructure, with sufficient resources and enthusiasm at every level to gather statistics and pass them on;
3. Governments' and authorities' willingness to permit disclosure of information that might be seen as a deterrent to tourism or as harmful to their image.

Reliable information about the distribution of disease is therefore most lacking from the countries of greatest interest to readers of this book: countries with plenty of disease but scarce medical resources; and where official statistics do exist, they almost always underestimate the true scale. Some countries under-report their cases of many diseases—perhaps so as not to harm their image or their tourist trade.

The tables that follow are a compromise that takes account of the fact that travelers nonetheless need access to this kind of information. They are based on WHO figures and a combination of other sources, with modifications when these are unconvincing or inadequate. Where official figures are absent, estimates have been sought from doctors working in the countries concerned or with specialist knowledge of particular diseases.

The figures given here do not correspond directly with the risk to individual travelers: they give a **rough indication** of the occurrence of particular diseases in the local population. There is often considerable variation in the distribution of disease **within** any one country, and all of the figures listed here are based on generalizations that cannot take account of this, or of differences in disease patterns between rural and urban areas. It is virtually impossible to make any meaningful generalization, for example, about a nonuniform land mass the size of the Commonwealth of Independent States (formerly the USSR) (which we have omitted from the tables), and the same probably applies to China, India, Brazil, and the Sudan.

The tables are far from flawless, and should be used with caution. In particular, they should **not** be used as a basis for important decisions, such as whether or not medical treatment should be sought after a dog bite.

We would like to acknowledge our gratitude to colleagues in some sixty countries (mostly Fellows of the Royal Society of Tropical Medicine and Hygiene) who have kindly given us the benefit of their opinion and local experience in amending the tables.

Some of the databases listed in Appendix 9 may be able to supply more specific local information about risks within countries and regions.

—Dr. Michael Barer and Dr. Richard Dawood

KEY

S = Similar or smaller number of cases per million population to those occurring in the USA; or no cases at all.

L = 3–10 times number of cases relative to the USA.
Or
Less than 10 cases per million population (where disease does not occur in the USA).

M = 11–100 times number of cases relative to the USA.
Or
11–100 cases per million (where disease does not occur in the USA).

H = Greater than 100 times number of cases relative to the USA.
Or
More than 100 cases per million population (where disease does not occur in the USA).

Africa (North)

	Cholera	Typhoid	Shigellosis	Amoebiasis	TB	Plague	Brucellosis	Diphtheria	Meningococcal infection	Polio	Yellow Fever	Dengue or other arboviruses	Viral hepatitis (A + B)	Rabies	Typhus	Malaria	Leishmaniasis	Trypanosomiasis	Syphilis	Gonorrhea	Schistosomiasis	Liver flukes	Hydatid disease	Tapeworms	Filariasis	Hookworm	Other intestinal worms
Algeria	H	H	L	M	H	S	M	H	M	M	S	S	H	H	S	M	H	S	S	S	L	S	H	L	S	L	L
Egypt	S	M	L	L	M	S	L	M	L	M	S	L	H	L	L	L	M	L	L	L	H	L	H	L	L	L	L
Libya	L	L	M	L	M	M	S	M	L	M	S	S	H	H	L	L	L	L	S	S	M	L	M	L	L	S	L
Mauritania	H	M	L	M	H	S	S	M	M	L	S	S	H	M	L	L	L	L	L	S	L	S	L	L	M	S	L
Morocco	M	L	M	M	S	S	M	L	M	S	S	H	L	L	M	S	L	L	H	S	M	L	S	S	L	S	L
Tunisia	M	M	L	M	M	S	S	L	L	M	S	S	H	H	L	L	M	S	S	L	L	L	M	L	S	L	L

Africa (Western)

	Cholera	Typhoid	Shigellosis	Amoebiasis	TB	Plague	Brucellosis	Diphtheria	Meningococcal infection	Polio	Yellow Fever	Dengue or other arboviruses	Viral hepatitis (A + B)	Rabies	Typhus	Malaria	Leishmaniasis	Trypanosomiasis	Syphilis	Gonorrhea	Schistosomiasis	Liver flukes	Hydatid disease	Tapeworms	Filariasis	Hookworm	Other intestinal worms
Benin	H	L	H	H	M	S	M	L	H	H	S	S	H	M	L	H	S	L	S	L	H	L	L	M	L	M	M
Burkina Faso	H	M	M	H	M	S	M	M	H	L	S	S	H	H	L	H	L	M	L	L	L	S	L	L	L	L	M
Cameroon	H	L	L	M	M	S	L	M	H	S	S	H	M	L	H	S	M	L	H	M	L	M	L	M	M	M	M
Cape Verde	H	L	L	L	M	S	L	L	H	M	S	S	M	H	H	S	L	H	H	H	M	L	M	L	M	L	H
Chad	H	H	M	H	M	S	M	M	M	L	M	M	L	M	H	L	M	L	S	L	L	L	L	L	M	L	L
Gambia	H	L	M	M	M	S	L	L	H	L	M	M	H	M	L	H	S	L	H	H	H	L	L	M	L	M	L
Ghana	H	H	M	M	M	S	L	S	H	H	M	M	S	H	S	L	S	H	H	S	L	S	H	H	S	L	H
Guinea	H	M	M	M	M	S	M	M	H	M	S	M	H	L	L	L	H	S	L	S	M	H	L	L	L	H	M
Guinea-Bissau	H	M	M	M	M	S	S	M	H	L	S	L	H	L	L	L	H	S	L	L	L	L	L	L	M	M	M
Ivory Coast	H	M	M	M	M	S	L	M	H	L	L	L	H	M	L	H	S	M	S	S	M	S	L	M	S	M	L
Liberia	H	M	M	M	M	S	L	M	H	M	L	L	H	L	H	S	L	S	M	L	L	L	L	M	L	M	M
Mali	H	M	L	M	M	S	L	M	H	H	S	S	H	H	L	H	L	L	L	M	L	M	L	L	L	H	L	M
Niger	H	L	L	M	M	S	L	M	H	M	M	M	H	H	L	H	S	M	M	M	M	H	L	L	L	H	L	L
Nigeria	H	L	H	H	M	S	M	L	M	L	S	H	H	L	H	S	M	S	M	H	L	L	H	L	L	H	M
Sao Tome and Principe	H	L	L	H	L	S	M	M	S	H	S	S	M	M	L	H	S	M	S	L	L	L	L	L	H	L	L
Senegal	H	M	L	H	M	S	L	H	H	H	M	M	H	H	M	L	H	S	L	M	S	L	L	L	M	L	L	M
Sierra Leone	H	H	M	M	H	S	L	S	H	L	L	H	L	L	M	L	H	S	L	S	H	H	H	S	S	L	H	M	M
Togo	H	L	L	H	M	S	L	L	H	H	S	S	H	H	L	H	S	M	S	S	H	L	L	L	H	M	M

Key   L: 'Low'   M: 'Medium'   H: 'High'   S: Similar or fewer cases relative to United States

Africa (Central and East)	Cholera	Typhoid	Shigellosis	Amoebiasis	TB	Plague	Brucellosis	Diphtheria	Meningococcal infection	Polio	Yellow Fever	Dengue or other arboviruses	Viral hepatitis (A + B)	Rabies	Typhus	Malaria	Leishmaniasis	Trypanosomiasis	Syphilis	Gonorrhea	Schistosomiasis	Liver flukes	Hydatid disease	Tapeworms	Filariasis	Hookworm	Other intestinal worms
Burundi	H	M	M	H	M	S	M	L	H	M	M	M	H	L	H	H	S	M	S	S	L	L	L	L	L	S	L
Central African Republic	H	M	M	H	M	S	L	M	H	M	M	M	H	M	L	H	L	M	S	L	L	L	L	L	M	L	S
Congo	H	M	M	M	M	S	M	M	H	L	M	M	H	M	M	H	S	M	L	L	M	L	L	L	M	M	L
Djibouti	H	M	H	H	M	S	S	M	H	H	L	L	H	M	L	H	L	L	S	L	L	L	L	L	L	M	L
Equatorial Guinea	H	M	M	H	M	S	S	M	H	M	M	M	M	L	H	S	M	L	S	L	S	L	L	L	L	L	L
Ethiopia	H	M	M	H	M	S	M	M	H	M	S	S	H	M	M	H	M	L	S	L	L	L	H	H	L	L	L
Gabon	H	M	L	M	M	S	L	L	H	M	S	S	H	L	M	H	S	S	S	L	L	L	L	L	L	L	L
Kenya	H	L	L	L	L	M	L	L	H	M	S	S	H	L	M	H	M	H	M	S	L	L	L	L	H	M	M
Malawi	H	M	M	L	M	S	L	L	H	L	S	S	H	M	L	H	S	M	S	L	H	L	L	L	M	H	M
Rwanda	H	M	H	H	M	S	L	L	H	H	S	S	H	M	L	H	S	M	M	L	M	S	L	L	M	L	L
Seychelles	S	S	S	L	M	S	S	M	L	M	M	H	M	L	L	S	S	M	M	L	L	L	L	L	M	L	L
Somalia	M	M	L	H	S	L	L	M	H	M	S	S	H	M	L	H	S	L	L	L	L	L	M	L	M	L	L
Sudan	H	M	M	L	M	S	L	H	H	H	S	S	M	L	M	L	H	M	M	S	H	L	M	M	M	M	M
Tanzania	H	L	L	M	M	H	L	L	L	H	S	S	H	L	M	H	S	S	M	L	L	L	L	L	L	L	L
Uganda	H	M	M	H	M	S	L	L	M	H	L	H	S	S	H	L	M	H	S	L	L	H	L	L	L	H	H
Zaire	H	M	M	M	M	H	L	M	H	L	L	L	H	M	H	H	S	M	L	S	L	L	L	L	L	H	L

Africa (Southern)	Cholera	Typhoid	Shigellosis	Amoebiasis	TB	Plague	Brucellosis	Diphtheria	Meningococcal infection	Polio	Yellow Fever	Dengue or other arboviruses	Viral hepatitis (A + B)	Rabies	Typhus	Malaria	Leishmaniasis	Trypanosomiasis	Syphilis	Gonorrhea	Schistosomiasis	Liver flukes	Hydatid disease	Tapeworms	Filariasis	Hookworm	Other intestinal worms
Angola	H	M	M	M	H	M	M	L	L	M	L	L	H	M	L	H	S	M	S	L	H	L	L	L	H	H	L
Botswana	H	L	L	M	H	S	L	L	L	L	S	S	H	M	L	M	S	M	L	S	L	L	M	H	M	L	H
Lesotho	H	M	L	S	H	L	S	L	L	L	S	L	H	M	L	S	S	S	M	M	S	S	S	H	S	S	H
Madagascar	H	L	M	L	H	H	S	M	L	M	S	S	H	M	L	H	S	S	S	L	L	L	L	L	L	L	H
Mauritius	S	M	L	L	L	S	S	S	L	S	M	S	S	L	S	L	M	S	S	S	S	H	L	L	L	L	L
Mozambique	H	S	L	M	H	L	M	L	L	M	S	M	H	L	H	S	M	S	S	M	L	L	M	M	H	H	H
Namibia	L	M	M	L	H	L	L	L	L	L	L	L	H	M	L	H	S	M	S	S	L	L	L	L	L	L	H
Reunion	S	M	L	H	L	S	L	M	S	L	S	S	M	M	L	S	S	L	M	S	L	L	L	M	L	S	L
South Africa	M	L	L	M	H	L	M	M	L	L	S	M	M	L	H	S	S	M	M	H	H	L	M	H	S	M	H
Swaziland	M	M	M	M	M	S	M	L	L	L	S	M	H	M	S	H	S	S	S	M	M	H	S	S	H	S	H
Zambia	H	L	M	M	H	S	L	M	L	M	S	S	H	L	H	S	H	M	L	L	M	L	L	M	M	H	H
Zimbabwe	H	L	L	L	M	L	L	L	L	L	S	S	H	L	H	S	H	L	M	H	L	S	M	H	L	M	H

Key L: 'Low'   M: 'Medium'   H: 'High'   S: Similar or fewer cases relative to United States

Asia: Near and Middle East	Cholera	Typhoid	Shigellosis	Amoebiasis	TB	Plague	Brucellosis	Diphtheria	Meningococcal infection	Polio	Yellow Fever	Dengue or other arboviruses	Viral hepatitis (A + B)	Rabies	Typhus	Malaria	Leishmaniasis	Trypanosomiasis	Syphilis	Gonorrhea	Schistosomiasis	Liver flukes	Hydatid disease	Tapeworms	Filariasis	Hookworm	Other intestinal worms
Afghanistan	S	M	M	M	M	S	H	M	S	L	S	S	H	M	M	L	M	S	S	S	L	S	M	L	L	H	H
Bahrain	L	H	M	H	L	S	L	L	S	H	S	S	M	H	M	H	M	S	S	L	L	S	L	L	L	L	M
Iran	H	H	H	M	L	S	H	L	S	L	S	S	M	L	S	H	H	S	S	S	M	S	M	M	M	S	M
Iraq	H	M	S	M	L	S	L	H	H	H	S	S	M	M	M	H	H	S	S	S	M	S	M	L	L	L	M
Israel	S	M	H	S	S	S	S	L	S	M	S	S	M	L	M	S	M	S	S	S	S	S	S	L	S	S	S
Jordan	L	M	M	M	L	S	S	L	S	L	S	S	M	S	S	L	L	L	S	S	S	L	S	M	S	M	M
Kuwait	S	H	M	M	M	S	H	L	H	L	S	S	H	S	L	S	M	S	S	S	S	S	M	L	S	S	L
Lebanon	H	M	L	L	L	S	L	L	L	M	S	S	M	L	L	S	L	S	S	S	L	L	M	S	L	L	L
Oman	L	M	S	L	M	S	L	H	H	H	S	S	M	M	H	M	S	S	L	M	S	L	L	L	L	L	L
Qatar	L	H	S	S	M	S	H	M	S	M	S	S	M	L	L	S	S	S	L	S	M	S	L	L	L	L	L
Saudi Arabia	L	M	L	M	L	S	M	M	H	L	S	S	H	S	L	M	M	S	S	S	M	S	M	L	M	L	M
Syrian Arab Republic	L	M	S	M	S	S	S	H	L	M	S	S	M	M	H	M	S	L	L	S	M	S	L	L	L	L	L
Turkey	L	M	M	M	L	S	L	M	L	M	S	S	M	M	M	H	L	S	S	S	L	L	H	M	L	S	H
United Arab Emirates	L	H	H	M	H	S	S	M	S	L	S	S	H	H	L	L	L	S	S	S	M	S	L	L	L	M	M
Yemen	L	M	S	M	H	S	S	H	H	L	S	S	M	H	M	H	M	S	S	S	M	S	H	L	M	L	H

Asia: Central and S. East	Cholera	Typhoid	Shigellosis	Amoebiasis	TB	Plague	Brucellosis	Diphtheria	Meningococcal infection	Polio	Yellow Fever	Dengue or other arboviruses	Viral hepatitis (A + B)	Rabies	Typhus	Malaria	Leishmaniasis	Trypanosomiasis	Syphilis	Gonorrhea	Schistosomiasis	Liver flukes	Hydatid disease	Tapeworms	Filariasis	Hookworm	Other intestinal worms
Bangladesh	H	M	H	H	M	S	S	M	H	L	S	M	H	H	M	H	L	S	S	L	S	S	L	L	L	M	M
Brunei	S	L	L	L	M	S	S	S	S	S	S	L	L	S	M	S	S	S	S	S	L	S	S	L	L	M	M
India	H	H	H	H	H	S	H	H	H	M	S	L	H	H	M	M	S	S	S	M	M	M	M	H	M	H	M
Indonesia	H	M	M	M	M	S	L	M	L	M	S	H	H	M	H	S	S	L	L	L	S	L	M	L	M	H	M
Malaysia	H	M	M	L	M	S	M	M	S	S	S	M	H	S	L	H	S	S	S	S	L	L	S	L	M	H	H
Mongolia	S	L	S	S	L	L	L	M	S	L	S	S	L	H	L	L	S	L	S	S	S	L	S	L	S	L	L
Myanmar	H	M	M	M	M	L	M	L	S	S	S	S	M	H	L	H	L	S	S	S	S	S	M	L	M	M	H
Nepal	H	M	L	M	L	M	S	S	M	H	S	S	L	H	M	L	L	L	S	S	S	L	L	L	L	L	H
Pakistan	M	H	H	H	M	S	H	H	H	H	S	M	H	H	M	H	M	S	S	S	L	M	M	M	M	H	H
Singapore	M	M	L	L	L	M	S	S	L	S	S	S	M	M	S	L	S	S	S	L	L	S	S	S	L	L	L
Sri Lanka	M	M	L	M	M	S	L	L	L	M	S	M	H	M	L	H	S	S	H	H	S	S	S	S	M	H	H
Thailand	M	M	H	M	M	S	M	S	M	S	M	M	L	H	S	S	M	M	M	M	M	L	H	H			

Key   L: 'Low'   M: 'Medium'   H: 'High'   S: Similar or fewer cases relative to United States

Asia: Far East	Cholera	Typhoid	Shigellosis	Amoebiasis	TB	Plague	Brucellosis	Diphtheria	Meningococcal infection	Polio	Yellow Fever	Dengue or other arboviruses	Viral hepatitis (A + B)	Rabies	Typhus	Malaria	Leishmaniasis	Trypanosomiasis	Syphilis	Gonorrhea	Schistosomiasis	Liver flukes	Hydatid disease	Tapeworms	Filariasis	Hookworm	Other intestinal worms
Cambodia	H	M	M	M	L	L	M	H	M	H	S	M	H	M	M	H	L	S	S	S	L	L	M	M	L	M	M
China	H	L	M	L	M	L	L	M	L	L	S	L	H	M	L	H	L	S	S	S	M	L	L	L	M	M	M
Hong Kong	L	L	M	L	H	S	L	L	S	L	S	L	H	M	L	S	L	S	L	M	L	M	L	L	L	L	L
Japan	L	S	L	L	L	S	L	L	S	L	S	L	L	S	L	S	L	S	S	S	S	L	L	L	L	L	L
Korea	H	L	S	L	M	L	M	M	M	L	S	L	H	L	M	S	L	S	S	L	L	M	M	L	L	L	L
Lao People's Dem Rep	L	L	L	M	M	S	M	H	L	S	M	M	M	L	M	L	S	L	L	L	L	L	L	L	L	L	L
Macau	L	L	M	S	H	L	L	L	L	L	S	L	H	L	L	S	L	S	L	M	L	M	L	L	L	L	L
Philippines	M	M	H	H	M	L	M	H	L	M	S	L	H	H	S	H	L	S	S	L	M	M	M	M	L	M	H
Taiwan	L	M	L	M	L	L	L	L	L	L	S	L	H	S	L	S	L	S	L	S	S	L	L	L	M	L	L
Vietnam	M	M	M	H	M	H	M	H	S	M	S	H	H	M	L	H	M	S	L	L	L	M	M	M	M	L	M

America (North and Central)	Cholera	Typhoid	Shigellosis	Amoebiasis	TB	Plague	Brucellosis	Diphtheria	Meningococcal infection	Polio	Yellow Fever	Dengue or other arboviruses	Viral hepatitis (A + B)	Rabies	Typhus	Malaria	Leishmaniasis	Trypanosomiasis	Syphilis	Gonorrhea	Schistosomiasis	Liver flukes	Hydatid disease	Tapeworms	Filariasis	Hookworm	Other intestinal worms
Belize	H	L	L	M	L	S	L	M	S	L	S	M	H	H	L	M	M	M	S	L	L	L	L	L	M	M	M
Canada	S	S	L	S	S	S	S	S	S	L	S	S	S	L	L	S	S	S	S	S	S	S	L	S	S	S	L
Costa Rica	H	L	S	H	S	S	L	M	S	L	S	L	M	M	L	H	H	L	L	M	L	L	M	M	M	M	H
El Salvador	H	M	M	H	L	S	L	M	S	L	S	L	H	H	L	M	L	L	L	L	L	L	L	L	L	M	M
Guatemala	H	M	H	M	M	S	L	M	S	M	S	L	H	M	L	H	M	L	L	S	L	L	L	M	M	M	M
Honduras	H	M	M	M	M	S	L	L	S	M	S	H	H	L	H	M	M	L	L	L	L	L	L	M	L	M	H
Mexico	H	M	M	H	S	S	S	L	S	M	S	M	H	H	L	H	L	L	S	S	L	S	M	M	L	M	H
Nicaragua	H	H	M	M	M	M	S	S	M	S	M	S	H	H	H	L	H	H	L	L	L	L	L	M	L	M	H
Panama	H	M	M	H	L	S	S	M	S	L	L	M	H	H	L	H	M	M	M	M	L	L	L	M	M	M	H

Key   L: 'Low'   M: 'Medium'   H: 'High'   S: Similar or fewer cases relative to United States

Americas: Caribbean

	Cholera	Typhoid	Shigellosis	Amoebiasis	TB	Plague	Brucellosis	Diphtheria	Meningococcal infection	Polio	Yellow Fever	Dengue/arboviruses	Viral hepatitis (A + B)	Rabies	Typhus	Malaria	Leishmaniasis	Trypanosomiasis	Syphilis	Gonorrhea	Schistosomiasis	Liver flukes	Hydatid disease	Tapeworms	Filariasis	Hookworm	Other intestinal worms
Antigua and Barbuda	S	L	L	L	S	S	S	S	S	S	S	M	M	S	S	S	S	S	L	L	M	L	L	L	L	M	M
Bahamas	S	S	M	L	S	S	S	S	S	S	S	M	M	S	S	S	S	S	S	M	M	S	S	L	L	L	M
Barbados	S	S	M	L	S	S	S	S	S	S	H	M	S	S	S	S	S	S	L	L	S	S	S	S	S	L	L
Bermuda	S	L	L	L	S	S	S	S	S	S	S	L	L	S	S	S	S	S	L	H	S	L	L	L	L	L	M
British Virgin Island	S	S	S	M	L	S	S	S	S	S	S	S	M	S	S	S	S	L	H	L	L	S	L	L	L	L	L
Cuba	S	S	M	H	S	S	L	M	S	S	S	S	S	M	S	S	S	L	L	L	M	S	L	L	M	M	M
Dominica	S	M	M	H	L	S	L	M	S	S	S	L	M	S	S	S	S	S	L	L	L	S	L	S	L	M	M
Dominican Rep	S	M	L	H	S	S	L	H	L	S	S	H	H	M	S	M	S	S	M	M	L	L	L	L	M	M	M
Grenada	S	L	L	L	S	S	S	S	S	S	S	L	M	L	S	S	S	S	L	L	S	L	L	L	L	M	M
Guadeloupe	S	L	L	L	S	S	L	S	S	S	S	L	M	S	S	S	S	S	L	L	S	L	L	L	L	M	M
Haiti	S	M	M	H	L	S	L	M	S	S	S	H	H	L	S	H	L	S	L	M	S	L	L	L	L	M	M
Jamaica	S	S	S	M	S	S	S	S	S	S	M	S	S	S	S	S	S	L	M	L	L	M	L	L	L	M	M
Martinique	S	L	L	L	L	S	S	S	S	S	S	L	M	S	S	S	S	S	L	L	S	L	L	L	L	M	M
Montserrat	S	S	S	M	S	S	S	S	S	S	S	M	M	S	S	S	S	S	H	H	M	L	L	L	L	M	M
Puerto Rico	S	S	M	L	S	S	S	S	S	S	S	H	M	L	S	S	S	L	L	L	L	L	L	L	L	L	M
St. Kitts and Nevis	S	S	S	L	S	S	S	S	S	S	S	M	M	S	S	S	S	L	M	L	L	M	L	L	L	M	M
St. Lucia	S	S	L	L	S	S	S	S	S	S	S	M	M	S	S	S	S	S	M	M	H	L	S	L	L	M	M
St. Vincent	S	L	L	L	S	S	S	S	S	S	S	L	M	S	S	S	S	L	L	S	L	S	L	S	L	M	M
Trinidad and Tobago	S	S	L	L	S	S	S	S	S	S	M	M	M	L	S	S	S	S	L	M	L	L	L	L	L	M	M

America (South)

	Cholera	Typhoid	Shigellosis	Amoebiasis	TB	Plague	Brucellosis	Diphtheria	Meningococcal infection	Polio	Yellow Fever	Dengue/arboviruses	Viral hepatitis (A + B)	Rabies	Typhus	Malaria	Leishmaniasis	Trypanosomiasis	Syphilis	Gonorrhea	Schistosomiasis	Liver flukes	Hydatid disease	Tapeworms	Filariasis	Hookworm	Other intestinal worms
Argentina	H	L	S	M	L	S	H	M	H	S	S	S	H	M	L	L	L	H	L	L	L	L	H	M	L	H	M
Bolivia	H	L	L	M	M	H	L	M	S	S	S	M	S	H	H	L	L	M	M	S	S	L	L	M	M	L	M
Brazil	H	M	L	H	H	H	L	M	H	S	L	L	H	L	S	H	M	H	M	M	H	L	L	M	L	H	H
Chile	H	M	L	L	S	S	S	S	M	S	S	S	S	M	S	L	S	L	L	S	L	L	L	M	M	S	M
Colombia	H	H	H	H	M	S	S	M	S	S	H	H	H	H	L	H	H	M	L	L	S	L	S	M	M	H	H
Ecuador	H	H	L	H	L	M	S	M	S	S	L	L	L	M	L	H	M	L	S	S	M	L	M	L	M	M	M
Falkland Islands	H	S	S	S	L	S	S	S	S	S	S	S	S	L	L	S	S	S	M	M	M	S	L	H	L	S	L
French Guiana	H	M	M	M	H	S	S	S	S	S	M	M	S	S	H	L	M	H	S	S	S	L	L	H	H	H
Guyana	H	M	M	L	M	S	S	L	S	L	L	M	L	H	M	M	S	S	M	M	L	M	M	H	H
Paraguay	H	L	M	M	M	S	S	M	L	S	S	S	H	M	L	M	M	L	L	S	M	L	M	M	L	H	M
Peru	H	L	H	M	M	M	M	H	M	S	S	L	L	H	M	L	H	M	L	S	S	L	M	L	M	L	S	H
Suriname	H	M	M	H	M	S	L	L	S	S	L	M	H	S	L	H	H	M	H	L	L	H	L	M	L	M	H	H
Uruguay	H	L	L	M	L	S	L	M	L	S	S	S	H	S	L	S	L	M	L	L	L	L	M	M	L	H	M
Venezuela	H	L	L	L	L	S	L	M	S	S	L	L	H	M	L	H	M	H	M	H	M	L	S	L	M	H	H

Key L: 'Low' M: 'Medium' H: 'High' S: Similar or fewer cases relative to United States

Oceania

	Cholera	Typhoid	Shigellosis	Amoebiasis	TB	Plague	Brucellosis	Diphtheria	Meningococcal infection	Polio	Yellow Fever	Dengue or other arboviruses	Viral hepatitis (A + B)	Rabies	Typhus	Malaria	Leishmaniasis	Trypanosomiasis	Syphilis	Gonorrhea	Schistosomiasis	Liver flukes	Hydatid disease	Tapeworms	Filariasis	Hookworm	Other intestinal worms
American Samoa	H	H	H	H	S	S	L	L	S	L	S	S	H	S	S	S	L	S	L	L	S	S	S	S	L	M	L
Australia	S	S	M	L	S	S	S	S	S	S	S	S	S	S	S	S	S	S	S	S	S	L	L	L	S	S	L
Cook Islands	S	S	S	S	H	S	L	S	M	L	S	S	M	S	S	S	L	S	L	M	S	S	S	S	L	L	L
Fiji	S	S	M	M	L	S	S	S	S	L	S	H	M	S	S	S	L	S	L	L	S	S	S	L	S	M	L
French Polynesia	S	M	M	M	M	S	S	S	L	L	S	H	M	S	S	S	L	S	M	L	S	S	S	S	M	M	H
Guam	S	S	L	M	M	S	S	L	L	L	S	S	S	S	S	M	S	L	M	S	S	S	S	S	M	M	M
Kiribati	S	L	L	M	H	S	S	L	S	L	S	S	M	S	S	S	L	S	L	S	S	S	S	S	M	M	M
New Caledonia	S	M	M	H	L	S	S	S	S	S	S	L	M	S	S	S	S	S	M	M	S	S	S	S	M	M	M
New Zealand	S	S	M	L	S	S	S	S	S	S	S	S	M	S	S	S	L	S	S	S	S	S	S	S	S	S	S
Pacific Islands	S	L	L	H	L	S	S	S	S	L	S	M	M	S	S	S	L	S	L	M	S	S	S	S	H	M	M
Papua New Guinea	S	M	M	H	H	S	S	S	L	S	H	H	S	H	S	S	L	L	S	S	S	S	S	S	H	H	H
Samoa	S	M	L	L	M	S	L	L	L	L	S	H	M	S	S	S	L	S	S	S	S	S	S	S	M	M	M
Solomon Islands	S	L	L	L	S	S	S	L	S	M	S	S	H	S	S	S	L	S	S	S	S	S	S	S	M	H	M
Tonga	S	H	M	M	H	S	S	L	S	S	S	H	M	S	S	S	L	S	L	S	S	S	S	S	M	M	M
Vanuatu	S	L	L	L	M	S	S	L	L	S	S	M	M	S	S	H	L	S	S	S	S	S	S	S	M	M	M
Wallis and Futuna Islands	S	L	L	H	M	S	S	S	S	S	S	H	M	S	S	S	L	S	L	S	S	S	S	S	H	H	H

Europe (selected countries)

	Cholera	Typhoid	Shigellosis	Amoebiasis	TB	Plague	Brucellosis	Diphtheria	Meningococcal infection	Polio	Yellow Fever	Dengue or other arboviruses	Viral hepatitis (A + B)	Rabies	Typhus	Malaria	Leishmaniasis	Trypanosomiasis	Syphilis	Gonorrhea	Schistosomiasis	Liver flukes	Hydatid disease	Tapeworms	Filariasis	Hookworm	Other intestinal worms
Bulgaria	S	S	H	L	S	S	L	S	S	S	S	S	M	S	L	S	S	S	S	S	S	S	S	L	S	S	S
Cyprus	S	L	S	S	S	S	M	L	L	S	S	S	L	S	M	S	L	S	L	L	S	S	L	S	S	S	L
Czechoslovakia	S	S	H	L	S	S	S	L	S	S	S	S	M	S	S	S	S	S	S	S	S	S	S	S	S	S	M
Denmark	S	S	L	M	S	S	S	S	S	S	S	S	S	S	S	S	S	S	S	S	L	S	S	M	L	S	S
Finland	S	S	M	M	S	S	S	S	S	S	S	S	S	S	S	S	S	S	S	L	S	S	S	L	S	S	S
Greece	S	M	S	L	L	S	M	S	S	S	S	S	L	S	L	S	S	S	S	S	L	H	S	L	L	S	S
Hungary	S	S	H	L	S	S	S	S	S	S	S	S	S	S	S	S	S	S	L	S	S	L	S	L	S	S	S
Iceland	S	S	S	S	S	S	S	S	L	S	S	S	S	S	S	S	S	S	L	S	S	L	L	L	S	S	S
Norway	S	S	S	S	S	S	S	S	M	S	S	S	S	S	S	S	S	S	S	S	S	S	L	S	S	S	S
Portugal	L	M	S	S	L	S	L	M	S	S	S	S	L	S	S	S	S	L	S	S	S	S	S	S	S	S	S
Romania	H	S	H	S	L	S	S	S	S	M	S	S	M	M	S	S	S	S	S	S	S	S	S	L	S	S	S
Spain	L	M	M	S	S	S	H	L	L	S	S	S	L	S	L	S	S	S	L	S	S	S	S	L	M	L	S
Sweden	S	S	L	S	S	S	S	S	S	S	S	S	S	S	S	S	S	S	S	S	L	S	S	S	S	S	S
Yugoslavia	S	L	H	L	S	L	L	L	S	S	S	S	H	L	L	L	S	S	S	S	L	L	M	S	S	S	S

Key   L: 'Low'   M: 'Medium'   H: 'High'   S: Similar or fewer cases relative to United States

CAN YOU DRINK THE WATER?

This is one of the questions that travelers most often ask; unfortunately, little reliable information is available to provide satisfactory answers. The bottom line must always be to be skeptical of claims about water purity; if there is any doubt, water should be from a reliable, bottled source, or boiled or purified.

Here is a listing of data derived from the opinions of medical and nursing staff from embassies of English-speaking countries, working in the countries concerned. It is based on results from a survey for Condé Nast *Traveler*, and reproduced by kind permission of its editor-in-chief, Thomas J. Wallace.

AFRICA	Water UNSAFE throughout country	Water considered SAFE in					Bottled water available
		Capital	Other main cities	Hotels and tourist areas	Rural areas	All over	
Algeria	x	regarded as unreliable even where chlorinated					yes
Benin	x						cities and towns
Botswana		x	x				Perrier *was* widely available
Burkina Faso	x						yes
Burundi	x						
Cameroon	x						yes
Central African Republic	x				some deep wells OK		costs $$$
Chad	x						yes
Congo	x	regarded as unreliable even where chlorinated					yes
Côte d'Ivoire	x	regarded as unreliable even where chlorinated					yes
Djibouti	x						not widely available
Egypt	x	some hotels claim to purify water—probably unreliable					yes
Ethiopia	x						cities only
Gabon		x					yes

(continued)

	Water UNSAFE throughout country	Water considered SAFE in					Bottled water available
AFRICA		Capital	Other main cities	Hotels and tourist areas	Rural areas	All over	
Ghana	×	regarded as unreliable even where chlorinated					cities and towns
Guinea	×						yes
Guinée Bissau	×						capital only
Kenya	×	regarded as unreliable even where chlorinated					cities only
Liberia	×						yes
Madagascar	×						cities only
Mali	×	regarded as unreliable even where chlorinated					cities and towns
Mauritania	×						cities only
Morocco		×					yes
Mozambique	×						yes
Niger	×	regarded as unreliable even where chlorinated					yes
Nigeria		×					yes
Rwanda	×						not available
Senegal		×					yes
Sierra Leone	×	regarded as unreliable even where chlorinated					yes
Somalia	×						yes
South Africa		×	×	×	×	×	yes
Sudan	×						variable supplies
Tanzania	×						capital only
Togo		×					yes
Tunisia	×	regarded as unreliable even where chlorinated					yes
Uganda	×						some hotels only
Zaire	×						yes
Zambia	×						yes
Zimbabwe		×	×	×			yes

Caribbean

	Water safety
Anguilla	B
Antigua	B
Aruba	T
Bahamas	B
Barbados	T
Barbuda	T/B
Bermuda	T
Bonaire	B
British Virgin Is.	T
Cuba	B
Curacao	T
Dominica	B
Dominican Republic	B
Grenada	B
Guadeloupe	B
Haiti	B
Jamaica	T
Martinique	T
Montserrat	B
Puerto Rico	T
Saba	B
St. Martin/St.Maarten	B/T
St. Vincent/Grenadines	B
St. Kitts/Nevis	B
St. Lucia	B
St. Eustatius	B
St. Barts	B
Trinidad/Tobago	T
U.S. Virgin Is.	B

T = tapwater considered safe in main tourist areas; B = bottled water advised.

Europe	Water UNSAFE throughout country	Water considered SAFE in					Bottled water available
		Capital	Other main cities	Hotels and tourist areas	Rural areas	All over	
Austria		×	×	×	×	×	yes
Belgium		×	×	×	×	×	yes
Bulgaria	spring water in spa towns said to be safe; tap water looks rusty and has a high lead content						
Commonwealth of Independent States (formerly the USSR)	×	often tastes horrible					soda water widely available; non-carbonated bottled water scarce
Czechoslovakia		×	×	×	× ·	×	yes
Denmark		×	×	×	×	×	yes no fluoride in water
Finland		×	×	×	×	×	yes
France		×	×	×	variable		yes
Germany		×	×	×	×	×	yes
Greece		×	×	×	water on islands unsafe		yes
Greenland		×	×	×	×	×	yes
Holland		×	×	×	×	×	yes
Hungary		×	×	×			yes
Iceland		×	×	×	×	×	cities and towns
Ireland		×	×	×	×	×	yes
Italy		×	×	×	variable		yes
Luxembourg		×	×	×	×	×	yes
Norway		×	×	× ·	×	×	cities and towns
Poland	tastes terrible, widely regarded as safe						yes
Portugal	×	regarded as unreliable even where chlorinated					yes
Romania	×						cities only; said to have high lead content
Spain		×	×				recent poisoning scare (bottles with plastic caps); widely available
Sweden		×	×	×	×	×	yes no fluoride in water
Switzerland		×	×	×	×	×	yes low fluoride
UK		×	×	×	×	×	yes
(former) Yugoslavia	×						no water very hard— shampoo won't lather

Americas	Water UNSAFE throughout country	Water considered SAFE in					Bottled water available
		Capital	Other main cities	Hotels and tourist areas	Rural areas	All over	
Argentina	×	regarded as unreliable even where chlorinated					yes
Belize		×					yes
Bolivia	×						cities only
Brazil	×	regarded as unreliable even where chlorinated					yes often tastes terrible
Canada		×	×	×	×	×	yes
Chile	×	regarded as unreliable even where chlorinated					yes tastes horrible
Colombia		×					cities only
Costa Rica	×						yes
Ecuador	×						yes
El Salvador	×						yes
Grenada	×						yes
Guatemala	×	regarded as unreliable even where chlorinated					yes
Guyana	×						limited availability
Honduras	×						yes
Mexico	×						yes
Nicaragua		×					very hard to find
Panama		×	×	×			yes
Paraguay		×	×	×			yes
Peru	×						cities and towns
Uruguay		×	×	×			cities and towns
Venezuela	×						yes

Asia/Pacific	Water UNSAFE throughout country	Water considered SAFE in					Bottled water available
		Capital	Other main cities	Hotels and tourist areas	Rural areas	All over	
Australia		×	×	×	×	×	yes
Bangladesh	×						
Burma	×						capital and tourist areas only
China	×	unreliable; considered safe in large hotels					yes
Fiji		×	×	×			not available
Hong Kong	×	regarded as unreliable even where chlorinated					yes
India	×						yes
Indonesia	×						'Aqua' brand considered safe
Japan		×	×	×	×	×	yes
Malaysia		×	×	×			yes
Marshall Is.	×						yes
Micronesia	×	regarded as unreliable even where chlorinated					cities (except when the ship is late!)
Nepal	×						cities only
New Zealand		×	×	×	×	×	yes
Pakistan	×						cities
Papua New Guinea		×	×	×			cities
Philippines	×	regarded as unreliable even where chlorinated					cities
Singapore		×	×	×	×	×	yes
Solomon Is.		×	×	×	×	×	not available
South Korea	×	unreliable; considered safe in large hotels					cities only
Sri Lanka	×						cities only
Thailand	×	regarded as unreliable even where chlorinated					yes
Western Samoa	×						hard to get

Middle East	Water UNSAFE throughout country	Water considered SAFE in					Bottled water available
		Capital	Other main cities	Hotels and tourist areas	Rural areas	All over	
Bahrain	×	regarded as unreliable even where chlorinated					cities and towns
Iraq		×	×				yes
Israel		×	×	×			yes
Jordan	×	regarded as unreliable even where chlorinated					yes
Kuwait		×	×	×	×	×	yes
Lebanon	×						
Oman	×	regarded as unreliable even where chlorinated					yes
Qatar		×	×	×	×	×	yes
Saudi Arabia	×	unreliable; considered safe in large hotels					cities
Turkey	×						yes
United Arab Emirates		×	×	×			
Yemen	×						

Appendix 5

SOME HINTS ON EATING ABROAD UNDER EXTREME CONDITIONS
OF BAD HYGIENE

1. **Choice of food**

   Diarrhea is preventable, not inevitable, but precautions often run counter to instinct. An attractive salad seems more healthful than a plate of French fries, and fresh fruit juice seems more healthful than sugary soda; in hot, poor countries, they are not. At home, we use "appetite appeal," not safety, to choose from a menu; they don't always go together. When traveling, it is hard to accept that we can't always eat what we want or what we have already paid for, especially when we feel tired and hungry. Cultivate the art of defensive eating!

   - If possible, choose food that *must* have been freshly cooked—e.g., omelette, French fries.
   - Freshly boiled food is always safe—e.g., rice, sweet corn.
   - Eat fruit or vegetables that are easily peeled or sliced open without contamination—e.g., bananas, citrus fruits, melon, papaya, avocado.
   - Eat food from sealed packs or cans (take emergency supplies!). Look for freshly baked bread (find the bakery).
   - Choose acceptably prepared local dishes rather than incompetently prepared imitation Western-style food.
   - Regard all cooked food as safe only when served hot.
   - Be prepared to send food back and to complain when appropriate.
   - Whenever possible, prepare your food yourself, or watch it being cooked.

2. **Don't eat**

   - Salads
   - Food that you do not *know* to have been freshly cooked, including hotel buffet food left out in warm temperatures
   - Food on which flies have settled or may have settled
   - Shellfish, crab, prawns, etc. (need eight minutes' vigorous boiling as an absolute minimum)

- Intricate dishes that have required much handling in preparation
- Unwashed (clean water) or unpeelable fruit or vegetables
- Ice cream and ices
- Dairy products made from unpasteurized milk. In some countries, not all "pasteurized" milk has really been pasteurized
- Rare meat, steak tartare, raw fish
- Unpeelable fruit (berries, grapes), or fruit peeled by others (fruit buffets)
- Food handled with dirty fingers
- Sauces and relishes left out on the table (hot sauces, however spicy, are not self-sterilizing!)

On a two-week vacation, you will probably be eating 42 meals prepared by others: the only way to protect yourself is to be selective about what you eat.

Beware of hospitality: if the food is not safe, refuse it. Where there is no alternative to unsafe food, smaller quantities are safer. Consider missing a meal; many Western travelers can afford to lose a little weight, and it is safer to do so by choice than from illness.

3. **Plates and cutlery**
These need to be washed with detergent, rinsed with clean water, and protected from flies.
   When this has not or cannot be done, and you suspect that they are contaminated, the risk can be reduced by rinsing with hot weak tea, a small amount of whisky, or by cleaning with an alcohol swab. Cutlery can be flamed with a candle or a cigarette lighter.
   Otherwise, don't eat the bottom layer of food on the plate—easy when food is served on a bed of rice. Alternatively, use paper plates and your own cutlery.

4. **Hands and fingers**
Should be washed at every opportunity. "Baby wipes" are often useful. Eat food that you have handled only if your hands are scrupulously clean; otherwise, use a clean tissue, the inside of a

clean plastic bag, or a piece of bread to handle food; or use your fingers, but discard any part of the food that you have handled.

5. **Drinks**
   Drinking water should be sterilized with iodine, or boiled. Hot tea is often easily available. Don't use ice. Bottled drinks should be opened in your presence—safest if carbonated. In the tropics, also try baby coconuts (they contain 1 pt. sweet water—bring your own straws). Don't drink fruit juices from street vendors; get into the habit of not using ice; don't use tap water—even for brushing teeth.

6. **Cups and glasses**
   Those that may be contaminated can be swilled out with hot tea or boiling water before use. Flies often settle on rims—pour away a little tea to rinse the rim of a teacup. Otherwise, use your own cup or water bottle, or drink bottled drinks directly from their bottle.

   Eating is supposed to be part of the travel experience. In Korea, local delicacies include dried fish heads, roasted locusts, sea slugs, toasted silkworms, snake and dog meat. In West Africa, you might be offered stir-fried termites; and in New Guinea, roasted palm grubs (they taste of caramel); in French Guiana, endangered species like black cayman ("caiman à l'orange"), red ibises, and anacondas are casually served in tourist hotels. In China, bear, deep-fried crunchy scorpion, and rat kebab are further possibilities. Some travelers regard health advice as an attempt to rob them of opportunities to try new foods: strict health grounds are not always the only reason for forgoing the pleasure. But no matter what food you are offered, and whether or not you are tempted to accept, the same principles of food hygiene always apply.

Appendix 6

This checklist is a summary of the main items to consider including in a medical kit for travel. It is unlikely that all of these items will be required: the area being visited, the availability of such items at your destination, and the length and nature of your trip will influence the exact requirement. Read Chapter 13 and the other relevant sections of this book before drawing up your own final list. (Brand names are listed in Chapter 13.)

I. First aid

Wound dressings	Band-Aids - Ace bandage SteriStrips sterile nonadherent pads tape—micropore —elastic
Antiseptics	powder spray—Betadine cream—Neosporin
Other first-aid items	alcohol wipes gauze bandage pads lancets safety pins scissors tweezers

2. Creams and lotions

Itch and bite	crotamiton* hydrocortisone 1 percent
Anti-fungal	miconazole cream/powder or clotrimazole cream/solution
Rubs	methyl salicylate trolamine salicylate

KEY
* = prescription required

| Cold sores and lips | acyclovir cream* |
| | lipsalve (Carmex, Chapstick) |

3. Tablets

Analgesics	acetaminophen
	aspirin
	ibuprofen
	codeine*
	hydrocodeine*

Antibiotics	trimethoprim/sulfamethoxazole*
	or
	co-amoxyclav*
	metronidazole*
	doxycycline*
	ciprofloxacin*

| Antimalarials | medication for prevention and treatment |
| | (see Chapter 13) |

Antihistamines	chlorpheniramine
	terfenadine*
	astemizole*

Motion sickness	promethazine
	cyclizine
	dimenhydrinate
	buclizine*
	scopolamine patches*

Treatment of diarrhea	electrolyte replacement
	anti-diarrheal—loperamide
	—bismuth sub-salicylate

4. Eye medication

sulfacetamide eyedrops*
garamycin eyedrops*

5. Other medicines

Vaginal infections   clotrimazole vaginal tablets
                              miconazole
Sleeping tablets (e.g., Temazepam*)
Vitamins
Antacid
Laxative (e.g., bran, senna)
Cold/sinus medication (e.g., Sinex, Otrivine)
Nausea medication (e.g., metoclopramide*)
Antiworm medication (e.g., mebendazole*)
Allergy emergency kit (e.g., Ana-Kit, Epipen)

6. Other items

HIV/AIDS-Hepatitis prevention kit (needles, syringes, etc.)
Sunscreens
Dental repair kit
Insect repellent
Water-purification kit
Toilet paper
Tampons
Spare eyeglasses/contact lenses

Appendix 7

POST-TROPICAL CHECKUP

The need for medical evaluation following return home from the tropics depends on where you have been, how long you spent there, and how closely exposed you have been to possible infection.

Dr. Martin S. Wolfe has been the tropical medicine specialist for the U.S. Department of State and the World Bank for 23 years, and has been involved with thousands of post-travel examinations on persons returning from the tropics.

Each year, almost 8 million Americans travel to the developing world. Increasingly, tourists are visiting exotic, remote parts of the world, sometimes for a period of weeks, and thus are at risk of exposure to diseases that are rare in the United States. At even greater risk for exotic infections are those who live or work in developing countries for prolonged periods.

WHO NEEDS A CHECKUP?

Post-travel evaluation is *not* necessary for the majority of short-term travelers who remain well during travel and following return. However, persons with a history of illness (especially diarrhea or fever) or who have been exposed to a high risk of disease while abroad even for a short period should undergo specific screening procedures after returning home.

Long-term travelers should undergo a post-travel examination even if they are asymptomatic, because the examination can sometimes reveal a cryptic treatable disease.

WHERE TO GO

Many American physicians are unfamiliar with exotic diseases and the sometimes subtle manifestations they may present. There is also a general lack of knowledge of the geographic distribution of exotic infections. If a returned individual's physician is not familiar with or comfortable with doing an evaluation for exotic disease, the traveler should seek care at a specialized travel clinic or major medical center (usually in the infectious-diseases section) familiar with tropical diseases. Appendix 8 lists centers in the United States with expertise in travel and tropical medicine.

SYMPTOMS AND SIGNS OF INFECTION

Symptoms of tropical diseases range from diarrhea, fever, jaundice, a rash, an itch, or skin swellings, to more vague and nonspecific symptoms like tiredness, loss of appetite, loss of weight, and feeling unwell. All of these require skilled evaluation, and this is especially urgent if there is any possibility of malaria. You should not wait for a checkup before reporting such symptoms to a physician.

You should tell the physician performing the examination about any illnesses that occurred while you were away, and any treatment you received—tests may be necessary to confirm that the treatment was fully successful.

TESTS

The following screening tests can be useful to detect evidence of disease in travelers who are symptom-free.

BLOOD TESTS

A complete blood count may provide evidence of infection (increased total white blood cell count), anemia (decrease in hemoglobin or hematocrit), or eosinophilia (increased eosinophils—a type of white blood cells—can be an indication of parasitic infections such as filariasis and schistosomiasis).

A blood antibody test is useful in determining possible infection in those with a history of possible exposure to schistosomiasis in infected areas; a positive test should prompt further parasitological examinations of the stool and/or urine. Schistosomiasis is acquired from swimming in or having contact with bodies of fresh water, and is especially common in tropical Africa, northeastern South America, and certain Caribbean islands. An antibody test is also available for filariasis, and a positive result can be confirmed by searching for parasites in the blood, tissue, or skin.

Any returning traveler who reports having sexual contact with a stranger or who has been injected with a nondisposable needle or syringe should have antibody screening for HIV infection, hepatitis B, and syphilis.

Tests of liver function can reveal evidence of recent or persistent

**SCREENING PROCEDURES TO BE CONSIDERED
FOR ASYMPTOMATIC RETURNING SHORT-TERM TRAVELERS**
Abbreviated history and physical examination
Complete blood count
Blood chemistry profile
Urinalysis
Hepatitis B surface antigen
VDRL or RPR (for syphilis)
HIV
Stool exam for ova and parasites
Stool culture for enteric bacterial pathogens
Glucose 6 phosphate dehydrogenase

inapparent viral hepatitis, or infection with other less common organisms.

URINE

Routine urinalysis is most useful in people who have been long-term residents abroad; the presence of red or white blood cells may suggest a parasitic or bacterial infection. For example, urinary schistosomiasis commonly causes asymptomatic urinary bleeding. Special tests are also available to detect eggs in schistosomiasis (see pp. 98–99).

STOOL EXAM

Most travelers who suffer from diarrhea recover completely, but in just under 10 percent of cases, more severe and prolonged symptoms may persist after return. The precise cause of these symptoms often is difficult to determine, although invasive bacteria and protozoal parasites are possible causes (see p. 29). A stool culture for bacteria, and stool examinations for parasites (to try to identify persisting organisms), should be performed in patients who return well but give a history of recent diarrhea while traveling. These tests can also serve as a check for cure in persons who have undergone specific treatment.

OTHER TESTS

Persons planning extensive foreign travel should have a pre-departure base-line tuberculin skin test (PPD), and should be re-tested annually while abroad and again on return home. Travelers

ROUTINE SCREENING PROCEDURES PERFORMED BIENNIALLY ON U.S. FOREIGN SERVICE PERSONNEL

History and physical examination
Vision test—intraocular pressure after age 40
Hearing test—screening, audiogram
Pulmonary function tests (as indicated)
Electrocardiogram (after age 40 or as indicated)
Flexible sigmoidoscopy (offered after age 50)
PPD skin test (or chest X ray as indicated)
PAP smear and pelvic exam (after age 21)
Mammogram (offered every two years, ages 40 to 50; required after age 50)
Stool Hemoccult (x3)
Complete blood count
Urinalysis
Blood chemistry profile
Blood type (pre-employment only)
Glucose 6 phosphate dehydrogenase (pre-employment only)
Hepatitis B antigen
HIV (after age 12)
VDRL or RPR (for syphilis)
Stool exams for ova and parasites (x3)
Schistosomiasis serology (returnees from endemic areas)

whose skin test converts to positive should have a chest X-ray, and drug prophylaxis should be considered.

The screening procedures to be considered for asymptomatic returning short-term travelers, particularly those in whom illness occurred during travel, are summarized on the previous page, and the above list shows the routine screening procedures that are performed on U.S. Foreign Service personnel at biennial intervals, and that should be considered for all persons returning from extended stays in developing countries.

ADVICE

A checkup also provides an opportunity to remind you to continue taking antimalarial tablets for at least four weeks after leaving a malarious area. Symptoms of malaria may still appear even though all screening tests are normal; report any symptoms promptly, and make sure your physician knows you have been living or traveling in a malarious region.

Appendix 8

IMMUNIZATION CENTERS, SPECIALIST CLINICS, GOVERNMENT
DEPARTMENTS, AND USEFUL ADDRESSES: SOURCES OF UP-TO-THE-
MINUTE INFORMATION AND ADVICE

UNITED STATES OF AMERICA

It is traditionally the responsibility of city, county, and state departments of health to provide information for the public about
immunization. Many still do this—for the price of a local call—and
they should also be consulted for information about the nearest
immunization clinic; health department clinics generally carry a
good stock of travel vaccines, including yellow fever.

Information can also be obtained from the following offices of
the U.S. Public Health Service:

New York: (718) 917-1685
Miami: (305) 526-2910
Chicago: (312) 686-2150
Los Angeles: (213) 215-2365
San Francisco: (415) 876-2872
Seattle: (206) 442-4519
Honolulu: (808) 541-2552

**The Voice Information System of the Centers for Disease Con-
trol and Prevention** can be accessed using a touch-tone phone, and
gives detailed information on current health advice tailored to your
destination. The advice is continuously updated. The CDC is fed-
erally funded, and is the major national source of information and
advice on infectious diseases. For a full briefing, first-time users can
expect to stay on the line for around 20 minutes—the service runs
24 hours a day (CDC staff are available to talk to, if required, 8:00
a.m.–4:30 p.m., Monday through Friday); the most economical time
to use the system is at night. The number is (404) 332-4559. Similar
information can also be obtained from the CDC by fax—especially
useful for more complicated information such as antimalarial regimes. Call (404) 332-4565, follow the prompts, and enter your
own fax number: you will receive a listing of the information available and can then request the information that matches your needs.
The service is excellent, and many local health departments have
started referring all callers to these services rather than attempting
to provide up-to-date information themselves.

Other Sources of Information

The Centers for Disease Control and Prevention (CDC), Atlanta, GA 30333, Tel. (404) 639-3311, also publishes *Health Information for International Travel* (see Further Reading), and is able to provide expert advice on infectious hazards of travel in cases of special difficulty.

U.S. State Department Citizens Emergency Center, Tel. (202) 647-5225, provides information about political and other risks abroad, and should be consulted if you intend to visit a part of the world where there is currently unrest or instability; also provides advice for travelers in distress. Using a touch-tone phone, you can select pre-recorded advisory information for any country; or you can speak directly with a State Department employee. This information is also available by modem via CompuServe (GO STATE) or direct on (202) 677-9225; the system is impressively easy to use. Twenty-four-hour assistance in an emergency is also available by calling the State Department's main number: (202) 634-3600.

The Superintendent of Documents is the source for government publications: (202) 512-0132.

Immunization Alert, 93 Timber Drive, Storrs, CT 06268, Tel. (800) 584-1999, (203) 487-0611, provides computerized health briefings, tailored to individual requirements and itineraries (prices from $10, also available by Fax).

Travax, (Shoreland Medical Marketing, Travel Health Information Services, 1417 N. Wauwatosa Avenue, Suite 201, Milwaukee, WI 53213-2646, Tel. (800) 755-2301, (608) 831-2331, Fax (414) 774-4060, also provides computerized health briefings, tailored to individual requirements and itineraries (prices from $10, also available by Fax).

Intercontinental Medical (ICM), 2720 Enterprise Parkway, Suite 106, Richmond, VA 23294, Tel. (800) ICM-8828, (804) 527-1094, Fax (804) 527-1941. For a fee of $28.50 (which covers an itinerary of 3 countries—add $3 for each additional country), ICM will mail travelers a printout of its own listing of physicians and hospitals in countries to be visited.

International Association of Medical Assistance to Travelers (IAMAT), 736 Center Street, Lewiston, NY 14092, publishes a listing of its network of physicians in different countries. The directory is free, though users are asked to contribute a donation to cover costs. IAMAT also sells mosquito nets.

World Status Map. Monthly summary of advisories and alerts (mainly political), available on subscription (also available on IBM-compatible computer diskette, or on-line). Box 466, Merrifield, VA 22116, Tel. (301) 564-8473 or (800) 322-4685.

TransSecur. Provides travel-security intelligence by phone; requires a touch-tone phone for access. Tel. (900) 884-4848.

Divers' Alert Network. Twenty-four-hour emergency telephone advice for divers with medical problems. Tel. (919) 684-8111.

International Society of Travel Medicine, c/o Dr. Hans Lobel, P.O. Box 15060, Atlanta, GA 30333-0060. Fax: (404) 488-4427. Recently formed international organization for doctors, nurses, and others interested in travel medicine.

Berna Products: call (800) 533-5899 in case of difficulty obtaining supplies of the oral typhoid vaccine.

Connaught: call (800) 822-2463 in case of difficulty obtaining supplies of the rabies, meningitis, or Japanese encephalitis vaccines.

Major travelers' clinics and centers specializing in tropical medicine†

ARIZONA
Travelers' Clinic, University of Arizona Health Sciences Center, (Department of Family and Community Medicine), Tucson, AZ 85724, Tel. (602) 626-7900

CALIFORNIA
Travel Clinic, UCSD Medical Center (Department of Family Medicine), 225 West Dickinson, San Diego, CA 92103, Tel. (619) 543-5787

UCLA Travelers' and Tropical Medicine Clinic, 10833 LeConte Ave., Los Angeles, CA 90024, Tel. (213) 825-9711

Travelers' Clinic, University of California, 350 Parnassus St., San Francisco, CA 94143, Tel. (415) 476-1872

COLORADO
Infectious Disease Division, University of Colorado Health Science Center, 4200 E. 9th Ave., Denver, CO 80262, Tel. (303) 320-7277

CONNECTICUT
International Travelers' Medical Service, University of Connecticut Health Center, Farmington, CT 06030, Tel. (203) 679-1000

† I am grateful to Dr. Leonard Marcus and the American Society of Tropical Medicine and Hygiene for assistance in obtaining some of these addresses.

Tropical Medicine and International Travelers' Clinic, Yale University School of Medicine, 20 York St., New Haven, CT 06504, Tel. (203) 785-2476 (Emergencies: (203) 785-2471)

DISTRICT OF COLUMBIA
Travelers' Clinic, George Washington University Medical Center, 2150 Pennsylvania Ave. N.W., Washington D.C., 20037, Tel. (202) 676-5558 or 676-8466

Travelers' Medical Service, 2141 K St. N.W., Washington, D.C. 20037, Tel. (202) 466-8109 or 331-0287

FLORIDA
Institute of Tropical Medicine, 1780 N.E. 168th St., North Miami Beach, FL 33162, Tel. (305) 947-1722

GEORGIA
Travelers' Medical Center, Emory University School of Medicine, Crawford Long Outpatient Center, 20 Linden Ave., Atlanta, GA 30365, Tel. (404) 686-5885

Travel Clinic, Piedmont Minor Emergency Clinic, 3115 Piedmont Rd., Atlanta, GA 30305, Tel. (404) 237-1755

HAWAII
Straub Clinic & Hospital, 888 S. King St., Honolulu, HA 96813, Tel. (808) 522-4511

ILLINOIS
Travel Clinic, University of Chicago Hospitals & Clinics, 5841 S. Maryland, Chicago, IL 60637, Tel. (312) 962-6112

KANSAS
Travel Medicine Clinic, University of Kansas Medical Center, 39th and Rainbow, Kansas City, KS 66103, Tel. (913) 588-3974

LOUISIANA
Department of Tropical Medicine, Tulane Medical Center, 1430 Tulane Ave., New Orleans, LA 70112, Tel. (504) 588-5199

MARYLAND
Travel Clinic, Johns Hopkins University, 550 N. Broadway, Baltimore, MD 21205, Tel. (301) 955-3934

MASSACHUSETTS
Division of Geographic Medicine and Infectious Diseases, New

England Medical Center Hospitals, 750 Washington St., Boston, MA 02111, Tel. (617) 956-7001

Travelers' Advice and Immunization Center, Massachusetts General Hospital, Boston, MA 02114, Tel. (617) 726-3906

Travelers' Health and Immunization Services, 148 Highland Ave., Newton, MA 02160, Tel. (617) 527-4003 or 366-0060

MICHIGAN
Travel Health Clinic, Henry Ford Hospital, 2799 West Grand Blvd., Detroit, MI 48202, Tel. (313) 876-2561

MISSOURI
Infectious Diseases Division, Washington University Medical Center, 216 S. Kings Hwy., St. Louis, MO 63110, Tel. (314) 454-7782

NEW YORK
International Health Care Services, Cornell Medical College, New York Hospital, 440 E. 69th St., New York, NY 10021, Tel. (212) 746-1601

International Health Clinic, Albert Einstein College of Medicine, 1300 Morris Park Ave., Bronx, NY 10461, Tel. (212) 430-2000

Travel Health Services, 50 E. 69th St., New York, NY 10021, Tel. (212) 734-3000

NORTH CAROLINA
Travel Clinic, Duke University Medical Center, 1700 Woodstock Rd., Durham, NC 27705, Tel. (919) 684-6832

OHIO
Travelers' Clinic, Division of Geographic Medicine, University Hospital of Cleveland, Cleveland, OH 44106, Tel. (216) 368-3496

PENNSYLVANIA
International Travel & Infectious Disease Service, Montefiore Hospital, 3459 Fifth Ave., Pittsburgh, PA 15213, Tel. (412) 648-6410

Travelers' Clinic, Milton S. Hershey Medical Center, Pennsylvania State University, Hershey, PA 17033, Tel. (717) 531-8885

Travelers' Health Center, Medical College of Pennsylvania, 3300 Henry Ave., Philadelphia, PA 19129, Tel. (215) 842-6465

TEXAS
University Center for Travel Medicine, 6410 Fannin, Houston, TX 77030-1501, Tel. (713) 797-4317

UTAH
Center for Infectious Diseases, Microbiology & Immunology, University of Utah School of Medicine, Salt Lake City, UT 84132, Tel. (801) 581-8811

WASHINGTON
Travelers' Medical and Immunization Clinic of Seattle, 509 Olive Way, Suite 1201, Seattle, WA 98101, Tel. (206) 624-6933
Travel and Tropical Medicine Clinic, University of Washington School of Medicine, University Hospital RC-02, 1959 N.E. Pacific St., Seattle, WA 98195, Tel. (206) 548-4888

WISCONSIN
International Travelers' Clinic, St. Luke's Hospital, 2900 W. Oklahoma, Milwaukee, WI 53215, Tel. (414) 649-6664

CANADA

To find your nearest immunization clinic, phone your local branch of Health and Welfare Canada. For a leaflet listing all clinics, phone or write to the Canadian Society for International Health (1565 Carling Ave., Ottawa, Ontario K1Z 8R1, Tel. (613) 728-5889).

Immunization: A Guide for International Travelers is published by Health and Welfare Canada; this leaflet is available free from its offices, and lists additional information sources, as well as immunization recommendations. It is updated annually.

There are tropical disease units at

Toronto General Hospital, Toronto, Ontario, M5G 1L7, Tel. (416) 595-3671
Vancouver General Hospital, Vancouver, BC V5Z 1M9, Tel. (604) 875-4148

Other sources of information

The Tropical Traveler, Hobbit Software Inc., P.O. Box 308, Victoria Station, Montreal, Quebec H3Z 2VB. Personalized computer health briefings in English or French.

UNITED KINGDOM

London's main vaccination centers are:
Hospital for Tropical Diseases Travel Clinic, 180–182 Tottenham
    Court Road, London W1P 9LE Tel. (071) 637-9899

British Airways Travel Clinics at 101 Cheapside, EC2V 6DT, Tel. (071) 606-2977; Gatwick London Terminal, Victoria Station, SW1W 9SJ, Tel. (071) 233-6661; 156 Regent St., W1R 5TA, Tel. (071) 439-9584; Hatton Cross (Heathrow Airport), Tel. (081) 562-5825

Thomas Cook Ltd., 45 Berkeley St., London W1A 1EB, Tel. (071) 499-4000

Trailfinders Ltd., 194 Kensington High St., London W8 7RG, Tel. (071) 938-3999

PPP Medical Center, New Cavendish St., London WC1, Tel. (071) 436-0224

Government sources

Information about vaccination requirements is available from:

International Relations Division, Department of Social Security, Alexander Fleming House, Elephant and Castle, London SE1 6BY, Tel. (071) 407-5522, Ext. 6749

Or see p. 50063 on PRESTEL. (There is free access to this service at most UK public libraries.)

Major UK centers specializing in tropical diseases

Hospital for Tropical Diseases, 4 St. Pancras Way, London NW1 OPE, Tel. (071) 387-4411

Liverpool School of Tropical Medicine, Pembroke Place, Liverpool L3 5QA, Tel. (051) 708-9393

Department of Communicable and Tropical Diseases, East Birmingham Hospital, Bordesley Green Road, Birmingham, B9 5ST, Tel. (021) 772-4311

Communicable Diseases (Scotland) Unit, Ruchill Hospital, Glasgow G20 9NB, Tel. (041) 946-7120

Other sources of information

The Malaria Reference Laboratory, at the London School of Hygiene and Tropical Medicine, Keppel St., London WC1E 7BR, Tel. (891) 600-350 provides free specialist advice about antimalarial precautions for individual countries, in the form of a recorded telephone message; it can also advise in cases of particular difficulty.

Medical Advisory Services for Travelers Abroad Ltd. (MASTA) is based at the London School of Hygiene and Tropical Medicine, Keppel St., London, WC1E 7HT, Tel. (071) 631-4408 Fax (071) 436-5389, provides computerized health printouts tailored to individual requirements; also supplies medical kits, impregnated mosquito nets, repellents, and water purifiers by mail order. Catalogue available, phone orders accepted.

The Foreign and Commonwealth Office, King Charles St., London SW1, Tel. (071) 270-3000, provides information about political risks abroad, and should be consulted if you intend to visit a part of the world where there is currently unrest or instability.

Hospital for Tropical Diseases Healthline, Tel. 0839-337733 Automated, recorded telephone advice service, tailored to your destination. Strongly recommended.

Other useful addresses

Nomad Travel Pharmacy, 3 Turnpike Lane, London N8 OPX. Tel. (081) 889-7014, Fax (081) 441-7208. Free advice service on medicines for travel; personalized medical kits for individual travelers and expeditions.

Expedition Advisory Center, Royal Geographical Society, 1 Kensington Gore, London SW7 2AR, Tel. (071) 589-5466. Huge variety of resources for travelers and expeditioners of all kinds. Organizes frequent lectures and seminars.

IRELAND

The free booklet *General Health Information for People Traveling Abroad* is published by the Health Promotion Unit of the Department of Health, Hawkins House, Dublin 2, Tel. 01-714711, and lists addresses and phone numbers of vaccination centers. Some main clinics:

Immunization Clinic, Royal College of Surgeons in Ireland, 84/85 Harcourt St., Dublin 2, Tel. 01-784422

Irish International Airlines Medical Center, Dublin Airport, Tel. 01-379900

Airport Medical Center, Shannon Airport, Co. Clare, Tel. 061-362491

Appendix 9

COMPUTERIZED HEALTH DATA BASES

The following computerized data bases provide access to information about changing health risks around the world, and are mainly intended for use by clinics and travel organizations that have to advise large numbers of travelers. No formal comparative studies have ever been undertaken between them, and the emphasis varies from one service to another; they each appear to be run by obsessive enthusiasts, however, which is a good sign!

USA

IMMUNIZATION ALERT
PC & Mac diskettes mailed weekly or monthly ($500 for monthly service, $750 for weekly service). See Appendix 8 for address.

TRAVAX
Runs on IBM-compatible PCs, updated weekly. Subscriptions cost $280–$1,000. See Appendix 8 for address. Not related to the UK service of the same name.

CANADA

CATIS
An expert system-based program. $475 annual subscription. Available from Travel and Inoculation Service, Toronto General Hospital, Toronto, Ontario.

THE TROPICAL TRAVELER
IBM-compatible system, available in English or French. Further information: Hobbit Software, P.O. Box 308, Victoria Station, Montreal, Quebec H3Z 2V8

UK

MASTA
Provides the data base used by the British Airways travel clinics. £850 annual fee for on-line access.

TRAVAX
An on-line service, provided by the Communicable Diseases (Scotland) Unit, Ruchill Hospital, Glasgow G20 9NB. (Tel. (041) 946-7120, Ext. 247 for information.) Service is free to general practitioners and noncommercial organizations.

FRANCE

EDISAN

Data base also includes information about local hospitals and doctors, medical evacuation, climate, environment, etc. Runs under Hypercard 2 on the Mac—needs at least 20MB. Initially $6,200, $1000 per year for annual update subscription. Limited edition (Micro Edisan) available in English, costs $540, $90 per year for update subscription. Information: CD Conseil, 18 Rue Le Sueur, Paris 75016.

FURTHER READING

Publications marked* are primarily written for doctors.

American Diabetes Association. *Travel Tips for Diabetics.* Available from the American Diabetes Association, 600 Fifth Avenue, New York, NY 10020.

American Medical Association Encyclopedia of Medicine. Random House, 1990. (Excellent, comprehensive home medical encyclopedia.)

American Red Cross. *Standard First Aid and Personal Safety* and *Advanced First Aid and Emergency Care.*

American Society of Tropical Medicine and Hygiene. *Health Hints for the Tropics,* 11th ed. Available from ASTM&H, 6436 31st St. N.W., Washington, DC 20015-2342.

Auerbach, P.S. *Medicine for the Outdoors.* Little, Brown, 1991.

Auerbach, P.S., and E.C. Geehr. *Management of Wilderness and Environmental Emergencies.* Collier Macmillan, 1989. (Five-star study of everything from plant and wildlife hazards to lightning, forest fires, and drowning.)*

Bezruchka, S. *A Guide to Trekking in Nepal.* Diadem, 1985. (How to do it safely.)

Bolz, F. *How to Be a Hostage and Live.* Lyle Stuart, New Jersey, 1987.

Centers for Disease Control and Prevention, Atlanta, Georgia. *Health Information for International Travel—*Supplement to *Morbidity & Mortality Weekly Report.* Published annually, in August. Available from the Superintendent of Documents, U.S. Govt. Printing Office, Washington DC 20402. (The official U.S. publication for physicians.)*

Collins, P. *Living in Troubled Lands.* Paladin Press, Boulder, CO, 1981

Condé Nast *Traveler* Magazine, New York. Carries travel health news items and features. Tel. (303) 665-1583 or (800) 777-0700 to subscribe.

DeHart, R.L. *Fundamentals of Aerospace Medicine.** Lea & Febiger, Philadelphia, 1985.

Diabetic Traveler. PO Box 8223 RW, Stamford, CT 06905, Tel. (203) 327-5832. USA. Quarterly newsletter.

Disabled Travelers' International Phrase Book. Disability Press. (Available from RADAR, 25 Mortimer Street, London WIN 8AB, UK.)

Diving Medicine, 2nd ed. (ed. A.A. Bove and J.C. Davis). W.B. Saunders, 1990.*

Edmonds, C. *Dangerous Marine Animals of the Indo-Pacific Region.* Wedneil Publications, Newport, Australia, 1975.*

FURTHER READING

Gilles, H.M., and D.A. Warrell. *Bruce Chwatt's Essential Malariology.* Edward Arnold, 1993. (New edition of a classic text, a definitive guide.)*

Gorman, S. (ed.) *The Travelers Handbook.* Wexas, 1991. (850 pages of useful travel info—essential reading, even if you're already a travel expert . . .)

A Guide to the Accessibility of Airport Terminals, Access Travel. Available from Airport Operators International, 1700 K Street NW, Washington DC 20006, USA. (For disabled travelers.)

Heath, D. and Williams, D.R. *High Altitude Medicine and Pathology.* Butterworth, 1989.*

Hatt, J. *The Tropical Traveller.* Penguin, 1993. (3rd edition of the best anthology of tropical travel tips around.)

IAMAT Directory. Available from IAMAT, 736 Center Street, Lewiston, NY 14092. (Names and addresses of English-speaking doctors all over the world.)

Jenkins, B.M. *Terrorism.* Butterworth Publishers, Stoneham, Massachusetts.

Jong, E.C. *The Travel and Tropical Medicine Manual.* Saunders, 1987.*

Journal of Wilderness Medicine. Wilderness Medical Society, Chapman & Hall.

Kohls, L.R. *Survival Kit for Overseas Living.* Intercultural Press, Yarmouth, Maine, 1984.

Lee, E.L. (ed.) *The Latin American Advisor: A Weekly Risk Management Newsletter for Decisions Makers and Global Daily Summary.* The Lee Group, Inc., 2044 Reynolds Street, Falls Church, VA 22043 Tel: (703) 237-2151; Fax (703) 237-0804.

Lobel, H.O., Steffen, R., Kozarsky, P.E. (eds.) *Travel Medicine 2: Proceedings of the 2nd Conference on International Travel Medicine, Atlanta 1991.* Available from International Society of Travel Medicine, PO Box 15060, Atlanta, Georgia, 30333-0060. (Published October 1992. More than 200 scientific papers on current issues in travel medicine—essential reading for any health professional with an interest in the subject.)*

Manson-Bahr, P.E.C. and Bell, D.R. *Manson's Tropical Diseases,* 19th ed. Baillière Tindall, 1987.*

The Medical Letter. Subscription newsletter for physicians, published fortnightly; gives periodic reviews of health information for travel. Available from 1000 Main St., New Rochelle, NY 1801.*

Melville, K.E.M. *Stay Alive in the Desert.* Roger Lascelles, London, 1984.

Motion and Space Sickness. G.H. Crampton (ed.), CRC Press, Boca Raton, FL, 1990.*

Nicholson, A.N. Hypnotics: their place in therapeutics. *Drugs,* **31,** 164-176, 1986.*

Nicholson, A.N., and others. Sleep after transmeridian flights. *Lancet,* **22,** November, 1205-8.*

Nicol, J. *Bites and Stings: The World of Venomous Animals.* David &

Charles, London, 1989. Includes listing of anti-venom suppliers, worldwide.

Peters, W. and Gilles, H.M. *Color Atlas of Tropical Medicine.* Wolfe Medical Atlases, 1989.*

Piet-Pelon, N. and Hornby, B. *Women's Guide to Overseas Living.* Intercultural Press, P.O. Box 760, Yarmouth, Maine, 04096. 1992.

Readers Digest *What to Do in an Emergency.* Reader's Digest Publications, 1986. (Covers almost every conceivable emergency, and even some inconceivable ones.)

Ryman, D. *Encyclopedia of Aromatherapy.* Piatkus Books, 1991. (Details use of aromatherapy to combat jet lag.)

Schull, C.R. *Common Medical Problems in the Tropics.* Macmillan, London, 1987. (Guide for health workers in developing countries.)

Scotti, A.J. *Executive Safety and International Terrorism: A Guide for Travelers.* Prentice-Hall, 1986.

Sutherland, S.K. *Australian Animal Toxins: The Creatures, Their Toxins, and Care of the Poisoned Patient.* Oxford University Press, Melbourne, 1983.*

Travel and Leisure magazine, New York. Carries travel health news items each month.

Travel Medicine Advisor. American Health Consultants Inc., PO Box 740056, Atlanta, Georgia.* (Looseleaf manual with periodic updates and bimonthly newsletter; the most valuable feature is the newsletter. Annual subscription approximately $150.)

Traveling Healthy. Bimonthly newsletter. Available from 104-48 70th Road, Forest Hills, NY 11375.

U.S. Dept. of Health, Education and Welfare. *The Ship's Medicine Chest and Medical Aid at Sea.* 1984. Available from the Superintendent of Documents, U.S. Govt. Printing Office, Washington DC 20402.

U.S. Dept. of State, Bureau of Consular Affairs. Issues many publications of interest to prospective travelers, including: *Your Trip Abroad; A Safe Trip Abroad; Tips for Travelers: the Caribbean, Central and South America, Cuba, Eastern Europe, Mexico, Middle East, People's Republic of China, Sub-Saharan Africa, Saudi Arabia, South Asia; The Citizens Emergency Center, Crisis Abroad; Travel Warning on Drugs Abroad; Travel Tips for Older Americans; Tips for Americans Residing Abroad; Key Officers of Foreign Service Posts* (names of key US officers abroad with addresses of all US embassies and consulates); *Background Notes, Country Information Notices,* and *Travel Advisory Memoranda.* Available from the Superintendent of Documents, U.S. Govt. Printing Office, Washington DC 20402. Tel. (202) 783-3238; some of these are also available from passport offices; in case of difficulty, write to the Bureau of Consular Affairs, Dept. of State, Washington DC 20402.

Walsh, A. *Able to Travel.* Prentice Hall, New York, 1993. (Personal experiences of travel from over 100 disabled travelers.)

Ward M.P., Milledge, J.S., and West, J.B. *High Altitude Medicine and Physiology*. Chapman and Hall Medical, 1989.*

Warrell, D.A. Venomous and poisonous animals. In *Tropical and Geographical Medicine* (ed. K.S. Warren and A.A.F. Mahmoud). McGraw-Hill, New York, 1990. (Excellent survey of the subject, in one of the best tropical medicine textbooks around.)*

Weiss, L. *Access to the World*. Henry Holt, New York, 1986. (Access guide for the disabled.)

Werner, D. *Where There Is No Doctor*. Macmillan 1985. (Available also from the Hesperian Foundation, PO Box 1692, Palo Alto, CA 94302, USA—intended for people in developing countries with little education, but contains much useful advice on management of common tropical conditions. Also available on microfiche.)

Wilson, M. E. *A World Guide to Infections*. OUP, 1991.

World AIDS. Panos Institute, 8 Alfred Place, London WC1E 7EB, UK. 1409 King Street, Alexandria, VA 22314 USA. (Worldwide news about AIDS.)

World Health Organization, Geneva. International travel and health: *Vaccination Requirements and Health Advice*. Published annually in the spring, available from the UN Bookshop, NY. (The official WHO listing of requirements and recommendations for travel, including global distribution of malaria and chloroquine resistance.)* *World Health Statistical Quarterly* and WHO *Weekly Epidemiological Record* periodically publish updated maps and assessments of the world malaria situation.* *Atlas of the Global Distribution of Schistosomiasis* (1987) shows all known geography of this disease, often listing cases by village. The ultimate reference. Other publications include: *Yellow Fever Vaccinating Centers for International Travel*; *International Medical Guide for Ships* (including *The Ship's Medicine Chest*); *The Rational Use of Drugs in the Management of Acute Diarrhea in Children; Prevention of Sexual Transmission of HIV*.

Yaffé, M. *Taking the Fear out of Flying*. Sterling Publishing Co, New York, 1987.

GLOSSARY

Acute: An acute illness is one that is sudden in onset, regardless of severity.

Antibody: A protein made by the body in response to anything that it recognizes as "foreign"—such as components of bacteria and viruses called antigens. Antibodies bind to antigens and inactivate them, and are "tailor-made" for each antigen. The principle of "active" immunization is based on the fact that exposure to a small amount of harmless antigen—present in a vaccine—stimulates the production of antibodies that remain ready for action when infection threatens. (Vaccines fool the immune system into believing that they are "the real thing.") (See also immune globulin.)

Antigen: Any substance capable of triggering an immune response. Such substances include components of bacteria, viruses, toxins, and vaccines. Hepatitis B surface antigen (HBsAg) is an antigen present in the blood of people who have had hepatitis B, and can be detected by laboratory tests.

Bacillus (plural Bacilli): "Rod-shaped" bacteria. Anthrax, Hansen's disease (leprosy), and TB are examples of diseases caused by bacilli.

Bacteria: Tiny organisms that consist of a single cell, and have a cell wall but no nucleus. There are a great many types, not all of which cause disease.

Chemoprophylaxis: The use of drugs to *prevent* disease.

Chronic: A chronic disease process is one that develops gradually or lasts a long time.

Contraindication: Any disease or condition that renders a proposed form of treatment or course of action undesirable.

Culture: Growth of microorganisms in the laboratory for testing and identification.

Cutaneous: Of the skin.

Diuretic: A drug that increases urine production.

Dysentery: Severe diarrhea with blood, mucus, and abdominal cramps.

Edema: Fluid in the tissues, causing swelling.

Embolism: The sudden blockage of an artery, usually by a blood clot that has traveled in the bloodstream from elsewhere in the body. A clot, or "thrombus," sometimes forms in the veins of the legs; "pulmonary embolism" occurs when it travels to, and blocks, the arteries of the lungs. Gas entering the bloodstream can have a similar effect—called "gas embolism."

Endemic: A disease that is constantly present to a greater or lesser degree in a particular area is termed endemic.

Esophagus: The gullet, or food passage from mouth to stomach.

Enterocytes: The cells that line the intestinal wall.

Host: Man, or any animal, that harbors a parasite.

HIV: Human immunodeficiency virus, the virus that causes AIDS.

Immune globulin: A protein possessing antibody activity. Immune globulins circulate in the bloodstream. "Passive" immunization consists simply of injecting a preparation of "ready-made" antibodies from donated blood into someone who does not have them, and is the principle on which passive immunization against hepatitis A is based.

Immunity: A state in which the individual is resistant to specific infections.

Incidence: The number of new cases of a disease in a given period.

Incubation period: The time between exposure to an infection and the appearance of the first symptoms; this can provide useful clues to the identity of an infectious disease.

Intradermal, intramuscular, intravenous: These terms refer to the position of the tip of the needle during an injection. An intradermal injection is given as close to the skin surface as possible. An intramuscular injection is given deep into a muscle—usually in the buttock. An intravenous injection is given into a vein, directly into the bloodstream.

Jaundice: Yellow discoloration of the skin and whites of the eyes, due to the presence in the blood of excess amounts of a substance called bilirubin, which is normally excreted by the liver into the bile. It occurs in hepatitis, other liver diseases, and sometimes malaria, and is a sign of reduced liver function. Non-medical people sometimes use this term to mean hepatitis.

Lesion: Sore, wound, ulcer, or area of tissue damage.

Lymph nodes (glands): Part of the immune system. Some can normally be felt as small lumps close to the skin in the neck, groin, and armpit. They may enlarge or become inflamed during an infection.

Microorganism: Any microscopic organism. Such organisms include viruses, bacteria, funguses and yeasts, protozoa, and rickettsiae.

Narcosis: Depression of the nervous system—by a drug or other agent, such as an excess of dissolved nitrogen in the blood (the latter is called nitrogen narcosis, which may occur in divers).

Papule: A small, circumscribed, solid elevation of the skin.

Parasite: An animal that lives within or upon man or any other animal (its host), and upon which it depends for nutrition and shelter—sometimes to the detriment of the host.

Pathogen, enteropathogen: Any disease-producing microorganism. Enteropathogens produce intestinal disease.

Physiological: Normal, or related to the way the body functions in health rather than in disease. Physiology is the science of the mechanisms of normal bodily function.

Prevalence: The total number of cases of a disease at a certain time in a given area.

Prophylaxis: A word that physicians use when they mean prevention!

Protozoa: The simplest organisms in the animal kingdom, each consisting of a single nucleated cell. Some of them cause disease. Malaria, amebic dysentery, sleeping sickness, trichomoniasis, and giardiasis are all caused by protozoa.

Psychotropic: Mind- or mood-altering.

Rickettsiae: A group of microorganisms that have many similarities to bacteria. They include the microorganisms that cause typhus.

Sputum: Phlegm; mucus secretions from the lung and respiratory passages.

Subcutaneous: Under all layers of the skin. Many immunizations are injected subcutaneously.

Thrombosis: Clotting of blood within a vein.

Toxin: A specific chemical produced by a living organism that damages or poisons another organism (e.g., man).

Trophozoite: The active, feeding, growing, disease-producing form of a protozoan parasite.

Ulcer: An inflamed defect following damage, at the surface of the skin, the stomach lining, or any other tissue surface.

Vector: A carrier of infection or of a parasite, from one host to the next.

Viruses: Tiny, particulate microorganisms, much smaller than bacteria and too small to be seen without the aid of the electron microscope. They live inside our cells, multiplying within them, and it is this characteristic which protects them from antibodies and drugs, and makes viral infections so difficult to treat.

Vitiligo: Patches of white, de-pigmented skin.

INDEX

Page numbers in **bold** refer
to tables.
Page numbers in *italics* refer
to illustrations.